T0226407

New Pipeline of Immunoregulatory Molecules and Biomarkers in Transplantation

Editor

INDIRA GULERIA

CLINICS IN LABORATORY MEDICINE

www.labmed.theclinics.com

Editor-in-Chief
MILENKO JOVAN TANASIJEVIC

March 2019 • Volume 39 • Number 1

ELSEVIER

1600 John F. Kennedy Boulevard • Suite 1800 • Philadelphia, Pennsylvania, 19103-2899

http://www.theclinics.com

CLINICS IN LABORATORY MEDICINE Volume 39, Number 1
March 2019 ISSN 0272-2712, ISBN-13: 978-0-323-66100-3

Editor: Stacy Eastman
Developmental Editor: Laura Fisher

Reprints. For copies of 100 or more, of articles in this publication, please contact the Commercial Reprints Department, Elsevier Inc., 360 Park Avenue South, New York, New York 10010-1710. Tel. 212-633-3874, Fax: 212-633-3820, E-mail: reprints@elsevier.com.

Clinics in Laboratory Medicine (ISSN 0272-2712) is published quarterly by Elsevier Inc., 360 Park Avenue South, New York, NY 10010-1710. Months of issue are March, June, September, and December. Business and Editorial offices: 1600 John F. Kennedy Blvd., Suite 1800, Philadelphia, PA 19103-2899. Periodicals postage paid at NewYork, NY and additional mailing offices. Subscription prices are $274.00 per year (US individuals), $541.00 per year (US institutions), $100.00 per year (US students), $349.00 per year (Canadian individuals), $657.00 per year (Canadian institutions), $185.00 per year (Canadian students), $404.00 per year (international individuals), $657.00 per year (international institutions), $185.00 (international students). Foreign air speed delivery is included in all Clinics subscription prices. All prices are subject to change without notice. POSTMASTER: Send address changes to *Clinics in Laboratory Medicine*, Elsevier Health Sciences Division, Subscription Customer Service, 3251 Riverport Lane, Maryland Heights, MO 63043. **Customer Service: 1-800-654-2452 (US). From outside of the US and Canada, call 1-314-447-8871. Fax: 1-314-447-8029. E-mail: journalscustomerservice-usa@elsevier.com (for print support) or journalsonlinesupport-usa@elsevier.com (for online support).**

Clinics in Laboratory Medicine is covered in *EMBASE/Exerpta Medica, MEDLINE/PubMed (Index Medicus), Cinahl, Current Contents/Clinical Medicine, BIOSIS and ISI/BIOMED.*

Contributors

EDITOR-IN-CHIEF

MILENKO JOVAN TANASIJEVIC, MD, MBA
Vice Chair for Clinical Pathology and Quality, Department of Pathology, Director of Clinical Laboratories, Brigham and Women's Hospital, Dana-Farber Cancer Institute, Associate Professor of Pathology, Harvard Medical School, Boston, Massachusetts, USA

EDITOR

INDIRA GULERIA, PhD, D (ABHI)
Assistant Professor of Medicine, Harvard Medical School, Associate Director, HLA Tissue Typing Laboratory, Associate Immunobiologist, Renal Transplant Program, Division of Renal Medicine, Transplantation Research Center, Brigham and Women's Hospital, Boston, Massachusetts, USA

AUTHORS

BASMAH S. AL DULAIJAN, MD
Transplantation Research Center, Renal Division, Brigham and Women's Hospital, Harvard Medical School, Boston, Massachusetts, USA

HAZIM ALLOS, MD
Transplantation Research Center, Renal Division, Brigham and Women's Hospital, Harvard Medical School, Boston, Massachusetts, USA

JAMIL AZZI, MD
Director, Renal Transplant Fellowship, Assistant Professor of Medicine, Transplantation Research Center, Associate Physician, Renal Division, Brigham and Women's Hospital, Harvard Medical School, Boston, Massachusetts, USA

MURUGABASKAR BALAN, PhD
Instructor, Division of Nephrology, Boston Children's Hospital, Boston, Massachusetts, USA

ALBANA BANO, MD
Transplantation Research Center, Renal Division, Brigham and Women's Hospital, Harvard Medical School, Boston, Massachusetts, USA

SAMIK CHAKRABORTY, PhD
Research Fellow, Division of Nephrology, Boston Children's Hospital, Boston, Massachusetts, USA

ANIL CHANDRAKER, MD, FASN
Associate Professor, Department of Medicine, Transplantation Research Center, Renal Division, Brigham and Women's Hospital, Harvard Medical School, Boston, Massachusetts, USA

ARAVIND CHERUKURI, MBBS (MD), MRCP, PhD
Section of Nephrology, Renal Fellow, Department of Medicine, Thomas E. Starzl
Transplantation Institute, University of Pittsburgh School of Medicine, Pittsburgh,
Pennsylvania, USA

JOHN CHOI, MD
Transplantation Research Center, Renal Division, Brigham and Women's Hospital,
Harvard Medical School, Boston, Massachusetts, USA

JONATHAN C. CHOY, PhD
Associate Professor, Department of Molecular Biology and Biochemistry, Centre for Cell
Biology, Development and Disease, Simon Fraser University, Burnaby, British Columbia,
Canada

NICHOLAS H. CHUN, MD
Translational Transplant Research Center, Assistant Professor, Department of Medicine,
Icahn School of Medicine at Mount Sinai, New York, New York, USA

MATTHEW F. CUSICK, PhD, D (ABHI)
Assistant Professor, Department of Surgery, HLA Laboratory Director, BCM Immune
Evaluation Laboratory, Houston, Texas, USA

QING DING, PhD
Research Assistant Professor, Department of Surgery, Thomas E. Starzl Transplantation
Institute, University of Pittsburgh School of Medicine, Pittsburgh, Pennsylvania, USA

IVICA GRGIC, MD
Department of Internal Medicine and Nephrology, University Hospital, Giessen and
Marburg, Philipps-University Marburg, Marburg, Germany

INDIRA GULERIA, PhD, D (ABHI)
Assistant Professor of Medicine, Harvard Medical School, Associate Director, HLA Tissue
Typing Laboratory, Associate Immunobiologist, Renal Transplant Program, Division of
Renal Medicine, Transplantation Research Center, Brigham and Women's Hospital,
Boston, Massachusetts, USA

PETER S. HEEGER, MD
Professor of Medicine and Immunology, Translational Transplant Research Center,
Department of Medicine, The Precision Institute of Immunology, Icahn School of
Medicine at Mount Sinai, New York, New York, USA

JULIAN K. HORWITZ, MD
General Surgery Resident, Translational Transplant Research Center, Department of
Surgery, Icahn School of Medicine at Mount Sinai, New York, New York, USA

PETER T. JINDRA, PhD, D (ABHI)
Assistant Professor, Department of Surgery, HLA Laboratory Director, BCM Immune
Evaluation Laboratory, Houston, Texas, USA

ZAHRAA KHAN, MD
Division of Nephrology and Hypertension, Departments of Medicine and Transplantation
Medicine, NewYork-Presbyterian–Weill Cornell Medicine, New York, New York, USA

MARTINA M. McGRATH, MD, MB, BCh
Transplantation Research Center, Renal Division, Brigham and Women's Hospital,
Harvard Medical School, Boston, Massachusetts, USA

KANISHKA MOHIB, PhD
Instructor, Department of Surgery, Research Instructor, Thomas E. Starzl Transplantation Institute, University of Pittsburgh School of Medicine, Pittsburgh, Pennsylvania, USA

THANGAMANI MUTHUKUMAR, MD
Associate Professor, Division of Nephrology and Hypertension, Departments of Medicine and Transplantation Medicine, Associate Program Director (Research), Renal Fellowship Program, NewYork-Presbyterian–Weill Cornell Medicine, New York, New York, USA

SOPHIE PACZESNY, MD, PhD
Nora Letzter Professor of Pediatrics and Professor of Microbiology and Immunology, Departments of Pediatrics and Microbiology Immunology, Melvin and Bren Simon Cancer Center, Indiana University School of Medicine, Indianapolis, Indiana, USA

SOUMITRO PAL, PhD
Associate Professor, Division of Nephrology, Boston Children's Hospital, Boston, Massachusetts, USA

KEVIN REY, BSc
Department of Molecular Biology and Biochemistry, Centre for Cell Biology, Development and Disease, Simon Fraser University, Burnaby, British Columbia, Canada

DAVID M. ROTHSTEIN, MD
Professor of Surgery, Medicine and Immunology, Thomas E. Starzl Transplantation Institute, University of Pittsburgh School of Medicine, Pittsburgh, Pennsylvania, USA

COURTNEY M. ROWAN, MD, MS
Assistant Professor, Department of Pediatrics, Division of Critical Care, Indiana University School of Medicine, Indianapolis, Indiana, USA

AKHIL SHARMA, MD
Clinical Instructor in Nephrology, Department of Medicine, Thomas E. Starzl Transplantation Institute, University of Pittsburgh School of Medicine, Pittsburgh, Pennsylvania, USA

HO SIK SHIN, MD, PhD
Renal Division, Department of Internal Medicine, Gospel Hospital, Kosin University College of Medicine, Busan, Republic of Korea

MANIKKAM SUTHANTHIRAN, MD
Stanton Griffis Distinguished Professor of Medicine, Chief, Division of Nephrology and Hypertension, Weill Cornell Medical College, Chief, Department of Transplantation Medicine, Department of Medicine New York-Presbyterian Hospital-Weill Cornell Medical Center, New York, New York, USA

OLGA A. TIMOFEEVA, PhD, D (ABHI)
Associate Professor, Pathology and Laboratory Medicine, Director of Molecular Pathology Laboratory, Co-Director of Immunogenetics Laboratory, Temple University and Hospital, Lewis Katz School of Medicine, Philadelphia, Pennsylvania, USA

SUDIPTA TRIPATHI, PhD
Instructor in Medicine, Associate Immunologist, Transplantation Research Center, Brigham and Women's Hospital, Harvard Medical School, Boston, Massachusetts, USA

MAYUKO UEHARA, MD, PhD
Transplantation Research Center, Renal Division, Brigham and Women's Hospital, Harvard Medical School, Boston, Massachusetts, USA

Contents

There has been a prolific amount of research dedicated to the T-regulatory cells (Tregs) and their role in achieving immune homeostasis. Here, the authors briefly discuss the known biology, utilization, and potential of Tregs, for current trials and future immunotherapy. Most current trials of Treg therapies include either ex vivo expanded Tregs transferred into the peripheral blood of patients with diseases of immunologic origin or interleukin 2 injected to stimulate Tregs directly. Ongoing trials designed to measure the clinical efficacy and safety profile of these novel therapeutic approaches have resulted in largely favorable outcomes in a variety of autoimmune and alloimmune diseases.

B cells shape the alloimmune response through polarized subsets. These cells inhibit or promote immune responses by expressing suppressive or proinflammatory cytokines. Their summed activity dictates the influence of B cells on the alloimmune response. We review the evidence for regulatory B cells and effector B cells in mice and humans, discuss current limitations in their phenotypic identification, and discuss regulatory B cells as a signature for clinical renal allograft tolerance and predictive markers for allograft outcomes. We discuss the effects of therapeutic agents on regulatory B cells and potential approaches to augment their numbers as a therapeutic tool.

The complement system, traditionally considered a component of innate immunity, is now recognized as a crucial mediator of the adaptive immune response in solid organ transplantation. Preclinical and early human trials have demonstrated the importance of complement effector mechanisms in driving allograft injury during specific antigraft immune responses, including ischemia-reperfusion injury, T-cell–mediated rejection, and antibody-mediated rejection, as well as a potential role for complement-derived risk stratification biomarkers. These data support the need for further testing of complement inhibitors in solid organ transplant recipients.

> This article reviews the current evidence to classify donor-specific antibodies (DSAs) using Food and Drug Administration–National Institutes of Health Biomarkers, EndpointS, and other Tools (BEST) resource terms as diagnostic, prognostic, predictive, monitoring, and risk biomarkers for graft rejection. The emphasis is on DSA characteristics, including the DSA levels determined by mean fluorescence intensity and/or titers, the ability to activate a complement cascade (C1q, C3d, and C4d binding), and specific IgG subclasses to define distinct roles of DSAs as biomarkers in clinical practice. In addition, technical limitation of DSA testing is discussed.

> Advances in the field of omics have led to a significant expansion in biomarkers identified for complications after hematopoietic stem cell transplantation (HSCT). Biomarkers can offer an effective method for early identification of a specific disease and can be used to guide therapies. Ongoing investigations to discover biomarkers for acute graft-versus-host disease as well as other post-HSCT complications may improve early diagnosis, prognosis, and the development of new therapeutic targets. The authors review the most recent and validated diagnostic, prognostic, predictive, and response to treatment biomarkers for early complications following HSCT consistent with 2014 NIH consensus on biomarker criteria.

> After more than 6 decades of clinical practice, the transplant community continues to research noninvasive biomarkers of solid organ injury to help improve patient care. In this review, we discuss the clinical usefulness of selective biomarkers and how they are processed at the laboratory. In addition, we organize these biomarkers based on specific aims and introduce innovative markers currently under investigation.

> Costimulation is a critical step in T-cell activation, and costimulatory blockade at the time of T cell activation leads to T-cell anergy and allograft tolerance in animal models of transplantation. CD28:B7 is the most important costimulatory pathway and the balance of signals between CD28 and cytotoxic T-lymphocyte associated protein 4 (CTLA-4) is a central determinant of transplant outcome. Form a clinical standpoint, CTLA-4 Ig is the only approved agent for costimulation blockade in transplantation. Advantages and disadvantages of its use are discussed. Progress in developing novel agents to target other pathways, including the promising CD40:CD154 pathway, is also discussed.

Murugabaskar Balan, Samik Chakraborty, and Soumitro Pal

Immunosuppression is essential to prevent graft rejection. However, immunosuppression impairs the ability of the host immune system to control viral infection and decreases tumor immunosurveillance. Therefore, immunosuppression after organ transplantation is a major risk factor for posttransplantation cancer. Notably, recent reports suggest that immunosuppressive agents can activate tumorigenic pathways independent of the involvement of the host immune system. In this review, we focus on cell-intrinsic tumorigenic pathways directly activated by immunosuppressive agents and discuss the much-described infection- and immune-mediated mechanisms of cancer development in organ transplant recipients.

Kevin Rey and Jonathan C. Choy

The microbiota is a community of microbes that colonizes body surfaces. It has many effects that influence immune activation and regulation. The success of organ transplantation is limited by rejection of grafts by the immune system so it is important to understand how immunologic responses are controlled in this setting. This review discusses the immunologic effects of the microbiota and how this microbial community may affect organ transplant rejection.

CLINICS IN LABORATORY MEDICINE

FORTHCOMING ISSUES

June 2019
Clinical Decision Support: Tools, Strategies, and Emerging Technologies
Anand S. Dighe, *Editor*

September 2019
Advances and Trends in Clinical Microbiology: The Next 20 Years
James E. Kirby, *Editor*

December 2019
Next Generation Sequencing and its Applications in Oncology Diagnostics
Jeffrey Gagan, *Editor*

RECENT ISSUES

December 2018
HLA and Disease
Julio C. Delgado and Eszter Lázár-Molnár, *Editors*

September 2018
Clinical Pathology
Geza S. Bodor, *Editor*

June 2018
Molecular Pathology: An Update
Martin H. Bluth, *Editor*

SERIES OF RELATED INTEREST

Surgical Pathology Clinics
Available at: https://www.surgpath.theclinics.com/

THE CLINICS ARE NOW AVAILABLE ONLINE!
Access your subscription at:
www.theclinics.com

Preface

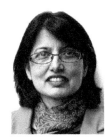

Indira Guleria, PhD, D (ABHI)
Editor

Having run a research laboratory for fifteen years with an emphasis on studying the role of regulatory costimulatory molecules in transplantation tolerance and witnessing tremendous growth in this field, as a guest editor for this issue of the *Clinics in Laboratory Medicine*, I instinctively chose to highlight advancements in the field of novel molecules and biomarkers in transplantation.

The focus during a transplant is to promote allograft tolerance and avoid allograft rejection. The article by Allos and colleagues on regulatory T cells, which have strong immunosuppressive characteristics, covers our evolving understanding of these cells and their inclusion in clinical trials. The article in this issue by Cherukuri and colleagues elegantly covers the regulatory B cells, which, through expression of immune-modulatory cytokine interleukin-10, can contribute to allograft acceptance and are showing great potential as a biomarker.

The article by Horwitz and colleagues on complement provides a remarkable description of the different mechanisms of complement-mediated injury and discusses the therapeutic role of complement inhibitors in solid organ transplant recipients. These studies tie in nicely with the article by Timofeeva on utilizing donor-specific antibodies, especially the ones with complement binding capabilities, as a biomarker for rejection of grafts. Using the 2014 National Institutes of Health consensus on biomarker criteria, Rowan and Paczesny describe Stimulation 2 to be the most validated and promising therapeutic target for acute graft-versus-host disease following stem cell transplantation. New emerging markers for solid organ transplant, such as measurement of donor-derived cell-free DNA and kidney solid organ response test, have been described in the article by Choi and colleagues. The article by Uehara and McGrath on the role of costimulatory molecules, which can modulate alloreactive T cells following transplantation. The role of gene variants in costimulatory molecules and cytokines associated with transplantation outcomes have been described in the article by Jindra and Cusick.

The article by Khan and colleagues presents an excellent description of the emerging role of miRNAs as robust biomarkers for assessing transplant outcomes following kidney transplantation. The miRNAs, along with exosomes, are expected

Clin Lab Med 39 (2019) xiii–xiv
https://doi.org/10.1016/j.cll.2018.12.001
0272-2712/19/© 2018 Published by Elsevier Inc.

labmed.theclinics.com

to evolve as biomarkers for assessing transplant rejection in other organs also. Interestingly, these biomarkers have also shown promise in predicting pregnancy disorders, as discussed in the article by Tripathi and Guleria on fetomaternal tolerance.

New developments in immunosuppressive agents that target T cells, B cells, plasma cells, and complement are outlined in the article by Shin and colleagues. It is hoped that these innovations will result in development of new safer alternatives that will supplant older immunosuppressive agents, including the commonly used calcineurin inhibitors that are associated with toxicity. Signaling molecules and molecular mechanisms involved in immunosuppressive agent-induced posttransplant cancer development are summarized in the article in this issue by Balan and colleagues.

Microbiota and their role in various human diseases is a fast developing area, and the article by Rey and Choy suggests a regulatory role for gut microbiota and discusses how this microbial community may affect organ transplant rejection.

I am very thankful and appreciative to all the leading experts in the field of solid organ and stem cell transplant, some of whom I have collaborated with in the past, who agreed to contribute an article for this issue.

Indira Guleria, PhD, D (ABHI)
Harvard Medical School
HLA Tissue Typing Laboratory
Renal Transplant Program
Division of Renal Medicine
Transplantation Research Center
Brigham and Women's Hospital
75 Francis Street
PBB 161G
Boston, MA 02115, USA

E-mail address:
iguleria@bics.bwh.harvard.edu

Regulatory T Cells for More Targeted Immunosuppressive Therapies

Hazim Allos, MD, Basmah S. Al Dulaijan, MD, John Choi, MD,
Jamil Azzi, MD*

KEYWORDS

- T-regulatory cells • FOXP3 • Immunotherapy

KEY POINTS

- Immune tolerance can be achieved via several different pathways, which can be subcategorized into 2 main subsets: cell-intrinsic and cell-extrinsic mechanisms.
- Avidly self-reactive lymphocytes can accomplish immunotolerance, in the broader sense, by undergoing programmed cell death, genetic rearrangements resulting in a distinctive antigen receptor, peripheral anergy in response to a self-antigen, and, finally, increased activation thresholds via increased expression of inhibitory molecules or activation-induced death.
- These components of the cell-intrinsic pathway for tolerance have been previously properly recognized and already greatly described.
- The CD4+ T-regulatory cell is the first cell subset to be recognized in the cell-extrinsic mechanism of immunotolerance.

INTRODUCTION

The adaptive immune system thrives on its foundational ability to create an almost innumerable repertoire of randomly assorted T-cell receptors (TCRs), including those toward self-antigens.[1] However, immune homeostasis is a multifaceted system of balanced biological checks that refrain from boisterous autoreactivity and exaggerated activity against pathogens. A lapse in this very delicate, and tightly regulated, homeostatic system in either aspect often results in dire consequences.[2] And, although the structure of immune reactivity has been extensively described in literature, immune regulation has only recently received explicit focus.

Disclosure: The authors have nothing to disclose.
Transplantation Research Center, Renal Division, Brigham and Women's Hospital, Harvard Medical School, Boston, MA, USA
* Corresponding author. Transplantation Research Center, Brigham and Women's Hospital, 221 Longwood Ave, Boston, MA 02115.
E-mail address: jazzi@rics.bwh.harvard.edu

Clin Lab Med 39 (2019) 1–13
https://doi.org/10.1016/j.cll.2018.11.001
0272-2712/19/© 2018 Elsevier Inc. All rights reserved.

labmed.theclinics.com

Immune tolerance can be achieved via several different pathways, which can be subcategorized into 2 main subsets: cell-intrinsic and cell-extrinsic mechanisms. Avidly self-reactive lymphocytes can accomplish immunotolerance, in the broader sense, by undergoing programmed cell death, genetic rearrangements resulting in a distinctive antigen receptor, peripheral anergy in response to a self-antigen and, finally, increased activation thresholds via increased expression of inhibitory molecules or activation-induced death.[3] These components of the cell-intrinsic pathway for tolerance have been previously properly recognized and already greatly described. The cell-extrinsic mechanisms have been mostly unnoticed until recently in 1972, Gershon and colleagues[4] had first provided evidence of a newly discovered, and imperative, player in the immunoregulatory system. The CD4+ T-regulatory cell (Treg) is the first cell subset to be recognized in the cell-extrinsic mechanism of immunotolerance.

DISCOVERY OF T-REGULATORY CELLS

It was first noted that depletion of T cells in adult rats by thymectomies, thereafter treated with low-dose x-ray irradiations, led to the development of autoimmune thyroiditis. When the normal immune cells were repleted, the disease reverted.[5,6] Similarly, Sakaguchi and colleagues[7] showed that thymectomy in neonatal mice at day 3 resulted in autoimmune oophoritis and that this was prevented by a single intraperitoneal injection of spleen cells or thymocytes from nonthymectomized mice. These results lead to the postulation that not only are self-reactive T cells capable of producing autoimmune phenomena present but "suppressor" T cells that counterbalance this inherent autoreactivity are also present. Sakaguchi and colleagues[8] showed that removal of a certain subpopulation of T cells, termed "Lyt+," from mice resulted in extensive autoimmunity. Reconstitution of this cell subset resulted in reversal of autoimmunity. Ultimately, these "Lyt+" cells were found to bear CD4+CD25^{high} (IL-2 receptor α [IL-2Rα] chain) and termed "T-regulatory cells." Furthermore, they were observed to lead to a diminution of self-, nonself, and allergic immune antigen responses.[9,10] However, because CD25 is also highly expressed in activated effector T cells, it is not a specific marker of Tregs. It was not until 2003 that the forkhead box transcription factor FOXP3 was found to be the specific marker of Tregs.[11,12]

The knowledge of FOXP3 stems from a rare monogenic disease; immunodysregulation, polyendocinopathy, enteropathy, X-linked syndrome (IPEX) is an X-linked autoimmune/inflammatory syndrome, caused by genetic defects in the FOXP3 gene. Characteristics of patients with IPEX are very similar to that of scurfy mice that lack Tregs.[13] This led to the vigorous study of FOXP3s' role in the Treg. Initial findings showed that FOXP3 coded for a transcriptional factor that is specifically expressed in naturally arising CD4+ Tregs. In addition, retroviral transfer of FOXP3 gene converts naïve T cells toward a Treg-like pathway.[14] These findings led to the conclusion that FOXP3 is the master gene that allows T cells to differentiate into functional Tregs.

A NONHOMOGENOUS POPULATION

The CD4+CD25 + CD127lowFOXP3+ Treg population constitutes approximately 5% to 15% of peripheral T-cell population and under close inspection can be divided into 22 distinct population based on differential surface marker expression.[15] However, broadly speaking, Tregs can be divided in 2 main types, denoted by their origin: thymus-derived Tregs and peripherally derived Tregs, also called natural Tregs (nTregs) and induced Tregs (iTregs), respectively.[16]

nTregs compromise most of the Treg population and respond chiefly to self-reactive T cells that have failed to undergo negative selection in the thymus. Naïve nTregs are characterized by CD44low, CD62Lhi, CXCR4low, and CCR7, allowing them to secondary lymphoid tissue. Local stimulation in the homed lymphoid organ creates a phenotypic switch to express a different array of chemokine receptors, with downregulation of CD62L and CCR7, allowing to traffic to the tissue of interest depending on which chemokine receptor had been expressed.[17–20] This switch marks the creation of a mature effector Treg, characterized by CCR7lowCD62LlowCD44hiKLRG1+, found in circulation and in tissues harboring immunologic activity.[21–23]

Peripherally, CD4+CD25− T-conventional cells (Tconvs) also have the capacity to become Tregs by induction; these are termed iTregs. There are several differences between nTregs and iTregs. First and foremost, iTregs have a broader TCR repertoire and the cells' differentiation requires their stimulation.[24] Varying conditions present themselves for iTreg differentiation and mainly include bacterial and viral infections, tumors, or in mucosal tissue in the context of oral tolerance.[25–27] However, expression of FOXP3 in these cells is highly unstable and these cells can revert back to Tconvs or even pathogenic Th memory cells once signals and cues, such as IL-2 and TGF-β, abate.[28]

It is worth mentioning that a distinct subset of Tregs was more recently found, the tissue-resident Tregs. Such Tregs have been identified in skin tissue, visceral adipose tissue, and muscle tissue.[29] Each of the tissues mentioned bears a specific Treg with different proportions, phenotypic marker expressions, cytokine secretions, and, therefore, function.[29] However, more research needs to be conducted on the nature of these Tregs and their impact on local tissue immune homeostasis and potential pathogenicity.

ESSENTIAL SIGNALS FOR TREG DEVELOPMENT AND MAINTENANCE

Maturation of T cells, in general, occurs first and foremost in the thymus. There, they undergo processes known as positive and negative selection. Positive selection occurs when a T cell's TCR has the ability to recognize major histocompatibility molecules, thereby allowing it to proceed in its maturation process. Negative selection then eliminates T cells via a process called clonal deletion if they bind, with high affinity, to self-protein antigens and are deemed autoreactive.[30] Physiologically, not all T cells with self-reactive high-affinity TCRs seem to be negatively selected. Indeed, it seems that the alternative pathway for autoreactive T cells is to shunt development into CD4+CD25 + Tregs.[31] However, because self-reactive TCRs are present on both negatively selected T cells and potential Tregs, there should be a secondary signal to induce the Treg pathway.

Tregs bear a high affinity IL-2R consisting of CD25(IL-2Rα), CD122 (IL-2Rβ), and CD132 (IL-2Rγ),[32] and, unsurprisingly, IL-2 is one of the major secondary signals essential for Treg differentiation. This observation stemmed from an experiment using mice that lack CD25, or IL-2 entirely, resulting in significant decrease in FOXP3+ nTreg population.[33] To a lesser degree, other γ-chain (γc) cytokines IL-7 and IL-15 are also deemed important for Treg differentiation and seemed to partially compensate for entire lack of IL-2, resulting in reduced but not absent FOXP3 Treg numbers.[34] Finally, TGF-βs' role in Treg development is somewhat unclear. TGF-βR–deficient mice were associated with the expression of proapoptotic proteins Bax, Bak, and Bim and concomitant low expression of Blc-2, resulting in high rates of apoptosis during negative selection and, furthermore, Bim ablation restores TGF-β signal deficiency.[35] These results suggested that TGF-β is not necessary to direct differentiation of nTregs but perhaps essential to maintain it.[35] Ultimately, the various interplay of the aforementioned cytokines, and their respective receptors, results in the phosphorylation of transcription factor STAT5, and, finally, induced expression of FOXP3.[36–38]

CD4+CD25−FOXP3− Tconvs are induced, and maintained, toward the Treg pathway by induction via TGF-β.[39,40] As previously mentioned, IL-2 is not absolutely necessary for the development of nTregs and can be replaced by other common γc cytokines, although by similarly conducted studies, it seems to be an irreplaceable signal that is crucial for iTregs.[39,41,42]

FOXP3 AND EPIGENETICS

FOXP3 is an X chromosome–encoded gene and is thought to be the master gene of the Tregs; its expression is induced after TCR stimulation and seems to mainly depend on the intensity of the stimulation.[31] As previously mentioned, IPEX is caused by genetic defects of FOXP3 and experimental scurfy mouse models share the characteristics.[13] Another study showed that because of random inactivation of the X chromosome in women heterozygous for FOXP3, FOXP3−/+ mice produce half the population of functional Tregs, and the other half dysfunctional, which further indicated that FOXP3s' presence is essential for the Treg population.[42] However, various studies have demonstrated that FOXP3 expression in cells is, albeit essential, not sufficient to produce fully functional Tregs. Lin and colleagues[43] demonstrated that mice expressing truncated FOXP3 maintained Treg phenotype but lacked full suppressive abilities. Therefore, there seems to be an independent and distinct factor that compromises a full Treg phenotype and function, in addition to FOXP3.

The FOXP3 locus is a conglomerate of 3 conserved noncoding sequences (CNS1–3) and a promotor region. The CNS are targets of epigenetic modifications causing either reduced or increased sterical hindrance, allowing either, respectively, increased or reduced transcription factor interaction and therefore gene expression.[44] An elucidating study by Ohkura and colleagues[45] demonstrated the role of epigenetics in fully functional Tregs, independent of the presence of FOXP3. According to the study there are 2 independent processes that occur in parallel in the course of Treg development that are necessary for a full-fledged Treg. Continuous TCR stimulation results in TCR-induced CpG hypomethylation of certain DNA regions, in the thymus and the periphery, and is required to obtain genome-wide Treg gene expression pattern. This hypomethylation pattern leads to higher stability and full phenotypic expression and is observed in nTregs and in vivo iTregs but not in vitro iTregs.[45]

SUPPRESSIVE STRATEGIES OF TREGS

Tregs use a variety of methods to impose their suppressive function, most of which are currently controversial and seem to depend on a variety of factors, such as nature of targeted suppression, context of immune response, and anatomic location of suppression. Direct suppression can occur in the absence of antigen-presenting cells (APCs) by direct cell-cell contact causing inhibition of TCR-stimulated IL-2 transcription.[46] Another postulated direct contact mechanism is via delivery of a highly expressed amount of cytoplasmic cAMP in Tregs to Tconvs by gap junctions.[47] Delivery of granzyme B and perforin, inducing apoptosis, seems to be another observed mechanism.[48,49] Tregs express high-affinity IL-2Rα (CD25) and, concurrent with this fact, it has been observed that Tregs competitively, and preferentially, bind IL-2 limiting the abundance for nonregulatory T cells.[50]

Tregs constitutively express cytotoxic T lymphocyte antigen 4 (CTLA-4), and there is evidence that Tregs use a CTLA-4–dependent manner to downregulate CD80/86 on APCs. This results in a limitation in antigen presentation and, therefore, activation of naïve T cells via CD28.[51] Perhaps most intuitively, Tregs secrete IL-10, which seems to be essential to keep immune responses at homeostasis in environmental interfaces such as the colon and lungs. IL-35 has been similarly implicated in tolerance in the gut. And, finally, TGF-β also seems to suppress Th1 responses.[52]

T-REGULATORY ADOPTIVE CELL TRANSFER THERAPY

The earliest therapies that implemented knowledge of Tregs' immunosuppressive abilities used transfer of Tregs into the peripheral blood of patients with varying conditions.

The first of these novel approaches was conducted by Trzonkowski and colleagues,[53] where ex vivo expanded Tregs were transferred into 2 cases of either acute or chronic graft-versus-host disease (GVHD). Despite triple suppressive therapy, insulin injections, bronchodilators, and multiple failed attempts of reduced dosing, the patient afflicted with chronic GVHD improved following transferred Treg therapy. Complete removal of one suppressive agent, insulin injections and bronchodilators, and reduction of prednisone was achieved as a direct consequence of Treg therapy. Moreover, 6 months posttransfer, percentages of Tregs remained high in peripheral blood (2.5% before transfer to 5%). In the case of acute GVHD, unfortunately, although modest improvements were initially seen, the lack of available Tregs halted further treatment.[53] Similarly, using umbilical cord blood as a source of Tregs, Brunstein and colleagues isolated,[54] expanded, and injected patients with acute GVHD at certain intervals. Results indicated that Treg infusion not only prevented GVHD manifestations but also inferred no increased risk of opportunistic infection or other obvious adverse effects. In another study involving 28 human leukocyte antigen (HLA)-haploidentical stem cell transplantation engrafted patients, 26 of 28 patients remained acute GVHD free, all remained chronic GVHD free, and CMV infection rates were significantly lower than with traditional therapies.[55]

Adoptive Treg transfer has also been used in autoimmune diseases, for example, in the setting of recently diagnosed diabetes mellitus type 1. Similarly, the results showed significantly decreased hemoglobin A1C levels; requirements of exogenous insulin, with 2 patients completely not requiring insulin; and increase in circulatory Tregs. And, moreover, no significant increased risk to infections or any adverse effects were observed.[56] A follow-up study also reported increased β-cell islet survival with repeated Treg administration over a course of 1 year.[57] However, a common limitation to all these studies is the questionable stability and eventual wane of the Treg populations in peripheral blood, and, therefore also their effects. Accordingly, more exploration of Treg stability and optimum conditions for persistence in peripheral blood is required to apply Tregs in immunotherapy more adequately.

This article elucidates, at least partially, a mechanism that explains this inherent Treg instability. On Treg activation, granzymes A and B are highly expressed and tend to leak out of compartmentalized granules, ultimately leading to cell intrinsic apoptosis. Blood samples drawn from renal transplant recipients undergoing rejection demonstrate an increase in chemokine receptors that home Tregs to the tissue-harboring inflammatory activity, receptors that are shared with inflammatory Th1 and Th17 cells, which mediate rejection. Similarly, increased granzyme B expression is seen in these Tregs as well.[58] Possibly, this may be a homeostatic phenomenon because the ability of antigen-specific T-cell clones to later be reactivated to the same antigen depends on an inflammatory milieu that Tregs directly counteract.[58]

T-REGULATORY CELL IL-2 IMMUNOTHERAPY

More recent trials for Treg immunotherapy stems from knowledge that IL-2 is imperative to the cell lines' integrity and maintenance in the periphery. CD4$^+$CD25$^+$ Tregs express all 3 components of the IL-2 receptor: CD25 (IL-2Rα), CD122 (IL-2Rβ), and CD132 (IL-2Rγ).[32] Complexes consisting of CD122 and CD132 create a low-affinity IL-2R; however, the trimeric complex present on Tregs constitutes a high-affinity IL-2R.[32] IL-2 has the ability to both expand and amplify the Treg or conventional T cells depending on concentration. Tregs and Tconvs are contradictory in function and have been shown to react differently under varying IL-2 concentrations.[59] Indeed, in vivo, low-dose IL-2 was shown to preferentially stimulate Tregs, likely because of their high-affinity trimeric IL-2R. In contrast, high-dose IL-2 stimulated Tconvs and Tregs, allowing for dual utilization of IL-2 for either immunosuppressive or immunopromoting functions, respectively.[59]

Initially, therapeutic approaches involved high-dose IL-2 administrations. Ahmadzadeh and colleagues[60] showed that high-dose IL-2 administration to patients with cancer resulted in a nearly 6-fold increase in circulatory Tregs, with substantial increase in FOXP3 expression. However, with further expanse of IL-2 immunotherapy trials, high-dose IL-2 administration was repeatedly associated with a multitude of adverse effects.

One of the earliest studies that clearly showed the safety profile and potential for efficacy of low-dose IL-2 therapy was conducted in Hepatitis C-induced vasculitis patients. Low-dose IL-2 administration to 10 patients resulted in clinical improvement in 80% of patients, increase in total percentage of Tregs, and the attenuation of overall inflammatory markers. Moreover, it was found to be clinically safe with adverse effects more commonly seen at the higher IL-2 doses.[61]

Koreth and colleagues[62] also demonstrated that low-dose IL-2 therapy preferentially expanded the Treg lines rather than conventional CD4+ T cells in patients with GVHD. Continued low-dose IL-2 administration was shown to be safe; it created sustained Treg expansion, with peak values at 4 weeks, and led to an overall reduction of GHVD manifestations. In another study that involved GVHD in allogeneic hematopoietic stem cell transplantation (HSCT) by Matsouka and colleagues,[63] the mechanisms of IL-2 therapy on Treg homeostasis was revealed, at least partially. The research group demonstrated that chronic GVHD is characterized by constitutive phosphorylation of Stat5 in Tconv with association of elevated levels of IL-7 and IL-15 and functional deficiency of IL-2. Low-dose IL-2 administration, over an 8-week period, resulted in discriminatory increase of Stat5 phosphorylation in Treg and a decrease in Tconv. Furthermore, IL-2 has been shown to induce a multitude of reactions from Tregs including increased thymic export, proliferation, and enhanced resistance to apoptosis.[63]

One of the major concerns of any suppressive immunotherapy resulting in an abated immune response is the potential for opportunistic infections. Kennedy-Nasser and colleagues, in a prospective cohort study, demonstrated the use of low-dose IL-2 therapy in allogeneic HSCT to treat GVHD. Patients were given low-dose IL-2 within a time frame of less than 30 days post-HSCT and continued for 6 to 12 weeks. No patient developed grade II–IV GVHD or grade 3/4 toxicities. More importantly, only 15% of the patients developed viral infections, compared with 63% of patients without IL-2 therapy, following standard protocol.[64] From this study, it seems that patients given low-dose IL-2 therapy seem to retain the ability to recognize and respond to viral antigens, unlike patients given standard post-HSCT protocol therapy. Two other studies in patients with GVHD further revealed the potential of low-dose IL-2 for efficacy and safety.[65,66]

IL-2 therapy has also been briefly studied in autoimmune diseases. Castela and colleagues[67] showed the potential of lowdose IL-2 therapy in patients with alopecia areata, with 4 out of 5 patients showing signs of clinical improvement. An objective

Table 1
Clinical trials with Tregs

Therapy Type	Disease Model	Effects	Source
Adoptive Treg transfer	Chronic GVHD	Reduced chronic GVHD manifestations; dose reduction of various immunosuppressive/symptomatic medications.	Trzonkowski et al,[53] 2009
	Prevention of acute GVHD	Prevention of GVHD manifestations; no increased risk of infection; no obvious adverse effects observed.	Brunstein et al,[54] 2011
	Prevention of acute GVHD	Umbilical cord isolated Tregs; prevention of acute GVHD in 26/28; prevention of chronic GVDH in 28/28; no increased risk of CMV infection.	Di Ianni et al,[55] 2011
	T1DM	Decreased HbA1c level; insulin dose reduction or complete withdrawal in 2 patients; increased Treg circulatory numbers; no increased risk of infections; no observable adverse effects.	Marek-Trzonkowska et al,[56] 2012
	T1DM	Follow-up study reporting increased β-islet cell survival with repeated Treg administration over 1 year.	Marek-Trzonkowska et al,[57] 2014
Low-dose IL-2 therapy	HCV-induced vasculitis	8/10 patients experienced clinical improvement; attenuation of inflammatory markers; increased total Treg percentages; safe with adverse effects observed at high-dose IL-2.	Saadoun et al,[61] 2011
	Chronic GVHD	Safe; sustained Treg expansion with peak values at 4 wk; decreased GVHD manifestations.	Koreth et al,[62] 2011
	Chronic GVHD	Molecular basis revealed discriminatory increase in Stat5 phosphorylation in Tregs and a decrease in Tconv numbers; increased Treg thymic export, proliferation, and resistance to apoptosis.	Matsuoka etal,[63] 2013
	Chronic GVHD	Decrease in GVHD manifestation development; no serious observable adverse effects; decrease in rate of viral infections compared with standard therapy.	Kennedy-Nasser et al,[64] 2014
	Chronic GVHD	Increased circulating Tregs; clinical improvements in >60% of patients with steroid refractory disease; no increased risk of infection.	Koreth et al,[65] 2016
	Chronic GVHD	Increased circulating Tregs first wk, normalization during second wk despite continued IL-2 administration; mildly decreased GVHD manifestations; safe.	Kim et al,[66] 2016
	Alopecia areata	4/5 patients showed clinical improvements; decreased CD8+ T-cell infiltration of scalp; increased circulatory Tregs; no major adverse effects observed.	Castela et al,[67] 2014
	Systemic lupus erythematosus	Decrease in disease manifestations; increased circulatory Tregs; decrease T follicular helper and TH17 cell percentages.	He et al,[68] 2016

(continued on next page)

Table 1
(continued)

Therapy Type	Disease Model	Effects	Source
Combined adoptive transfer & low-dose IL-2	Chronic GVHD	Increased circulatory Tregs; observable clinical improvement and/or stabilization.	Theil et al,[69] 2015

Abbreviations: HbA1c, hemoglobin A1C; T1DM, type 1 diabetes mellitus.

decrease in CD8+ T cells infiltration in scalp biopsies, increase in circulatory Tregs, and no major signs of toxicity were also observed. In the more systemically affected autoimmune diseases, He and colleagues[68] showed that the utilization of recombinant human IL-2 in systemic lupus erythematosus, over the course of 2 weeks, resulted in significant decrease in disease manifestations, increase in Treg circulatory cells, and a drop in T follicular helper and TH17 cell percentages.

More interestingly, a recent clinical trial conducted a partial evaluation of the combined effect of adoptive Treg transfer and simultaneous IL-2 injections in patients with chronic GVHD. The 3 patients who received this regime showed increased counts in circulating Tregs and clinical improvements and/or stabilization.[69] **Table 1** summarizes various clinical trials involving Tregs. Clearly more research is required to draw conclusions; nonetheless combined therapy may prove to show more favorable results.

Key Points

- History of Tregs
- Treg biology and function
- Ex vivo expanded and transfusion Treg therapy trials
- IL-2 therapy trials

SUMMARY

Cellular therapy using ex vivo expanded Tregs and immunotherapy using IL-2 to directly stimulate Tregs in vivo is the result of years of conglomerated research into the novel aspects of the immune system. Current trials are largely favorable in efficacy and with paucity of adverse effects shows a great potential compared with traditional therapies. However, further research into efficacy, safety, and, particularly, questions of stability of the Treg population in vivo, is required to fully approach Tregs as bona fide therapies in immune-originated diseases.

REFERENCES

1. Sprent J, Webb SR. Intrathymic and extrathymic clonal deletion of T cells. Curr Opin Immunol 1995;7(2):196–205.
2. Vijay KK, Ohashi PS, Sartor RB, et al. Dysregulation of immune homeostasis in autoimmune diseases. Nat Med 2012;18(1):42.
3. Sakaguchi S, Yamaguchi T, Nomura T, et al. Regulatory T cells and immune tolerance. Cell 2008;133(5):775–87.
4. Gershon RK, Cohen P, Hencin R, et al. Suppressor T cells. J Immunol 1972; 108(3):586.
5. Penhale WJ, Farmer A, Irvine WJ. Thyroiditis in T cell-depleted rats. Influence of strain, radiation dose, adjuvants and antilymphocyte serum. Clin Exp Immunol 1975;21(3):362–75.
6. Penhale WJ, Irvine WJ, Inglis JR, et al. Thyroiditis in T cell-depleted rats: suppression of the autoallergic response by reconstitution with normal lymphoid cells. Clin Exp Immunol 1976;25(1):6–16.
7. Sakaguchi S, Takahashi T, Nishizuka Y. Study on cellular events in postthymectomy autoimmune oophoritis in mice. II. Requirement of Lyt-1 cells in normal female mice for the prevention of oophoritis. J Exp Med 1982;156(6): 1577–86.
8. Sakaguchi S, Fukuma K, Kuribayashi K, et al. Organ-specific autoimmune diseases induced in mice by elimination of T cell subset. I. Evidence for the active

participation of T cells in natural self-tolerance; deficit of a T cell subset as a possible cause of autoimmune disease. J Exp Med 1985;161(1):72–87.

9. Sakaguchi S, Sakaguchi N, Asano M, et al. Immunologic self-tolerance maintained by activated T cells expressing IL-2 receptor alpha-chains (CD25). Breakdown of a single mechanism of self-tolerance causes various autoimmune diseases. J Immunol 1995;155(3):1151–64.

10. Palomares O, Yaman G, Azkur AK, et al. Role of Treg in immune regulation of allergic diseases. Eur J Immunol 2010;40(5):1232–40.

11. Zheng Y, Chaudhry A, Kas A, et al. Regulatory T-cell suppressor program co-opts transcription factor IRF4 to control T(H)2 responses. Nature 2009;458(7236): 351–6.

12. Yu F, Sharma S, Edwards J, et al. Dynamic expression of transcription factors T-bet and GATA-3 by regulatory T cells maintains immunotolerance. Nat Immunol 2015;16(2):197–206.

13. Sakaguchi S. The origin of FOXP3-expressing CD4+ regulatory T cells: thymus or periphery. J Clin Invest 2003;112(9):1310–2.

14. Hori S, Nomura T, Sakaguchi S. Control of regulatory T cell development by the transcription factor Foxp3. Science 2003;299(5609):1057–61.

15. Mason GM, Lowe K, Melchiotti R, et al. Phenotypic complexity of the human regulatory T cell compartment revealed by mass cytometry. J Immunol 2015;195(5): 2030–7.

16. Nie J, Li YY, Zheng SG, et al. FOXP3(+) treg cells and gender bias in autoimmune diseases. Front Immunol 2015;6:493.

17. Yuan X, Cheng G, Malek TR. The importance of regulatory T-cell heterogeneity in maintaining self-tolerance. Immunol Rev 2014;259(1):103–14.

18. Sather BD, Treuting P, Perdue N, et al. Altering the distribution of Foxp3(+) regulatory T cells results in tissue-specific inflammatory disease. J Exp Med 2007; 204(6):1335–47.

19. Svensson M, Marsal J, Ericsson A, et al. CCL25 mediates the localization of recently activated CD8αβ+ lymphocytes to the small-intestinal mucosa. J Clin Invest 2002;110(8):1113–21.

20. Hamann A, Andrew DP, Jablonski-Westrich D, et al. Role of alpha 4-integrins in lymphocyte homing to mucosal tissues in vivo. J Immunol 1994;152(7):3282.

21. Lee JH, Kang SG, Kim CH. FoxP3+ T cells undergo conventional first switch to lymphoid tissue homing receptors in thymus but accelerated second switch to nonlymphoid tissue homing receptors in secondary lymphoid tissues. J Immunol 2006;178(1):301–11.

22. Huehn J, Siegmund K, Lehmann JC, et al. Developmental stage, phenotype, and migration distinguish naive- and effector/memory-like CD4+ regulatory T cells. J Exp Med 2004;199(3):303–13.

23. Beyersdorf N, Ding X, Tietze JK, et al. Characterization of mouse CD4 T cell subsets defined by expression of KLRG1. Eur J Immunol 2007;37(12):3445–54.

24. Haribhai D, Williams JB, Jia S, et al. A requisite role for induced regulatory T cells in tolerance based on expanding antigen receptor diversity. Immunity 2011;35(1): 109–22.

25. Curotto de Lafaille MA, Lafaille JJ. Natural and adaptive foxp3+ regulatory T cells: more of the same or a division of labor? Immunity 2009;30(5):626–35.

26. Liu VC, Wong LY, Jang T, et al. Tumor evasion of the immune system by converting CD4+CD25- T cells into CD4+CD25+ T regulatory cells: role of tumor-derived TGF-. J Immunol 2007;178(5):2883–92.

27. Josefowicz SZ, Niec RE, Kim HY, et al. Extrathymically generated regulatory T cells control mucosal TH2 inflammation. Nature 2012;482(7385):395–9.
28. Zhou X, Bailey-Bucktrout SL, Jeker LT, et al. Instability of the transcription factor Foxp3 leads to the generation of pathogenic memory T cells in vivo. Nat Immunol 2009;10(9):1000–7.
29. Zhou X, Tang J, Cao H, et al. Tissue resident regulatory T cells: novel therapeutic targets for human disease. Cell Mol Immunol 2015;12(5):543–52.
30. Sebzda E, Mariathasan S, Ohteki T, et al. Selection of the T cell repertoire. Annu Rev Immunol 1999;17(1):829–74.
31. Jordan MS, Boesteanu A, Reed AJ, et al. Thymic selection of CD4+CD25+ regulatory T cells induced by an agonist self-peptide. Nat Immunol 2001;2(4):301–6.
32. Shevach EM. Application of IL-2 therapy to target T regulatory cell function. Trends Immunol 2012;33(12):626–32.
33. Fontenot JD, Rasmussen JP, Gavin MA, et al. A function for interleukin 2 in Foxp3-expressing regulatory T cells. Nat Immunol 2005;6(11):1142–51.
34. Burchill MA, Yang J, Vogtenhuber C, et al. IL-2 receptor -dependent STAT5 activation is required for the development of Foxp3+ regulatory T cells. J Immunol 2006;178(1):280–90.
35. Ouyang W, Beckett O, Ma Q, et al. Transforming growth factor-beta signaling curbs thymic negative selection promoting regulatory T cell development. Immunity 2010;32(5):642–53.
36. Burchill MA, Yang J, Vang KB, et al. Linked T cell receptor and cytokine signaling govern the development of the regulatory T cell repertoire. Immunity 2008;28(1):112–21.
37. Lio CW, Hsieh CS. A two-step process for thymic regulatory T cell development. Immunity 2008;28(1):100–11.
38. Koch MA, Tucker-Heard G, Perdue NR, et al. The transcription factor T-bet controls regulatory T cell homeostasis and function during type 1 inflammation. Nat Immunol 2009;10(6):595–602.
39. Chen W, Jin W, Hardegen N, et al. Conversion of peripheral CD4+CD25- naive T cells to CD4+CD25+ regulatory T cells by TGF-beta induction of transcription factor Foxp3. J Exp Med 2003;198(12):1875–86.
40. Marie JC, Letterio JJ, Gavin M, et al. TGF-beta1 maintains suppressor function and Foxp3 expression in CD4+CD25+ regulatory T cells. J Exp Med 2005;201(7):1061–7.
41. Davidson TS, DiPaolo RJ, Andersson J, et al. Cutting edge: IL-2 is essential for TGF- -mediated induction of Foxp3+ T regulatory cells. J Immunol 2007;178(7):4022–6.
42. Zheng Y, Rudensky AY. Foxp3 in control of the regulatory T cell lineage. Nat Immunol 2007;8(5):457–62.
43. Lin W, Haribhai D, Relland LM, et al. Regulatory T cell development in the absence of functional Foxp3. Nat Immunol 2007;8(4):359–68.
44. Huehn J, Beyer M. Epigenetic and transcriptional control of Foxp3+ regulatory T cells. Semin Immunol 2015;27(1):10–8.
45. Ohkura N, Hamaguchi M, Morikawa H, et al. T cell receptor stimulation-induced epigenetic changes and Foxp3 expression are independent and complementary events required for Treg cell development. Immunity 2012;37(5):785–99.
46. Thornton AM, Shevach EM. CD4+CD25+ immunoregulatory T cells suppress polyclonal T cell activation in vitro by inhibiting interleukin 2 production. J Exp Med 1998;188(2):287–96.

47. Bopp T, Becker C, Klein M, et al. Cyclic adenosine monophosphate is a key component of regulatory T cell-mediated suppression. J Exp Med 2007;204(6): 1303–10.

48. Gondek DC, Lu LF, Quezada SA, et al. Cutting edge: contact-mediated suppression by CD4+CD25+ regulatory cells involves a granzyme B-dependent, perforin-independent mechanism. J Immunol 2005;174(4):1783–6.

49. Grossman WJ, Verbsky JW, Barchet W, et al. Human T regulatory cells can use the perforin pathway to cause autologous target cell death. Immunity 2004; 21(4):589–601.

50. Pandiyan P, Zheng L, Ishihara S, et al. CD4+CD25+Foxp3+ regulatory T cells induce cytokine deprivation-mediated apoptosis of effector CD4+ T cells. Nat Immunol 2007;8(12):1353–62.

51. Wing K, Onishi Y, Prieto-Martin P, et al. CTLA-4 control over Foxp3+ regulatory T cell function. Science 2008;322(5899):271–5.

52. Josefowicz SZ, Lu LF, Rudensky AY. Regulatory T cells: mechanisms of differentiation and function. Annu Rev Immunol 2012;30:531–64.

53. Trzonkowski P, Bieniaszewska M, Juścińska J, et al. First-in-man clinical results of the treatment of patients with graft versus host disease with human ex vivo expanded CD4+CD25+CD127− T regulatory cells. Clin Immunol 2009;133(1): 22–6.

54. Brunstein CG, Miller JS, Cao Q, et al. Infusion of ex vivo expanded T regulatory cells in adults transplanted with umbilical cord blood: safety profile and detection kinetics. Blood 2011;117(3):1061.

55. Di Ianni M, Falzetti F, Carotti A, et al. Immunoselection and clinical use of T regulatory cells in HLA-haploidentical stem cell transplantation. Best Pract Res Clin Haematol 2011;24(3):459–66.

56. Marek-Trzonkowska N, Mysliwiec M, Dobyszuk A, et al. Administration of CD4+CD25highCD127- regulatory T cells preserves β-cell function in type 1 diabetes in children. Diabetes Care 2012;35(9):1817.

57. Marek-Trzonkowska N, Myśliwiec M, Dobyszuk A, et al. Therapy of type 1 diabetes with CD4(+)CD25(high)CD127-regulatory T cells prolongs survival of pancreatic islets - results of one year follow-up. Clin Immunol 2014;153(1):23–30.

58. Sula Karreci E, Eskandari SK, Dotiwala F, et al. Human regulatory T cells undergo self-inflicted damage via granzyme pathways upon activation. JCI Insight 2017; 2(21) [pii:91599].

59. Boyman O, Sprent J. The role of interleukin-2 during homeostasis and activation of the immune system. Nat Rev Immunol 2012;12(3):180–90.

60. Ahmadzadeh M, Rosenberg SA. IL-2 administration increases CD4+ CD25(hi) Foxp3+ regulatory T cells in cancer patients. Blood 2006;107(6):2409–14.

61. Saadoun D, Rosenzwajg M, Joly F, et al. Regulatory T-cell responses to low-dose interleukin-2 in HCV-induced vasculitis. N Engl J Med 2011;365(22):2067–77.

62. Koreth J, Matsuoka K, Kim HT, et al. Interleukin-2 and regulatory T cells in graft-versus-host disease. N Engl J Med 2011;365(22):2055–66.

63. Matsuoka K, Koreth J, Kim HT, et al. Low-dose interleukin-2 therapy restores regulatory T cell homeostasis in patients with chronic graft-versus-host disease. Sci Transl Med 2013;5(179):179ra43.

64. Kennedy-Nasser AA, Ku S, Castillo-Caro P, et al. Ultra low-dose IL-2 for GVHD prophylaxis after allogeneic hematopoietic stem cell transplantation mediates expansion of regulatory T cells without diminishing antiviral and antileukemic activity. Clin Cancer Res 2014;20(8):2215–25.

65. Koreth J, Kim HT, Jones KT, et al. Efficacy, durability, and response predictors of low-dose interleukin-2 therapy for chronic graft-versus-host disease. Blood 2016; 128(1):130–7.

66. Kim N, Jeon YW, Nam YS, et al. Therapeutic potential of low-dose IL-2 in a chronic GVHD patient by in vivo expansion of regulatory T cells. Cytokine 2016; 78:22–6.

67. Castela E, Le Duff F, Butori C, et al. Effects of low-dose recombinant interleukin 2 to promote t-regulatory cells in alopecia areata. JAMA Dermatol 2014;150(7): 748–51.

68. He J, Zhang X, Wei Y, et al. Low-dose interleukin-2 treatment selectively modulates CD4(+) T cell subsets in patients with systemic lupus erythematosus. Nat Med 2016;22(9):991–3.

69. Theil A, Tuve S, Oelschlägel U, et al. Adoptive transfer of allogeneic regulatory T cells into patients with chronic graft-versus-host disease. Cytotherapy 2015; 17(4):473–86.

Regulatory and Effector B Cells: A New Path Toward Biomarkers and Therapeutic Targets to Improve Transplant Outcomes?

Aravind Cherukuri, MBBS (MD), MRCP, PhD[a], Qing Ding, PhD[b],
Akhil Sharma, MD[a], Kanishka Mohib, PhD[b],
David M. Rothstein, MD[c],*

KEYWORDS

- Regulatory B cells • Effector B cells • IL-10 • TNF-α • Transplant tolerance
- Biomarker • Human • Mouse

KEY POINTS

- No specific phenotypic marker exists for regulatory B cells or effector B cells in either animal models or in humans.
- Regulatory B cells are frequently identified by the expression of their signature cytokine, IL-10.
- Relative expression of IL-10 to tumor necrosis factor-α in immature B cells in peripheral blood is a good marker for human regulatory B cell or regulatory B cell versus effector B cell activity.
- Regulatory B cells may serve as a marker of human renal allograft tolerance and may be able to predict transplant outcomes.
- Strategies to expand regulatory B cells in vivo and ex vivo exist, suggesting that regulatory B cells may have therapeutic potential in clinical transplantation.

Disclosure Statement: Dr. Rothstein get fund support from NIH grants AI114587 , AI129880 and American Society of Transplantation TIRN grant on Biomarker Discovery and Validation.
[a] Section of Nephrology, Department of Medicine, University of Pittsburgh, Thomas E. Starzl Transplantation Institute, University of Pittsburgh School of Medicine, 200 Lothrop Street, W1545 Biomedical Science Tower, Pittsburgh, PA 15261, USA; [b] Department of Surgery, University of Pittsburgh, Thomas E. Starzl Transplantation Institute, University of Pittsburgh School of Medicine, 200 Lothrop Street, W1545 Biomedical Science Tower, Pittsburgh, PA 15261, USA; [c] Departments of Surgery, Medicine and Immunology, Thomas E. Starzl Transplantation Institute, University of Pittsburgh Medical Center, 200 Lothrop Street, W1545 Biomedical Science Tower, Pittsburgh, PA 15261, USA
* Corresponding author.
E-mail address: rothsteindm@upmc.edu

INTRODUCTION

In addition to antibody secretion, B cells shape the immune response through antigen presentation, costimulation, and cytokine production.[1-3] In this regard, distinctly polarized B-cell subsets expressing either proinflammatory or antiinflammatory cytokines respectively, can promote or inhibit adaptive and innate immunity.[2-5] For example, regulatory B cells (Bregs), inhibit autoimmune diseases and transplant rejection, and promote tumor growth.[1-4,6,7] Although their suppressive function is mainly attributed to the expression of the immunomodulatory cytokine, IL-10, Bregs also use other suppressive cytokines and mechanisms, including IL-35, Fas ligand, PD-L1, transforming growth factor-β, and granzyme B.[8-17] Although initially identified in mice, evidence now suggests that Bregs also play a significant role in human disease and transplantation.[8-17] In contrast, effector B cells (Beff) expressing proinflammatory cytokines such as IL-6, IL-17, tumor necrosis factor (TNF)-α, and interferon (IFN)-γ, can profoundly augment antimicrobial responses, autoimmunity, and transplant rejection.[2-5,18-20] Although the central focus of this review is on Bregs and the important role they play in experimental and clinical transplantation, the net modulating effect of B cells on the alloimmune response is likely a summation of the opposing activities of both Bregs and Beff cells, and both are addressed herein.

B-CELL DEPLETION STUDIES MAKE A CASE FOR BOTH REGULATORY B CELLS AND EFFECTOR B CELLS

B-cell depletion in humans with anti-CD20 can reduce inflammatory T-cell responses and rapidly ameliorate rheumatoid arthritis, diabetes mellitus, and multiple sclerosis (MS), without affecting autoantibody levels,[18,21-23] suggesting a proinflammatory role.[2-4,24-27] In contrast, B-cell depletion can also promote inflammatory T-cell responses, exacerbate autoimmunity, and promote renal allograft rejection,[28-31] suggesting a regulatory role. Murine models confirm this duality. For example, in murine models of inflammatory bowel disease or contact hypersensitivity, B-cell deficiency or depletion can worsen autoimmunity.[32-35] In EAE (a murine model of MS), B-cell depletion can either worsen or ameliorate disease depending on the timing. Moreover, B-cell deficiency can either augment or inhibit antitumor responses and tumor growth.[27,36-40] As detailed elsewhere in this article, Breg/Beff cell ratios (based on cytokine expression) are decreased in MS and strongly predict outcomes in renal transplantation.[11,41,42] These findings strongly suggest that B cells can play both a regulatory or proinflammatory effector role and the influence of B cells on immune response in a given patient is likely a summation of the opposing activity of both Bregs and Beff cells. If such cells could be targeted independently, the immune response might be augmented or inhibited, as required by the clinical setting.

THE PROBLEM IN DEFINING REGULATORY B CELLS AND EFFECTOR B CELLS: THE LACK OF A SPECIFIC PHENOTYPE

There are no phenotypic markers or transcription factors that specifically identify either Bregs or Beff cells. Rather, Bregs and Beff cells are defined by their expression of either antiinflammatory or proinflammatory cytokines. Thus, at present, Bregs are best characterized by the expression of their signature cytokine, IL-10. However, IL-10 is expressed at very low frequency (approximately 1%) in the overall B-cell population.[6,33-35] As a result, multiple B-cell phenotypes that are enriched for IL-10$^+$ B cells have been used as a surrogate for Bregs to elucidate their biology and function. For example, in mice, CD1d$^+$ B cells in the gut were initially shown to transfer IL-10–dependent inhibition of intestinal inflammation.[33] Subsequent studies found that a number of other subsets, including CD1d[hi] CD5[+] ("B10") and CD21[hi]CD23[hi]CD24[hi] (T2-marginal zone precursors) B cells, were enriched for IL-10 expression and again transferred IL-10–dependent amelioration of murine EAE and systemic lupus erythematosus (SLE).[35,43] Importantly, although enriched, IL-10[+] B cells comprise a minority of cells (eg, 15%) within each of these B-cell subsets. Furthermore, the IL-10[+] B cells in each of these small phenotypic subsets, comprise only 10% to 20% of all IL-10[+] B cells in secondary lymphoid organs. Even though the frequency of IL-10[+] expression is low in the remaining 80% to 90% of B cells, these make up the large majority of IL-10[+] B cells. However, the frequency of IL-10[+] cells in these B-cell subsets is too low to demonstrate activity in B-cell transfer models. Another challenge that impedes better understanding of the role of Bregs cells in health and disease, is the IL-10 secretion itself. Owing to low levels of expression, IL-10 is usually only observed after in vitro stimulation of B cells.[6,33–35] This limits the ability to perform meaningful transfer experiments with freshly isolated IL-10[+] cells, examine their function, or perform transcriptional analysis with an aim to uncover a unifying marker or understand their downstream function, without prior stimulation.

In summary, current Breg phenotypes actually represent the subsets most enriched for IL-10 expression in any given disease model, and this may be influenced by the type of stimulation used to elicit IL-10 expression. Importantly, these individual subsets are not specific, nor are they necessarily representative of most IL-10[+] Bregs. Although there are a growing number of examples where Bregs use mechanisms other than IL-10 to suppress immune responses, such Bregs are poorly understood and their relation to IL-10[+] Bregs is unknown.

More recently, TIM-1[+] and CD9[+] B cells were found to be more inclusive markers for Bregs.[6,44] Although still not specific (IL-10[+] B cells comprising only approximately 15%–20% of TIM-1[+] or CD9[+] populations), each of these subsets encompass approximately 75%–85% of all IL-10[+] B cells.[6,44] Notably, TIM-1 and CD9 have functional roles, as they have been shown to positively or negatively regulate IL-10 expression respectively (discussed elsewhere in this article).[6,44–47] Both TIM-1[+] and CD9[+] populations contain IL-10[+] B cells belonging to each of the different canonical B-cell subsets, including transitional 1 and 2 (T1, T2), marginal zone, marginal zone precursors, follicular, and plasma cells.[6,44] The frequency of IL-10 expression varies significantly, as does the size of each subset.[6,44,48,49] Our recent findings examining unstimulated B cells isolated from IL-10 reporter mice, show that plasma, follicular, and marginal zone B cells each contain 25% to 30% of IL-10[+] B cells. It will be important to determine whether IL-10[+] B cells belonging to different subsets exhibit distinct functions.

B cells can also express various proinflammatory cytokines. Although various phenotypic markers have been used to identify IL-10[+] Bregs, far less is known about the phenotypic identity of proinflammatory Beff cells, hampering our ability to understand Beff biology. Harris and colleagues[50] first demonstrated that B cells, dubbed "Be1," could be polarized in vitro to express IFN-γ. Since then, "innate-like B cells" have been shown to express various proinflammatory cytokines that contribute to rapid host responses to microbial infections. Examples include IL-2 (Polygyrus; T helper [Th] type 2 response), IL-17 (*Trypanosoma cruzii*; reduced parasitemia), and IFN-γ (*Listeria*; monocyte activation and *Salmonella*, Th type 1 responses).[5,51,52] Of these, a small subset of CD11a[Hi]FcγRIII[Hi] B cells, which rapidly and transiently expresses IFN-γ in response to Toll-like receptor ligands, remains the only identified innate-like subset of Be1/Beff cells.[5,51,52]

In addition to the innate-like Beff cells described, proinflammatory B cells are also active in more protracted autoimmune and tumor settings.[11,41] For example, loss of B-cell IL-6 reduces Th1 and Th17 responses, reducing the severity of EAE.[4,20,53] Additionally, loss of B cell IFN-γ reduces Th1 responses, resulting in increased Tregs and resistance to proteoglycan-induced arthritis.[4,20,53] The phenotype of these Beff cells was previously unknown. In this regard, we recently showed that another TIM-family member, TIM-4, is a broad marker for Be1 cells that are enriched for IFN-γ and low in IL-10 expression (and encompass the innate-like CD11a^{Hi}FcγRIII^{Hi} subset). TIM-4$^+$ B cells promote Th1 polarization while reducing Tregs and regulatory cytokines such as IL-10. As such, they enhance allograft rejection and reduce tumor growth and metastasis in an IFN-γ–dependent manner.[45] B cells also play a requisite role in chronic rejection of murine cardiac allografts.[54] Although the phenotype and exact mechanism are unknown, this role is not antibody mediated and is driven by both antigen presentation and maintenance of splenic lymphoid architecture required for productive immunity.

HUMAN REGULATORY B CELLS AND EFFECTOR B CELLS

Based on the studies of Bregs in mice, various groups set out to identify subsets of human B cells enriched for IL-10 expression that might be defective in autoimmune settings. Although no specific phenotype was discovered, Blair and colleagues[17] found that IL-10$^+$ B cells were enriched in the CD24^{hi}CD38^{hi} immature B cell (TrB) subset. Moreover, TrB cells from patients with SLE were defective in IL-10 expression when stimulated through the CD40 pathway, compared with normal subjects. Subsequently, Iwata and colleagues[8] showed that human CD24^{hi}CD27$^+$ memory B cells expressed the most IL-10, but no defects in IL-10 expression were seen in a variety of autoimmune subjects, including patients with SLE.[55] Since then, various additional phenotypes have been reported to enrich for IL-10$^+$ human B cells, including TNFR2$^+$, CD25^{hi}CD71^{hi}CD73$^-$, CD27$^+$CD43$^+$CD11b$^+$, and TIM1$^+$ B cells, and CD27^{int}CD38^{hi} plasmablasts, and each of these subsets has been shown to suppress proinflammatory T-cell responses in vitro.[8,17,48,56–59] Of note, there is a significant overlap between some of these subsets. For example, TNFR2$^+$ and TIM1$^+$ B cells are both enriched in IgM$^+$ memory B cells and TrBs.[57,58]

As in mice, only a small proportion of B cells within each of these human subpopulations actually express IL-10, and IL-10 is expressed by multiple B-cell subsets. Indeed, we found that several major B-cell subsets (eg, TrB, Memory, and naïve) all express IL-10 at relatively high frequencies (10%–15%).[11] Importantly, we found that B cells within these same subsets also coexpress inflammatory cytokines like TNF-α, and that the ratio of IL-10/TNF-α correlated best with in vitro regulatory activity. Thus, TrBs (high IL-10/TNF-α ratio) were able to suppress T-cell inflammatory cytokine expression in vitro, whereas neither memory nor naïve B cells (low IL-10/TNF-α ratios) could not. However, both naïve B cells and memory B cells became suppressive in vitro when TNF-α was neutralized, and conversely, TrBs lost their suppressive activity when IL-10 was neutralized. Finally, although IL-10 alone was unchanged, the TrB IL-10/TNF-α ratio decreased with acute renal allograft rejection. These data highlight the limitations of current makers, demonstrate the importance of measuring cytokines rather than just phenotype, and, importantly, suggest that Bregs and Beff cells might both contribute to outcomes. These findings are supported by studies in patients with MS. B cells from patients with MS expressed lower IL-10 with high TNF-α expression. Importantly, the ratio of B cell IL-10/TNF-α expression correlated with disease relapses. However, the phenotype of the cells that express either IL-10 or TNF-α was not examined.[18,41]

In summary, none of the current phenotypic markers for human Breg populations are specific. They identify subpopulations enriched for IL-10, but are not necessarily representative of the majority of IL-10$^+$ B cells that might also exhibit potent Breg activity. Further, even more poorly defined Beff cells are present in the same canonical B-cell subsets and may counteract Breg activity and influence the outcomes observed.[6,45] Thus, we believe that the balance of IL-10/TNF-α, expressed particularly by immature TrBs, is a better read-out of Breg (or Breg/Beff) activity than either B-cell subsets or IL-10 alone.

REGULATORY B CELLS AND CLINICAL TRANSPLANTATION: IS THERE A REGULATORY B CELL SIGNATURE OF OPERATIONAL TOLERANCE?

Evidence accumulating over the last 2 decades strongly supports a potent immuno-modulatory role for B cells in clinical transplantation. Bregs have been extensively studied in the context of operational kidney transplant tolerance (defined as patients with stable renal function despite withdrawal of immunosuppression). Several studies have shown an increase in TrBs and/or IL-10$^+$ B cells in peripheral blood of operationally tolerant renal transplant patients when compared with patients with stable function on immunosuppression, or those with chronic rejection.[9,60–62] A similar B-cell signature was also noted in patients rendered tolerant via induction of mixed chimerism, and this phenotype remained stable over time.[63] It must be emphasized that these studies failed to detect differences in TrBs or their IL-10 expression between tolerant patients and healthy subjects, and subsequent studies have shown that the differences seen in tolerant versus stable transplant patients might be due to immunosuppression itself.[64,65] Moreover, because these studies were not prospective, it is unknown whether these changes in TrBs could predict tolerance in patients before withdrawal of immunosuppression.

TrBs from operationally tolerant patients have been shown to be more suppressive of autologous T-cell responses than those from stable patients still on immunosuppression.[61] In this regard, Nova-Lamperti and colleagues[61] showed that B cells from tolerant patients exhibited high CD40 expression, low CD86 expression, and low Erk phosphorylation upon BCR engagement, when compared with both stable patients on immunosuppression and healthy volunteers. All 3 mechanisms were related to increased B-cell IL-10.[61,62] Another study showed that B cells that secrete granzyme B in vitro were specifically increased in operationally tolerant patients when compared with both stable patients on maintenance immunosuppression and healthy volunteers.[12] These cells exhibited a plasma cell phenotype (CD138^{hi}) and inhibited T-cell IL-21 secretion, whereas other T-cell proinflammatory cytokines including TNF-α and IFN-γ remained unaffected.[12] Despite the excitement over these potentially important findings, it should be noted that the B-cell signature of tolerance with predominance of Bregs, is seen in only kidney transplantation. Specifically, it is not found in other organs such as the liver, where patients prospectively undergo immunosuppression withdrawal.[9,60–62]

REGULATORY B CELLS AND CLINICAL TRANSPLANTATION: CAN REGULATORY B CELLS PREDICT TRANSPLANT OUTCOMES?

In the vastly more common nontolerance setting, Bregs seem to play an important role in inhibiting rejection and promoting good outcomes. As previously mentioned, B-cell depletion in the peritransplant period can markedly increase the rate of acute renal allograft rejection and, in cardiac allograft recipients, it may be associated with an increased rate of cardiac transplant vasculopathy. This suggests that Bregs, inadvertently depleted by anti-CD20, may play a critical protective role in the peri-transplant period in transplant patients with standard immunologic risk.[31,66] In contrast, rituximab (anti-CD20) has been added successfully to plasmapheresis and intravenous immunoglobulin in peritransplant desensitization protocols in HLA-incompatible transplantation.[67] Interestingly, B-cell repopulation after rituximab treatment of such high-risk patients is characterized by an increase in allospecific TrBs, a decrease in allospecific memory B cells, and no increase in acute rejection. This finding suggests that allospecific TrBs could contribute to improved outcomes in HLA-incompatible transplant recipients.[68] This scenario is reminiscent of MS, which is responsive to B-cell depletion therapy. Although patients with MS exhibit high TNF-α and low IL-10 in their peripheral B cells, this aberrant cytokine ratio is corrected in newly emerging B cells after rituximab therapy. Taken together, these studies suggest that the immunologic status of a given patient may reflect the relative proportion of Bregs/Beffs, and therefore affect the relative depletion of these 2 subpopulations after B-cell depletion therapy. In renal transplant patients at standard risk, there may be a relatively a higher proportion of Bregs than Beffs, and B-cell depletion jeopardizes engraftment of the kidney allograft. In autoimmune or allosensitized patients, Beffs may predominate, and B-cell depletion will likely have a salutary effect on engraftment/autoimmunity.

In several small, single-center studies, a greater number of TrBs in peripheral blood was independently associated with protection from rejection and positively correlated with estimated glomerular filtration rate and superior graft survival in kidney transplantation.[69–72] For example, we showed that a lesser number of TrBs 2 years after renal transplantation was associated with higher rates of rejection and donor-specific antibody (DSA), and a lower estimated glomerular filtration rate at 2 years, along with a significant decline in estimated glomerular filtration rate from 6 months to 2 years.[72] Subsequently, Shabir and colleagues[70] showed that higher TrB frequency in the first year was associated with protection from acute rejection over a 5-year follow-up period. In contrast, a low TrB frequency was associated with a significantly increased risk of rejection. Finally, in a small prospective study, patients with acute renal allograft rejection were subsequently found to have an increase in CD86[+] B cells and plasmablasts and a significant reduction in TrBs and granzyme B[+] B cells at 1 year.[73]

Although these studies may be informative, cytokine expression by B cells/subsets was not examined. This limits our ability to understand the underlying changes in Bregs/Beff that occur in various clinical settings that could improve accuracy, understanding, and ultimately treatment strategies. In this regard, we examined 47 patients 2 to 20 years after transplantation who had for-cause renal transplant biopsies.[11] Patients with graft dysfunction who experienced rejection exhibited a decrease in TrB number and frequency compared with patients with graft dysfunction without rejection, a comparable group of stable patients, or healthy controls. However, the TrB IL-10:TNF-α ratio was specifically decreased and showed the strongest association in patients with graft dysfunction and rejection. Moreover, the TrB IL-10:TNF-α ratio was highly correlated with in vitro Breg function. Indeed, TrBs from patients experiencing rejection specifically lost their in vitro regulatory activity. Importantly, at the time of the late for-cause biopsy the TrB IL-10:TNF-α ratio (but not IL-10 alone) could strongly predict the presence of rejection (receiver operator characteristics area under the curve, 0.82; $P<.0001$).[11] Moreover, among patients exhibiting rejection, patients with a higher TrB IL-10/TNF-α ratio exhibited significantly better allograft survival over the following 3 years. Taken together, these findings again implicate the balance between Bregs and Beffs as a possible driving force for adverse transplant outcomes.

Of note, most patients in this study suffered from chronic antibody-mediated rejection. These findings are generally supported by Nouël and colleagues,[74] who showed that B cells from patients with chronic antibody-mediated rejection exhibit a decreased number of TrBs and lose suppressive capacity in vitro compared with B cells from healthy volunteers or those with stable allograft function. However, we believe that the TrB cytokine ratio adds valuable information related to diagnosis, prognosis, and Breg/Beff function in the setting of allograft rejection versus quiescence.

These studies were extended by showing that the ratio of T1/T2 transitional B cells closely reflects the changes in the TrB IL-10:TNF-α ratio and might serve as a simpler marker for Breg/Beff activity. Importantly, a low T1/T2 ratio in stable patients 2-year after transplantation was independently associated with and strongly predicted graft outcomes over a 5-year follow-up period (receiver operator characteristics area under the curve, >0.8; P<.0005), whereas clinical parameters including delayed graft function, creatinine, and DSA were not predictive (receiver operator characteristics area under the curve range, 0.56–0.66).[75] Based on promising results in patients with late rejection and stable function at 2 years, we are now prospectively examining the TrB cytokine ratio in the early posttransplant period as a predictive biomarker for subsequent rejection and outcomes.

Bregs, especially TrBs, have also been studied in stem cell transplant settings. For example, TrBs constitute a majority of B cells in the cord blood and are enriched for IL-10[+] B cells that suppress in vitro T-cell proliferation and proinflammatory cytokine expression.[76] Importantly, in patients who received cord blood transplants, the development of graft-versus-host disease was associated with a sharp decrease in IL-10[+] B cells among the reconstituting B cells, and B cells from such patients lose their ability to suppress allogeneic T cells in vitro.[77] Similarly, putative Breg subsets (TrB and IgM[+] memory B cells) were also reduced in number and lost in vitro Breg activity in stem cell transplant recipients with chronic graft-versus-host disease.[76] Taken together, these studies suggest that Bregs, or the balance of Bregs/Beffs, may help to establish an important immunologic set point. Moreover, they might potentially serve as strong biomarkers that can aid clinical decisions in transplantation.

EFFECTS OF THERAPEUTIC AGENTS ON REGULATORY B CELLS

Given the potentially important role of Bregs in modulating alloresponses, promoting a state of allograft tolerance, and preventing allograft rejection, it is important to consider the impact of drugs routinely used to treat transplant patients on Breg number, function, and their ability to promote allograft survival. A variety of immunosuppressive agents targeting T cells also inhibit or deplete B cells and potentially affect Breg number. For example, alemtuzumab (anti-CD52) profoundly depletes peripheral B cells along with T cells. B-cell reconstitution after alemtuzumab is predominantly composed of immature TrBs and is associated with a prolonged suppression of memory B cells. Interestingly, a decreased number of TrBs in the reconstituting B-cell pool after alemtuzumab induction was associated with increased rejection and DSA detection along with poor allograft function.[72,78–80] In comparison, thymoglobulin leads to B-cell depletion, although its effect on memory B cells may be less pronounced.[80–82] In contrast, basiliximab (anti-CD25) induction does not deplete peripheral B cells, but may result in a phenotype dominated by memory cells.[83] Rituximab (anti-CD20), which has been used both as an induction agent especially in HLA-incompatible transplant recipients and to treat antibody-mediated rejection, results in a significant long-lasting B-cell depletion, particularly of naïve B cells and possibly memory B cells.[84] As noted elsewhere in this discussion, wholesale B-cell depletion with rituximab may have variable effects on autoimmune and transplant recipients, perhaps depending on their immunologic status and relative Breg/Beff ratio. Finally, glucocorticoids, used both in induction and maintenance regimens, may affect B-cell function by promoting apoptosis within the specific B-cell subsets.[64,85] This decreases B-cell numbers, particularly within the TrB subset. Interestingly, despite the routine use of glucocorticoids for the treatment of acute allograft rejection, early ex vivo studies suggest that, in therapeutic dose ranges, they actually enhance antibody production.[86,87]

Almost all commonly used maintenance immunosuppressive agents in transplantation influence B cells and may directly or indirectly affect Bregs. For example, cyclosporine reduces TrBs with less effect on memory or mature B cells.[69] Mycophenolic acid has been shown to cause a dose-dependent decrease in B-cell IL-10 and decreased expression of CD80 and CD86.[88,89] Further, mammalian target of rapamycin inhibitors are associated with a reduction in TrB numbers and an increase in $CD27^+$ memory B cells.[90] Finally, belatacept, a selective T-cell costimulation blocker, may promote a more Bregs phenotype with increased IL-10$^+$ B cells, higher TrB cell frequency, and reduced B-cell differentiation into plasmablasts, when compared with calcineurin inhbitor therapy.[91,92] A recent study has demonstrated that addition of belumimab (anti-BLyS, a B-cell survival factor) to tacrolimus, mycophenolate, and prednisolone in basiliximab-induced renal transplant recipients led to a significant increase in the ratio of B-cell IL-10/IL-6 in the first 3 months after transplantation. However, the clinical implications of this finding remain to be studied.[93] As mentioned elsewhere in this article, a recent analysis of operationally tolerant kidney transplant recipients reported that the TrB number is decreased with the use of either prednisolone or azathioprine and, conversely, withdrawal of steroids was associated with a significant increase in their number.[64] The fact that almost all immunosuppressive agents routinely used in the clinical management of transplant patients influence B cells, and specifically Bregs, has potentially important diagnostic and therapeutic implications. More studies are needed to understand which combinations might promote, rather than inhibit, IL-10$^+$ B cells. Moreover, studies examining B-cell subsets, including Bregs, as prognostic or diagnostic markers in transplantation, must carefully consider the effects of these agents on B-cell phenotype and the potential for the resultant bias.

STRATEGIES TO EXPAND REGULATORY B CELLS IN HUMANS

Given evidence for their beneficial role in murine and human transplantation, expansion of Bregs and inhibition of Beffs, could be an important protolerogenic strategy. Murine studies suggest that specific expansion of Bregs or inhibition of Beffs may be possible. In this regard, TIM-1 and CD9, both broad markers for IL-10$^+$ Bregs, have been shown to have functional roles in mice. For example, TIM-1 positively regulates IL-10 expression by B cells and treatment of mice with an anti–TIM-1 antibody (RMT1-10) results in a 2- to 4-fold expansion of IL-10$^+$ Bregs, which are essential for prolonged allograft survival.[6,45–47,94] Moreover, a loss-of-function TIM-1 mutation decreases both basal Bregs and promotes allograft rejection.[46,47] This finding suggests that the binding of apoptotic cells to TIM-1, a phosphatidylserine receptor, may be important for maintaining basal Breg levels. Moreover, apoptotic cells increase IL-10$^+$ Bregs in vitro and in vivo through TIM-1 binding, and can inhibit collagen-induced arthritis.[45,46,95] TIM-1 is enriched on human IL-10$^+$ B cells, suggesting a therapeutic potential.

Other factors negatively regulate Breg expansion. For example, CD9-deficient mice have almost double the number of IL-10$^+$ B cells, indicating an inhibitory effect of CD9 on Breg expansion.[44] Similarly, CD22 negatively regulates BCR signaling and inhibits

IL-10 expression.[96] Finally, Breg frequency is decreased in the presence of inflammatory cytokines such as IFN-γ and TNF-α.[11,45] Although the mechanisms are unclear, this suggests a reciprocal relationship between Bregs and Beff. In this regard, anti–TIM-4 is a potent tolerogenic agent in murine allograft models and its tolerogenic activity is wholly dependent on the presence of TIM-4$^+$ B cells.[45] Anti–TIM-4 inhibits IFN-γ expression by TIM-4$^+$ Beff cells and this leads to a reciprocal increase in IL-10 expression by TIM-1$^+$ Bregs, although the mechanisms are unclear.

In humans, a variety of agents, including IFN-β, fingolimod, liquinimod, tocilizumab, and infliximab, which are used to treat autoimmune disorders, may enhance Breg numbers and/or activity.[14,97–104] Additionally, other agents such as vitamin D, retinoic acid, and sotrastaurin can induce ex vivo B-cell proliferation and ensuing IL-10$^+$ Breg expansion might contribute to their therapeutic efficacy.[88,105,106] Many such drugs have not been examined in the transplant arena.

Another approach to Breg-based therapy uses adoptive therapy of Bregs expanded ex vivo. It has been noted in mice that various cytokines induced in inflammatory settings, including IL-1β, IL-4, IL-6, IL-21, IL-35, and IFN-α can expand Bregs in vitro or in vivo.[6,14,107–109] Remarkably, in vitro culture using IL-4 and IL-21 along with CD40L/BAFF-expressing feeder cells was shown to expand murine Bregs up to 1 million-fold.[109] Transfer of these ex vivo expanded Bregs ameliorated EAE, proving that their regulatory activity was retained. Similarly, transitional B cells from healthy human donors can be expanded with IFN-α and CpG-C ex vivo and retain their IL-10 expression, phenotype, and Breg activity.[14] Importantly, this same approach was unsuccessful using B cells from patients with SLE. In an in vivo setting, Bregs may interact with other cell types that could provide cytokines that promote their expansion, such as macrophages (IL-1-β, IL-6), Tfh (IL-21), B cells (IL-35), and pDCs (IFN-α).[14,109]

SUMMARY

Bregs and Beffs exhibit a potent ability to modulate immune response and could potentially alter the course of various autoimmune, alloimmune, and infectious processes. Accumulating evidence suggests that increased Breg frequency and intact Breg function correlates strongly with the development of a tolerant clinical state, reduced rejection episodes, and improved long-term allograft survival. Therefore, strategies that specifically aim to expand Bregs or enhance their function, or conversely inhibit/deplete Beffs, represent promising therapeutic options to improve transplant outcomes. This aim is hindered by our limited understanding of Breg and Beff biology, and limited knowledge of their development, induction, and in vivo effector function. This limitation is compounded by a lack of specific markers that would allow us to identify these cell populations for monitoring, or as targets for depletion. Nonetheless, protocols that can expand B cells (in vivo or in vitro) that are highly enriched for IL-10, while expressing low levels of proinflammatory cytokines, have potential to reset the immune set point and improve clinical outcomes. Finally, given that alterations within the Breg subsets may precede rejection episodes, Bregs may play a promising role as biomarkers to guide preemptive treatment of at-risk transplant recipients.

REFERENCES

1. Mauri C, Menon M. The expanding family of regulatory B cells. Int Immunol 2015;27:479–86.
2. Shen P, Fillatreau S. Antibody-independent functions of B cells: a focus on cytokines. Nat Rev Immunol 2015;15:441–51.

3. Lund FE, Randall TD. Effector and regulatory B cells: modulators of CD4+ T cell immunity. Nat Rev Immunol 2010;10:236–47.
4. Fillatreau S. Pathogenic functions of B cells in autoimmune diseases: IFN-gamma production joins the criminal gang. Eur J Immunol 2015;45:966–70.
5. Bao Y, Liu X, Han C, et al. Identification of IFN-γ-producing innate B cells. Cell Res 2014;24:161–76.
6. Ding Q, Yeung M, Camirand G, et al. Regulatory B cells are identified by expression of TIM-1 and can be induced through TIM-1 ligation to promote tolerance in mice. J Clin Invest 2011;121:3645–56.
7. Balkwill F, Montfort A, Capasso M. B regulatory cells in cancer. Trends Immunol 2013;34:169–73.
8. Iwata Y, Matsushita T, Horikawa M, et al. Characterization of a rare IL-10-competent B-cell subset in humans that parallels mouse regulatory B10 cells. Blood 2011;117:530–41.
9. Newell KA, Asare A, Kirk AD, et al. Identification of a B cell signature associated with renal transplant tolerance in humans. J Clin Invest 2010;120:1836–47.
10. Sagoo P, Perucha E, Sawitzki B, et al. Development of a cross-platform biomarker signature to detect renal transplant tolerance in humans. J Clin Invest 2010;120:1848–61.
11. Cherukuri A, Rothstein DM, Clark B, et al. Immunologic human renal allograft injury associates with an altered IL-10/TNF-α expression ratio in regulatory B cells. J Am Soc Nephrol 2014;25:1575–85.
12. Chesneau M, Michel L, Dugast E, et al. Tolerant kidney transplant patients produce B cells with regulatory properties. J Am Soc Nephrol 2015;26:2588–98.
13. Pallier A, Hillion S, Danger R, et al. Patients with drug-free long-term graft function display increased numbers of peripheral B cells with a memory and inhibitory phenotype. Kidney Int 2010;78:503–13.
14. Menon M, Blair PA, Isenberg DA, et al. A regulatory feedback between plasmacytoid dendritic cells and regulatory B cells is aberrant in systemic lupus erythematosus. Immunity 2016;44:683–97.
15. Noh J, Lee JH, Noh G, et al. Characterisation of allergen-specific responses of IL-10-producing regulatory B cells (Br1) in Cow Milk Allergy. Cell Immunol 2010; 264:143–9.
16. Siewe B, Stapleton JT, Martinson J, et al. Regulatory B cell frequency correlates with markers of HIV disease progression and attenuates anti-HIV CD8+ T cell function in vitro. J Leukoc Biol 2013;93:811–8.
17. Blair PA, Noreña LY, Flores-Borja F, et al. CD19(+)CD24(hi)CD38(hi) B cells exhibit regulatory capacity in healthy individuals but are functionally impaired in systemic Lupus Erythematosus patients. Immunity 2010;32:129–40.
18. Lino AC, Dorner T, Bar-Or A, et al. Cytokine-producing B cells: a translational view on their roles in human and mouse autoimmune diseases. Immunol Rev 2016;269:130–44.
19. Barr TA, Brown S, Mastroeni P, et al. TLR and B cell receptor signals to B cells differentially program primary and memory Th1 responses to Salmonella enterica. J Immunol 2010;185:2783–9.
20. Olalekan SA, Cao Y, Hamel KM, et al. B cells expressing IFN-gamma suppress Treg-cell differentiation and promote autoimmune experimental arthritis. Eur J Immunol 2015;45:988–98.
21. Roll P, Dorner T, Tony HP. Anti-CD20 therapy in patients with rheumatoid arthritis: predictors of response and B cell subset regeneration after repeated treatment. Arthritis Rheum 2008;58:1566–75.

22. Cambridge G, Perry HC, Nogueira L, et al. The effect of B-cell depletion therapy on serological evidence of B-cell and plasmablast activation in patients with rheumatoid arthritis over multiple cycles of rituximab treatment. J Autoimmun 2014;50:67–76.

23. Martin F, Chan AC. B cell immunobiology in disease: evolving concepts from the clinic. Annu Rev Immunol 2006;24:467–96.

24. Hu CY, Rodriguez-Pinto D, Du W, et al. Treatment with CD20-specific antibody prevents and reverses autoimmune diabetes in mice. J Clin Invest 2007;117: 3857–67.

25. Edwards JC, Szczepanski L, Szechinski J, et al. Efficacy of B-cell-targeted therapy with rituximab in patients with rheumatoid arthritis. N Engl J Med 2004;350: 2572–81.

26. Bouaziz JD, Yanaba K, Venturi GM, et al. Therapeutic B cell depletion impairs adaptive and autoreactive CD4+ T cell activation in mice. Proc Natl Acad Sci U S A 2007;104:20878–83.

27. Matsushita T, Yanaba K, Bouaziz JD, et al. Regulatory B cells inhibit EAE initiation in mice while other B cells promote disease progression. J Clin Invest 2008; 118:3420–30.

28. Kappos L, Hartung HP, Freedman MS, et al. Atacicept in multiple sclerosis (ATAMS): a randomised, placebo-controlled, double-blind, phase 2 trial. Lancet Neurol 2014;13:353–63.

29. Thaunat O, Morelon E, Defrance T. Am"B"valent: anti-CD20 antibodies unravel the dual role of B cells in immunopathogenesis. Blood 2010;116:515–21.

30. Bouaziz JD, Yanaba K, Tedder TF. Regulatory B cells as inhibitors of immune responses and inflammation. Immunol Rev 2008;224:201–14.

31. Clatworthy MR, Watson CJ, Plotnek G, et al. B-cell-depleting induction therapy and acute cellular rejection. N Engl J Med 2009;360:2683–5.

32. Watanabe R, Fujimoto M, Ishiura N, et al. CD19 expression in B cells is important for suppression of contact hypersensitivity. Am J Pathol 2007;171:560–70.

33. Mizoguchi A, Mizoguchi E, Takedatsu H, et al. Chronic intestinal inflammatory condition generates IL-10-producing regulatory B cell subset characterized by CD1d upregulation. Immunity 2002;16:219–30.

34. Fillatreau S, Sweenie CH, McGeachy MJ, et al. B cells regulate autoimmunity by provision of IL-10. Nat Immunol 2002;3:944–50.

35. Yanaba K, Bouaziz JD, Haas KM, et al. A regulatory B cell subset with a unique CD1dhiCD5+ phenotype controls T cell-dependent inflammatory responses. Immunity 2008;28:639–50.

36. Shah S, Divekar AA, Hilchey SP, et al. Increased rejection of primary tumors in mice lacking B cells: inhibition of anti-tumor CTL and TH1 cytokine responses by B cells. Int J Cancer 2005;117:574–86.

37. Qin Z, Richter G, Schüler T, et al. B cells inhibit induction of T cell-dependent tumor immunity. Nat Med 1998;4:627–30.

38. DiLillo DJ, Yanaba K, Tedder TF. B cells are required for optimal CD4+ and CD8+ T cell tumor immunity: therapeutic B cell depletion enhances B16 melanoma growth in mice. J Immunol 2010;184:4006–16.

39. Schultz KR, Klarnet JP, Gieni RS, et al. The role of B cells for in vivo T cell responses to a Friend virus-induced leukemia. Science 1990;249:921–3.

40. Nelson BH. CD20+ B cells: the other tumor-infiltrating lymphocytes. J Immunol 2010;185:4977–82.

41. Bar-Or A, Fawaz L, Fan B, et al. Abnormal B-cell cytokine responses a trigger of T-cell-mediated disease in MS? Ann Neurol 2010;67:452–61.

42. Cherukuri A, Salama AD, Carter CR, et al. Human transitional B cell T1/T2 ratio is a new marker for allograft deteriotration in kidney transplant recipients. Kidney Int 2017;91:183–95 *denotes equal contribution.

43. Blair PA, Chavez-Rueda KA, Evans JG, et al. Selective targeting of B cells with agonistic anti-CD40 is an efficacious strategy for the generation of induced regulatory T2-like B cells and for the suppression of lupus in MRL/lpr mice. J Immunol 2009;182:3492–502.

44. Sun J, Wang J, Pefanis E, et al. Transcriptomics identify CD9 as a marker of murine IL-10-competent regulatory B cells. Cell Rep 2015;13:1110–7.

45. Ding Q, Mohib K, Kuchroo VK, et al. TIM-4 identifies IFN-gamma-expressing proinflammatory B effector 1 cells that promote tumor and allograft rejection. J Immunol 2017;199:2585–95.

46. Xiao S, Brooks CR, Sobel RA, et al. Tim-1 is essential for induction and maintenance of IL-10 in regulatory B cells and their regulation of tissue inflammation. J Immunol 2015;194:1602–8.

47. Yeung MY, Ding Q, Brooks CR, et al. TIM-1 signaling is required for maintenance and induction of regulatory B cells. Am J Transplant 2015;15:942–53.

48. Matsumoto M, Baba A, Yokota T, et al. Interleukin-10-producing plasmablasts exert regulatory function in autoimmune inflammation. Immunity 2014;41: 1040–51.

49. Shen P, Roch T, Lampropoulou V, et al. IL-35-producing B cells are critical regulators of immunity during autoimmune and infectious diseases. Nature 2014; 507:366–70.

50. Harris DP, Goodrich S, Gerth AJ, et al. Regulation of IFN-gamma production by B effector 1 cells: essential roles for T-bet and the IFN-gamma receptor. J Immunol 2005;174(11):6781–90.

51. Bermejo DA, Jackson SW, Gorosito-Serran M, et al. Trypanosoma cruzi trans-sialidase initiates a program independent of the transcription factors RORγt and Ahr that leads to IL-17 production by activated B cells. Nat Immunol 2013;14:514–22.

52. Wojciechowski W, Harris DP, Sprague F, et al. Cytokine-producing effector B cells regulate type 2 immunity to H. polygyrus. Immunity 2009;30:421–33.

53. Barr TA, Shen P, Brown S, et al. B cell depletion therapy ameliorates autoimmune disease through ablation of IL-6-producing B cells. J Exp Med 2012;209: 1001–10.

54. Zeng Q, Ng YH, Singh T, et al. B cells mediate chronic allograft rejection independently of antibody production. J Clin Invest 2014;124:1052–6.

55. Mauri C, Menon M. Human regulatory B cells in health and disease: therapeutic potential. J Clin Invest 2017;127:772–9.

56. van de Veen W, Stanic B, Yaman G, et al. IgG4 production is confined to human IL-10-producing regulatory B cells that suppress antigen-specific immune responses. J Allergy Clin Immunol 2013;131:1204–12.

57. Aravena O, Ferrier A, Menon M, et al. TIM-1 defines a human regulatory B cell population that is altered in frequency and function in systemic sclerosis patients. Arthritis Res Ther 2017;19:8.

58. Ticha O, Moos L, Wajant H, et al. Expression of tumor necrosis factor receptor 2 characterizes TLR9-driven formation of interleukin-10-producing B cells. Front Immunol 2017;8:1951.

59. Griffin DO, Rothstein TL. Human "orchestrator" CD11b(+) B1 cells spontaneously secrete interleukin-10 and regulate T-cell activity. Mol Med 2012;18: 1003–8.

60. Chesneau M, Pallier A, Braza F, et al. Unique B cell differentiation profile in tolerant kidney transplant patients. Am J Transplant 2014;14:144–55.
61. Nova-Lamperti E, Fanelli G, Becker PD, et al. IL-10-produced by human transitional B-cells down-regulates CD86 expression on B-cells leading to inhibition of CD4+T-cell responses. Sci Rep 2016;6:20044.
62. Nova-Lamperti E, Chana P, Mobillo P, et al. Increased CD40 ligation and reduced BCR signalling leads to higher IL-10 production in B cells from tolerant kidney transplant patients. Transplantation 2017;101:541–7.
63. Newell KA, Asare A, Sanz I, et al. Longitudinal studies of a B cell-derived signature of tolerance in renal transplant recipients. Am J Transplant 2015;15:2908–20.
64. Rebollo-Mesa I, Nova-Lamperti E, Mobillo P, et al. Biomarkers of tolerance in kidney transplantation: are we predicting tolerance or response to immunosuppressive treatment? Am J Transplant 2016;16:3443–57.
65. Markmann JF. Signatures of tolerance or immunosuppression? Am J Transplant 2016;16:3320–1.
66. Vidic AS, Edwards R, Toll LB, et al. Rituximab induction and risk of cardiac allograft vasculopathy, rejection and death. J Heart Lung Transplant 2017;36:S88.
67. Vo AA, Lukovsky M, Toyoda M, et al. Rituximab and intravenous immune globulin for desensitization during renal transplantation. N Engl J Med 2008;359:242–51.
68. Kopchaliiska D, Zachary AA, Montgomery RA, et al. Reconstitution of peripheral allospecific CD19+ B-cell subsets after B-lymphocyte depletion therapy in renal transplant patients. Transplantation 2009;87:1394–401.
69. Tebbe B, Wilde B, Ye Z, et al. Renal transplant recipients treated with calcineurin-inhibitors lack circulating immature transitional CD19+ CD24hiCD38hi regulatory B-lymphocytes. PLoS One 2016;11:e0153170.
70. Shabir S, Girdlestone J, Briggs D, et al. Transitional B lymphocytes are associated with protection from kidney allograft rejection: a prospective study. Am J Transplant 2015;15:1384–91.
71. Svachova V, Sekerkova A, Hruba P, et al. Dynamic changes of B-cell compartments in kidney transplantation: lack of transitional B cells is associated with allograft rejection. Transpl Int 2016;29:540–8.
72. Cherukuri A, Salama AD, Carter C, et al. An analysis of lymphocyte phenotype after steroid avoidance with either alemtuzumab or basiliximab induction in renal transplantation. Am J Transplant 2012;12:919–31.
73. Schlosser HA, Thelen M, Dieplinger G, et al. Prospective analyses of circulating B cell subsets in ABO-compatible and ABO-incompatible kidney transplant recipients. Am J Transplant 2017;17:542–50.
74. Nouël A, Ségalen I, Jamin C, et al. B cells display an abnormal distribution and an impaired suppressive function in patients with chronic antibody-mediated rejection. Kidney Int 2014;85:590–9.
75. Cherukuri A, Salama AD, Carter CR, et al. Reduced human transitional B cell T1/T2 ratio is associated with subsequent deterioration in renal allograft function. Kidney Int 2017;91:183–95.
76. Khoder A, Sarvaria A, Alsuliman A, et al. Regulatory B cells are enriched within the IgM memory and transitional subsets in healthy donors but are deficient in chronic GVHD. Blood 2014;124:2034–45.
77. Sarvaria A, Basar R, Mehta RS, et al. IL-10+ regulatory B cells are enriched in cord blood and may protect against cGVHD after cord blood transplantation. Blood 2016;128:1346–61.

78. Heidt S, Hester J, Shankar S, et al. B cell repopulation after alemtuzumab induction-transient increase in transitional B cells and long-term dominance of naïve B cells. Am J Transplant 2012;12:1784–92.

79. Todeschini M, Cortinovis M, Perico N, et al. In kidney transplant patients, alemtuzumab but not basiliximab/low-dose rabbit anti-thymocyte globulin induces B cell depletion and regeneration, which associates with a high incidence of de novo donor-specific anti-HLA antibody development. J Immunol 2013;191:2818–28.

80. Toso C, Edgar R, Pawlick R, et al. Effect of different induction strategies on effector, regulatory and memory lymphocyte sub-populations in clinical islet transplantation. Transpl Int 2009;22:182–91.

81. Kho MM, Bouvy AP, Cadogan M, et al. The effect of low and ultra-low dosages Thymoglobulin on peripheral T, B and NK cells in kidney transplant recipients. Transpl Immunol 2012;26:186–90.

82. Zand MS, Vo T, Huggins J, et al. Polyclonal rabbit antithymocyte globulin triggers B-cell and plasma cell apoptosis by multiple pathways. Transplantation 2005;79:1507–15.

83. Longshan L, Dongwei L, Qian F, et al. Dynamic analysis of B-cell subsets in de novo living related kidney transplantation with induction therapy of basiliximab. Transplant Proc 2014;46:363–7.

84. Kamburova EG, Koenen HJ, Boon L, et al. In vitro effects of rituximab on the proliferation, activation and differentiation of human B cells. Am J Transplant 2012;12:341–50.

85. Kovacs WJ. To B or not to B? Glucocorticoid impact on B lymphocyte fate and function. Endocrinology 2014;155:339–42.

86. Grayson J, Dooley NJ, Koski IR, et al. Immunoglobulin production induced in vitro by glucocorticoid hormones: T cell-dependent stimulation of immunoglobulin production without B cell proliferation in cultures of human peripheral blood lymphocytes. J Clin Invest 1981;68:1539–47.

87. Fauci AS, Pratt KR, Whalen G. Activation of human B lymphocytes. IV. Regulatory effects of corticosteroids on the triggering signal in the plaque-forming cell response of human peripheral blood B lymphocytes to polyclonal activation. J Immunol 1977;119:598–603.

88. Matz M, Lehnert M, Lorkowski C, et al. Effects of sotrastaurin, mycophenolic acid and everolimus on human B-lymphocyte function and activation. Transpl Int 2012;25:1106–16.

89. Joly MS, Martin RP, Mitra-Kaushik S, et al. Transient low-dose methotrexate generates B regulatory cells that mediate antigen-specific tolerance to alglucosidase alfa. J Immunol 2014;193:3947–58.

90. Latorre I, Esteve-Sole A, Redondo D, et al. Calcineurin and mTOR inhibitors have opposing effects on regulatory T cells while reducing regulatory B cell populations in kidney transplant recipients. Transpl Immunol 2016;35:1–6.

91. Leibler C, Matignon M, Pilon C, et al. Kidney transplant recipients treated with belatacept exhibit increased naïve and transitional B cells. Am J Transplant 2014;14:1173–82.

92. Furuzawa-Carballeda J, Bostock IC, Lima G, et al. Immunophenotyping of peripheral immunoregulatory as well as Th17A and Th22 cell subpopulations in kidney transplant recipients under belatacept or cyclosporine treatment. Transpl Immunol 2014;30:107–13.

93. Banham GD, Flint SM, Torpey N, et al. Belimumab in kidney transplantation: an experimental medicine, randomised, placebo-controlled phase 2 trial. Lancet 2018. https://doi.org/10.1016/S0140-6736(18)30984-X.

94. Lee KM, Kim JI, Stott R, et al. Anti-CD45RB/anti-TIM-1-induced tolerance requires regulatory B cells. Am J Transplant 2012;12:2072–8.

95. Gray M, Miles K, Salter D, et al. Apoptotic cells protect mice from autoimmune inflammation by the induction of regulatory B cells. Proc Natl Acad Sci U S A 2007;104:14080–5.

96. Yanaba K, Bouaziz JD, Matsushita T, et al. The development and function of regulatory B cells expressing IL-10 (B10 cells) requires antigen receptor diversity and TLR signals. J Immunol 2009;182:7459–72.

97. Schubert RD, Hu Y, Kumar G, et al. IFN-β treatment requires B cells for efficacy in neuroautoimmunity. J Immunol 2015;194:2110–6.

98. Toubi E, Nussbaum S, Staun-Ram E, et al. Laquinimod modulates B cells and their regulatory effects on T cells in multiple sclerosis. J Neuroimmunol 2012; 251:45–54.

99. Grützke B, Hucke S, Gross CC, et al. Fingolimod treatment promotes regulatory phenotype and function of B cells. Ann Clin Transl Neurol 2015;2:119–30.

100. Snir A, Kessel A, Haj T, et al. Anti-IL-6 receptor antibody (tocilizumab): a B cell targeting therapy. Clin Exp Rheumatol 2011;29:697–700.

101. Assier E, Boissier MC, Dayer JM. Interleukin-6: from identification of the cytokine to development of targeted treatments. Joint Bone Spine 2010;77:532–6.

102. Bankó Z, Pozsgay J, Gáti T, et al. Regulatory B cells in rheumatoid arthritis: alterations in patients receiving anti-TNF therapy. Clin Immunol 2017;184:63–9.

103. Anolik JH, Ravikumar R, Barnard J, et al. Cutting edge: anti-tumor necrosis factor therapy in rheumatoid arthritis inhibits memory B lymphocytes via effects on lymphoid germinal centers and follicular dendritic cell networks. J Immunol 2008;180:688–92.

104. Wang QT, Wu YJ, Huang B, et al. Etanercept attenuates collagen-induced arthritis by modulating the association between BAFFR expression and the production of splenic memory B cells. Pharmacol Res 2013;68:38–45.

105. Heine G, Niesner U, Chang HD, et al. 1,25-dihydroxyvitamin D(3) promotes IL-10 production in human B cells. Eur J Immunol 2008;38:2210–8.

106. Di Caro V, Phillips B, Engman C, et al. Involvement of suppressive B-lymphocytes in the mechanism of tolerogenic dendritic cell reversal of type 1 diabetes in NOD mice. PLoS One 2014;9:e83575.

107. Rosser EC, Oleinika K, Tonon S, et al. Regulatory B cells are induced by gut microbiota-driven interleukin-1β and interleukin-6 production. Nat Med 2014; 20:1334–9.

108. Wang RX, Yu CR, Dambuza IM, et al. Interleukin-35 induces regulatory B cells that suppress autoimmune disease. Nat Med 2014;20:633–41.

109. Yoshizaki A, Miyagaki T, DiLillo DJ, et al. Regulatory B cells control T-cell autoimmunity through IL-21-dependent cognate interactions. Nature 2012;491: 264–8.

Complement and Transplantation

From New Mechanisms to Potential Biomarkers and Novel Treatment Strategies

Julian K. Horwitz, MD[a,b], Nicholas H. Chun, MD[a,c], Peter S. Heeger, MD[a,c,d],*

KEYWORDS

- Complement • T cells • Antibody-mediated rejection • Ischemia-reperfusion injury

KEY POINTS

- Complement activation, via the lectin and classical pathways, is an important mediator of ischemia-reperfusion injury.
- Local production of complement by immune cells induces antigen-presenting cell maturation and effector T-cell expansion, while inhibiting regulatory T-cell generation.
- Donor-specific antibody (DSA)-mediated complement activation initiates a proinflammatory gene program in donor endothelial cells.
- Serum-based complement components have the potential to serve as biomarkers for allograft rejection.

INTRODUCTION

The complement system is traditionally considered a component of the innate immune system. In the context of transplantation, evidence published since the late 1990s has expanded understanding of links between complement and adaptive immunity,

Disclosures: The authors have nothing to disclose.

Funding: The work was supported by NIH, NIAID grants R01 AI071185 and R01 AI132405 awarded to P.S. Heeger and K08 AI135101 to N.H. Chun.

[a] Translational Transplant Research Center, Icahn School of Medicine at Mount Sinai, One Gustave L Levy Place, New York, NY 10029, USA; [b] Department of Surgery, Icahn School of Medicine at Mount Sinai, One Gustave L Levy Place, New York, NY 10029, USA; [c] Department of Medicine, Icahn School of Medicine at Mount Sinai, One Gustave L Levy Place, New York, NY 10029, USA; [d] The Precision Institute of Immunology, Icahn School of Medicine at Mount Sinai, One Gustave L Levy Place, New York, NY 10029, USA

* Corresponding author. Translational Transplant Research Center, Department of Medicine, Icahn School of Medicine at Mount Sinai, Annenberg Building Box 1243, One Gustave L Levy Place, New York, NY 10029.

E-mail address: peter.heeger@mssm.edu

including alloimmune responses and transplant injury. Among many pathogenic functions in transplantation, complement participates in ischemia-reperfusion (I/R) injury, controls the strength of the donor-reactive T-cell immune response, and acts as an effector for antibody-initiated allograft injury. This article reviews the biology of the complement system and discusses current concepts regarding how complement contributes to the pathogenesis of transplant injury. How the discovery of these fundamental mechanisms has led to development and testing of (1) novel treatment strategies that could limit allograft injury and improve the health of transplant recipients and (2) complement-derived biomarkers for post-transplant risk stratification is also discussed.

BIOLOGY OF THE COMPLEMENT SYSTEM

The complement system is composed of more than 30 soluble and membrane-bound proteins, including zymogens, receptors, and regulators. The individual complement components can be categorized by their ability to initiate, amplify, or regulate the complement cascade and/or perform effector functions (**Fig. 1**).

Complement activation can be initiated via the classical pathway, the lectin pathway, and the alternative pathway.[1] The classical pathway is activated when C1q, as part of the C1qrs complex, binds to the Fc regions of IgG or IgM. The activated C1qrs complex then cleaves C4 and C2, forming the membrane-bound C4bC2b C3 convertase, which enzymatically cleaves C3 into C3a (an anaphylatoxin) and C3b. In the lectin pathway, mannose-binding lectins (MBLs), as well as collectins and ficolins, function as pattern recognition receptors and bind bacterial carbohydrate and/or lipid motifs. MBLs can also directly recognize neoantigens expressed by injured or apoptotic cells,[2] a mechanism pathogenically linked to I/R injury (discussed later). Once bound, the lectin binding proteins function as opsonins and also interact with MBL-associated serine proteases (MASPs). On binding to MBL, MASP-1 and MASP-2 act analogously to the C1qrs complex, the MBL/MASP-1/2 complex that cleaves C4 and C2 to generate C4bC2b C3 convertases. In the alternative pathway, complement activation occurs continuously and spontaneously at low levels, through a process commonly referred to as *tickover*. This process is initiated by spontaneous hydrolysis of C3, forming $C3(H_2O)$, which permits binding of factor B. Factor D–mediated cleavage of $C3(H_2O)$ –bound factor B forms the initial C3 convertase, $C3(H_2O)Bb$, which cleaves C3 into C3a and C3b. C3b then associates with Bb to form the membrane-bound C3bBb alternative pathway C3 convertase. Once C3 convertases are formed by any of the 3 activation pathways, the alternative pathway amplifies complement activation by using the locally produced C3b molecules to form more C3 convertases.

The surface-bound, multimeric, C3 convertases can bind additional C3b molecules to yield the C5 convertases, C4bC2bC3b and C3bBbC3b (see **Fig. 1**). These enzymes cleave C5 into C5a (another anaphylatoxin) and C5b, the latter initiating the formation of the C5b-9 membrane attack complex (MAC).[3] The MAC forms a pore in cell membranes, which promotes cytolysis in non-nucleated cells (including bacteria and red blood cells). MACs inserted into nucleated cells generally induce cellular activation,[4] rather than lysis, and/or promote tissue injury.[5] Soluble and surface-bound split products, including C3a, C3b, iC3b, C3dg, and C5a, mediate separate but overlapping effector functions.[6] C3a and C5a ligate their respective receptors C3aR1 and C5aR1, 7-transmembrane–spanning, G-protein–coupled receptors (GPCRs) expressed on various cell types to mediate chemotaxis, cytokine release, antigen-presenting cell (APC) activation, and T-cell activation and expansion (discussed later).[7–10] C3b, iC3b, and C3dg bind to various complement receptors, functioning as opsonins.

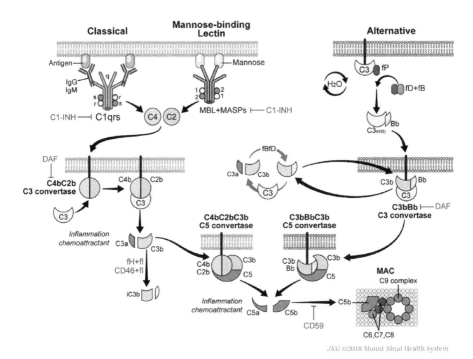

Fig. 1. Overview of the complement cascade and its regulators. Complement activation can be initiated by the classical pathway triggered by cross-linking cell-bound subclasses of IgG and IgM antibodies, the MBL pathway triggered by carbohydrates present on bacteria surface, and the alternative pathway that undergoes spontaneous activation on cell surfaces. All 3 pathways converge into 1 key amplification step to form multimeric C3 convertases, which cleave C3 to C3a and C3b, the latter forming additional C3 convertases (amplification) and then initiating formation of the C5 convertase. Subsequently, C5 cleavage yields C5a and C5b, ultimately forming the MAC (C5b-9) on the target cells. Complement activation/amplification is restrained on self-cells by several membrane-bound and soluble regulatory proteins (*red*). See text for further details. Surface-expressed regulators include DAF, which accelerates the decay of cell-surface assembled C3 convertases; MCP, a cofactor for factor I (fI) that inactivates C3b to iC3b; and CD59 (protectin, inhibits formation of the MAC). Factor H (fH) is a soluble complement regulator that exhibits both DAF and cofactor activity. C1-INH inhibits C1qrs and MBL-MASP complexes, limiting classical pathway and MBL pathway activation, respectively.

Under physiologic conditions, multiple regulatory mechanisms throughout the cascade prevent injury to self-cells but permit complement activation on pathogens that do not express complement regulators[6] (see **Fig. 1**). The C1-inhibitor (C1-INH) inactivates the C1qrs complex, as well as the MBL/MASP-1/MASP-2 complex, to prevent classical and lectin pathway activation. Decay-accelerating factor (DAF [CD55]), a glycophosphatidylinositol (GPI)-anchored, cell surface–expressed protein, accelerates the decay of the C3 convertases, thereby limiting amplification of the complement cascade. Soluble factor H and surface-expressed membrane cofactor protein (MCP [CD46]) are cofactors for factor I that cleave C3b into iC3b, a mechanism that irreversibly disassociates C3 convertases. Downstream, ubiquitously expressed carboxypeptidases rapidly inactivate the C3a and C5a anaphylatoxins while the surface expressed, GPI-anchored protein CD59 (protectin) prevents the formation of MACs.

Although the liver produces the majority of the circulating (plasma) complement components, complement proteins are locally produced by multiple other cell types, including endothelial cells, parenchymal cells (eg, tubular cells in the kidney[11]), and immune cells, including T cells and APCs.[12]

COMPLEMENT AND ISCHEMIA-REPERFUSION INJURY

Static cold storage of donor organs induces tissue hypoxia, mitochondrial damage, and ATP depletion, which, on reperfusion, results in the generation of free oxygen radicals and organ damage, commonly referred to as I/R injury.[13] In kidney transplantation, I/R injury presents clinically as delayed graft function (DGF). Extensive experimental evidence now supports a crucial role for complement in this process (**Fig. 2**). I/R-induced injury to endothelial cells results in surface expression of neoantigens that can be recognized by MBL[14–16] or collectins.[17] Subsequent complement activation yields C3a and C5a that bind to their respective receptors on endothelial cells (among other cell types). These ligations crucially mediate I/R injury[18–20] (see **Fig. 2**). Data from animal models also suggest that donor brain death up-regulates complement activation in renal allografts prior to procurement, which provides the dominant source of complement driving I/R injury.[21,22] The elucidation of these mechanisms has resulted in novel strategies aimed at preventing I/R injury and DGF. Chun and colleagues[23] showed in 2018 that peritransplant treatment with C1-INH (to block MBL and classical pathway complement activation) overcame prolonged cold ischemia-induced, complement-dependent, I/R injury, and cardiac allograft rejection in a mouse model. Subsequent work by Jordan and colleagues[24] translationally showed that C1-INH administration can limit DGF and improve kidney function in human recipients of deceased donor kidneys. C1-INH also improved lung function in a small cohort of lung transplant patients with early, primary graft dysfunction (a form of I/R injury),[25] further highlighting the utility of this treatment strategy.

In another approach targeting complement-dependent injury, investigators treated donor lungs with a nebulized C3a receptor (C3aR1) antagonist to ameliorate brain death-associated I/R injury in a murine lung transplant model.[26] Additionally,

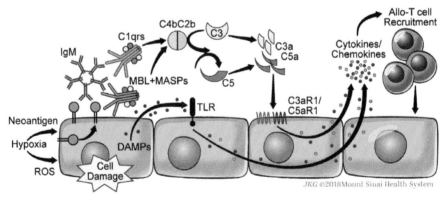

Fig. 2. Mechanisms through which complement mediates I/R injury. Hypoxia induces surface expression of neoantigens that are recognized by natural, preformed IgM and MBL (and/or collectins), which then initiate complement activation. After reperfusion, the generation of reactive oxygen species (ROS) is associated with graft-derived complement production and activation as well as the release of damage-associated molecular patterns (DAMPs). Subsequent Toll-like receptor (TLR) signaling synergizes with and amplifies complement activation, together yielding C3a and C5a. These anaphylatoxins signal through their 7-transmembrane spanning GPCRs on endothelial cells (among other cellular targets), inducing cytokine/chemokine release and facilitating T-cell infiltration into the allograft.

mirococept (APT070), a lipid-tailed C3 convertase inhibitor that can be perfused into donor organs and inserts into the endothelial cell membranes within the allograft, has been shown to prevent kidney I/R injury in rodents[27] and to improve early islet allograft inflammation in a humanized mouse model.[28] Studies testing efficacy of mirococept to prevent DGF in human recipients of deceased donor kidneys are ongoing.[29] In contrast to the positive effects of C1-INH alluded to previously, a recent prospective randomized trial testing anti-C5 monoclonal antibody (mAb), eculizumab, in kidney transplantation showed no effect in preventing DGF,[30] suggesting that prevention of DGF requires proximal complement inhibition (at or prior to the C3 convertase step).

COMPLEMENT AND T-CELL–MEDIATED REJECTION

Building on the paradigm-shifting observation that C3-deficiency prolongs murine renal allograft survival,[31] work from several groups revealed an unanticipated role for immune cell–derived complement as a regulator of T cells, including T cells reactive to transplant antigens (**Fig. 3**). These studies showed that during cognate interactions between CD4[+] T cells and APCs, both cell types down-regulate surface expression of DAF and secrete alternative pathway complement components, which together result in local production of C3a and C5a. The interacting partners also up-regulate surface expression C3aR1 and C5aR1 during activation.[32] Subsequent autocrine and paracrine C3a/C3aR1 and C5a/C5aR1 signaling via the phosphatidylinositol 3-kinase gamma pathway induces alloreactive, effector T-cell proliferation/differentiation and

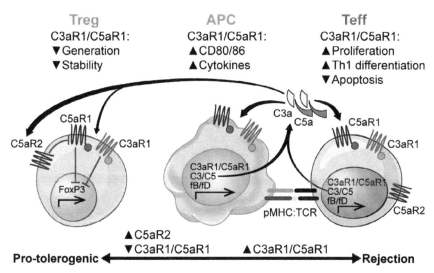

Fig. 3. Mechanisms through which complement modulates T-cell–mediated rejection. Cognate interactions between APCs and T cells yield immune cell–derived complement production, which activates through the alternative pathway to yield C3a and C5a. The anaphylatoxins bind to their respective receptors (C3aR1 and C5aR1) on the interacting partners to induce APC maturation and effector T-cell proliferation/expansion, survival, and differentiation. The same signals simultaneously inhibit the generation, stability, and function of Tregs in part by inhibiting Foxp3 expression. Because C5aR2 binds C5a but lacks a GPCR signaling motif, C5aR2 expression on T cells limits the ability of free C5a to bind to C5aR1 and thus facilitates Treg induction by limiting C5a/C5aR1 ligations.

inhibits T-cell apoptosis. Simultaneously, immune cell–derived C3a/C5a ligations with their receptors on APCs induce up-regulation of costimulatory molecules and cytokines[32] to further amplify the effector T-cell response. Remarkably, Sheen and colleagues[33] showed in 2017 that Toll-like receptor–induced APC activation, a process believed crucial for protective immune responses against pathogens and for pathogenic immune responses directed at transplanted organs, requires immune cell production of complement and subsequent C3a/C3aR1 and C5a/C5aR1 ligations on the APC.

Analogous processes apply to human T-cell/APC interactions. C3a and C5a are locally produced during in vitro cultures of human T cells and allogeneic dendritic cells, resulting in alloreactive T-cell activation and expansion.[34,35] Separate work from the Kemper laboratory[36] showed a distinct role for complement in human T-cell immunity by demonstrating that the intracellular production of complement cleavage products, including C5a, is crucially involved in human T-cell activation, in part via activation of the inflammasome. Consistent with a role for complement as a modulator of human T cells, patients genetically deficient in C3 have impaired type 1 helper T cell differentiation.[37]

In contrast to complement-dependent promotion of effector T-cell responses, immune cell–derived, locally produced C3a/C5a inhibits the generation and stability of regulatory T cells (Tregs) in mice and humans[9,10,38] (see **Fig. 3**), which contribute to augmenting the antigen-specific effector T-cell response. The inhibitory effects of C3aR1/C5aR1 signaling on Treg generation are modulated by T-cell–expressed C5aR2 that binds C5a but lacks the intracellular signaling domain to initiate GPCR signaling.[39] Evidence suggests that in T cells, C5aR2 functions to bind C5a and prevent C5a from binding to and activating C5aR1. Verghese and colleagues[40] showed in 2018 that absence of C5aR2 limits, while transgenic overexpression of C5aR2 enhances, in vivo Treg generation, independent of C5aR1 expression on the T cells.

Mechanistic experiments showed that C3aR1/C5aR1-initiated signaling, which is prevented by overexpression of C5aR2,[3] results in AKT-dependent phosphorylation of the transcription factor Foxo1, preventing its nuclear translocation and subsequently limiting FoxP3 transcription.[10] Conversely, disrupting C3aR1/C5aR1 signaling on T cells genetically or pharmacologically[10,38] augments Treg generation, stabilizes FoxP3 expression, and is protolerogenic.

Complement regulation of T-cell immunity is broadly relevant and applies in the context of infectious pathogens,[41] autoimmune diseases,[42] and T-cell–driven transplant rejection. As examples of the latter, absence of DAF (lifts restraint on production of C3a and C5a[43]) accelerates cardiac allograft rejection[44] whereas anti-C5 mAb,[45] C5aR1 antagonism,[46] or absence of C3aR1 signaling[47] reduces T-cell priming and improves allograft survival in mice. Similarly, Treg-dependent allograft survival/tolerance is facilitated by blocking C3aR1/C5aR1 signaling[9] or augmenting C5aR2 expression on immune cells.[40] Together with the observations that these mechanisms apply to human T cells,[34] the data support the need to test the clinical impact of complement inhibition on T-cell-mediated allograft rejection in humans.

COMPLEMENT AND ANTIBODY-MEDIATED TRANSPLANT INJURY

Complement has established effects on antibody production and function. Complement receptor 1 (CR1 [CD35]) and complement receptor 2 (CR2 [CD21]) bind to antigen-bound C3b and C3dg, respectively, the latter lowering the threshold for B-cell activation and promoting antigen retention by follicular dendritic cells.[48,49] C3-deficient mice fail to produce high-affinity IgG responses against major histocompatibility antigens in skin grafts,[50] confirming its relevance to transplantation.

In addition to complement's role in donor-specific antibody (DSA) production, complement activation has been shown to be an important effector mechanism of antibody-initiated allograft injury in murine models[51] and in human transplant recipients[52,53] (**Fig. 4**). DSA can activate complement via the classical pathway, ultimately inducing graft inflammation and injury through C3a/C5a production and MAC formation.[52] Although MAC formation mediates lysis in non-nucleated cells, terminal complement activation on donor human endothelial cells induces noncanonical nuclear factor (NF)-κB signaling, initiating a proinflammatory gene program that facilitates recruitment of alloreactive T cells required for the development of allograft injury.[54]

Building on these fundamental observations, clinicians have studied the efficacy of eculizumab, an anti-human C5 mAb, to prevent and/or treat antibody-mediated rejection (ABMR) in human transplant recipients. Eculizumab plus plasma exchange reduced the incidence of ABMR in 26 sensitized kidney transplant recipients compared with a control group,[55] and it successfully treated ABMR in a small cohort,[56] although it failed to demonstrate efficacy in another case series.[57] Cases of ABMR resistant to eculizumab[55] suggest that complement components proximal to the C5 convertase and/or noncomplement (eg, Fc receptor)-dependent effector mechanisms can contribute to the antibody-initiated pathology. A pilot study of C1-INH, which blocks activation of the classical and MBL pathways (see **Fig. 1**), suggests efficacy for treatment of ABMR,[58] but larger -scale studies are needed.

COMPLEMENT AND TRANSPLANT REJECTION BIOMARKERS

With the recognition that complement activation is a critical mediator of I/R injury, T-cell–mediated rejection, and ABMR, investigators have begun to test whether complement-derived biomarkers could be useful as prognostic risk-assessment tools in transplantation. To this end, research on potential biomarkers has focused on 3 broad areas: single-nucleotide polymorphisms (SNPs) in complement genes, measures of complement-binding capacity of DSA, and detection of serum-based complement components.

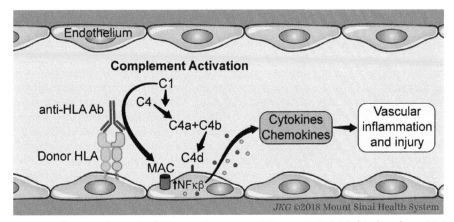

Fig. 4. Mechanisms through which complement modulates ABMR. DSAs bind to donor HLA on endothelial cells and initiate complement activation via the classical pathway, leading to complement deposition, local C3a/C5a production, and MAC formation. The latter causes noncanonical NF-κB signaling that initiates a proinflammatory gene program, enhancing recruitment of alloreactive T cells and development of vascular injury.

Both functional and nonfunctional SNPs have been identified in complement components throughout the cascade, including within the complement regulators. Their functional effects and relevance to renal transplant outcomes are summarized in a 2017 review.[59] Recipient SNPs in C5 (rs17611, increases serum C5a levels) and C5aR1 (rs4804049, nonfunctional) have been linked to worse renal allograft function at 1 year post-transplant and allograft failure, respectively. Similarly, two C3 SNPs (rs10411506 and rs2230205) correlate with ABMR in renal transplant recipients.[60] Because donor-expressed complement regulatory proteins could confer protection from DSA,[61] investigators have hypothesized that donor SNPs within regulators could also be used to assess post-transplant risk. A donor CD59 promoter polymorphism (rs147788946) is associated with an increased rate of early acute rejection in renal allografts[62] and a higher incidence of chronic rejection among lung transplant recipients.[63] Going forward, sufficiently powered validation studies will be crucial in ultimately determining whether treatment strategies should be individualized based on expression of the various SNPs.

DSA-associated allograft injury is in part dependent on complement-mediated effector functions, so the prognostic value of the complement-binding capacity of anti-HLA antibodies has become an important question in transplantation. A 2013 cohort study of 1016 kidney transplant recipients suggested that patients with C1q-binding (C1q$^+$) DSA have elevated rates of ABMR compared with C1q$^-$ DSA$^+$ patients (48% vs 16%).[64] Similar associations were documented in heart[65] and in lung[66] transplant recipients. In another cohort study of 70 renal transplant patients who developed de novo DSA (dnDSA), C1q binding was correlated with post-dnDSA graft loss.[67] The investigators of this study also demonstrated, however, that C1q positivity correlated with DSA titer and mean fluorescence intensity, suggesting that C1q binding may simply reflect the strength of the serum DSA and may not add significant prognostic information beyond standard DSA testing.

A noninvasive, serum-based biomarker for allograft rejection could help avoid unnecessary biopsies and lead to earlier treatment, potentially improving transplant outcomes. Although no such validated biomarker currently exists in transplantation, there are complement-related candidates. Soluble CD59 (sCD59), which is associated with cellular damage, including post–myocardial infarction,[68] was found elevated in a cohort of patients who developed bronchiolitis obliterans syndrome (BOS) after lung transplantation.[69] Importantly, serum sCD59 concentrations were elevated prior to the clinical diagnosis of BOS in these patients, and sCD59 was determined to be an independent predictor for the development of BOS. In another study, investigators demonstrated a correlation between serum C4d$^+$ (a marker of classical pathway complement activation) microvesicles and ABMR in a cohort of kidney transplant patients[70]; treatment of their ABMR was associated with an improvement in estimated glomerular filtration rate and a reduction in C4d$^+$ microvesicle concentration. With regard to acute cellular rejection, a 2018 study found an association between circulating immune complexes, specific for complement factor H, and acute cellular rejection in liver transplant recipients.[71] These intriguing findings support the need for further testing of complement biomarkers and/or complement biomarker profiles aimed at individualizing risk stratification and treatment algorithms for transplant patients.

CONCLUDING REMARKS

The complement system, traditionally considered a component of innate immunity, is now recognized as a crucial mediator of the adaptive immune response in solid organ transplantation. Preclinical and early human trials have begun to elucidate how specific complement components modulate the various forms of post-transplant anti-graft immune responses (eg, I/R injury, T-cell–mediated cellular rejection, and ABMR). These data, together with the pharmaceutical industry's increasing interest in developing complement inhibitors,[72] support the need to test whether complement inhibition, potentially guided by complement-derived risk assessing biomarkers, can improve allograft survival and patient-centered outcomes in transplantation.

REFERENCES

1. Walport MJ. Complement. First of two parts. N Engl J Med 2001;344(14): 1058–66.
2. Takahashi K, Ip WE, Michelow IC, et al. The mannose-binding lectin: a prototypic pattern recognition molecule. Curr Opin Immunol 2006;18(1):16–23.
3. Bamberg CE, Mackay CR, Lee H, et al. The C5a receptor (C5aR) C5L2 is a modulator of C5aR-mediated signal transduction. J Biol Chem 2010;285(10): 7633–44.
4. Park P, Haas M, Cunningham PN, et al. Inhibiting the complement system does not reduce injury in renal ischemia reperfusion. J Am Soc Nephrol 2001;12(7): 1383–90.
5. Adler S, Baker PJ, Johnson RJ, et al. Complement membrane attack complex stimulates production of reactive oxygen metabolites by cultured rat mesangial cells. J Clin Invest 1986;77(3):762–7.
6. Ricklin D, Hajishengallis G, Yang K, et al. Complement: a key system for immune surveillance and homeostasis. Nat Immunol 2010;11(9):785–97.
7. Guo RF, Ward PA. Role of C5a in inflammatory responses. Annu Rev Immunol 2005;23:821–52.
8. Klos A, Tenner AJ, Johswich KO, et al. The role of the anaphylatoxins in health and disease. Mol Immunol 2009;46(14):2753–66.
9. Kwan WH, van der Touw W, Paz-Artal E, et al. Signaling through C5a receptor and C3a receptor diminishes function of murine natural regulatory T cells. J Exp Med 2013;210(2):257–68.
10. van der Touw W, Cravedi P, Kwan WH, et al. Cutting edge: receptors for C3a and C5a modulate stability of alloantigen-reactive induced regulatory T cells. J Immunol 2013;190(12):5921–5.
11. Peake PW, O'Grady S, Pussell BA, et al. C3a is made by proximal tubular HK-2 cells and activates them via the C3a receptor. Kidney Int 1999;56(5):1729–36.
12. Lalli PN, Strainic MG, Yang M, et al. Locally produced C5a binds to T cell-expressed C5aR to enhance effector T-cell expansion by limiting antigen-induced apoptosis. Blood 2008;112(5):1759–66.
13. Siedlecki A, Irish W, Brennan DC. Delayed graft function in the kidney transplant. Am J Transplant 2011;11(11):2279–96.
14. Zhang M, Carroll MC. Natural IgM-mediated innate autoimmunity: a new target for early intervention of ischemia-reperfusion injury. Expert Opin Biol Ther 2007; 7(10):1575–82.
15. Haas MS, Alicot EM, Schuerpf F, et al. Blockade of self-reactive IgM significantly reduces injury in a murine model of acute myocardial infarction. Cardiovasc Res 2010;87(4):618–27.
16. Busche MN, Pavlov V, Takahashi K, et al. Myocardial ischemia and reperfusion injury is dependent on both IgM and mannose-binding lectin. Am J Physiol Heart Circ Physiol 2009;297(5):H1853–9.

17. Nauser CL, Farrar CA, Sacks SH. Complement recognition pathways in renal transplantation. J Am Soc Nephrol 2017;28(9):2571–8.

18. Thurman JM, Ljubanovic D, Edelstein CL, et al. Lack of a functional alternative complement pathway ameliorates ischemic acute renal failure in mice. J Immunol 2003;170(3):1517–23.

19. De Vries B, Matthijsen RA, Wolfs TG, et al. Inhibition of complement factor C5 protects against renal ischemia-reperfusion injury: inhibition of late apoptosis and inflammation. Transplantation 2003;75(3):375–82.

20. Peng Q, Li K, Smyth LA, et al. C3a and C5a promote renal ischemia-reperfusion injury. J Am Soc Nephrol 2012;23(9):1474–85.

21. Farrar CA, Zhou W, Lin T, et al. Local extravascular pool of C3 is a determinant of postischemic acute renal failure. FASEB J 2006;20(2):217–26.

22. Atkinson C, Floerchinger B, Qiao F, et al. Donor brain death exacerbates complement-dependent ischemia/reperfusion injury in transplanted hearts. Circulation 2013;127(12):1290–9.

23. Chun N, Fairchild RL, Li Y, et al. Complement dependence of murine costimulatory blockade-resistant cellular cardiac allograft rejection. Am J Transplant 2017; 17(11):2810–9.

24. Jordan SC, Choi J, Aubert O, et al. A phase I/II, double-blind, placebo-controlled study assessing safety and efficacy of C1 esterase inhibitor for prevention of delayed graft function in deceased donor kidney transplant recipients. Am J Transplant 2018. https://doi.org/10.1111/ajt.14767.

25. Sommer W, Tudorache I, Kuhn C, et al. C1-esterase-inhibitor for primary graft dysfunction in lung transplantation. Transplantation 2014;97(11):1185–91.

26. Cheng Q, Patel K, Lei B, et al. Donor pretreatment with nebulized complement C3a receptor antagonist mitigates brain-death induced immunological injury post-lung transplant. Am J Transplant 2018;18(10):2417–28.

27. Patel H, Smith RA, Sacks SH, et al. Therapeutic strategy with a membrane-localizing complement regulator to increase the number of usable donor organs after prolonged cold storage. J Am Soc Nephrol 2006;17(4):1102–11.

28. Xiao F, Ma L, Zhao M, et al. APT070 (mirococept), a membrane-localizing C3 convertase inhibitor, attenuates early human islet allograft damage in vitro and in vivo in a humanized mouse model. Br J Pharmacol 2016;173(3):575–87.

29. Kassimatis T, Qasem A, Douiri A, et al. A double-blind randomised controlled investigation into the efficacy of Mirococept (APT070) for preventing ischaemia reperfusion injury in the kidney allograft (EMPIRIKAL): study protocol for a randomised controlled trial. Trials 2017;18(1):255.

30. Heeger P, Akalin E, Baweja M, et al. Lack of efficacy of eculizumab for prevention of delayed graft function (DGF) in deceased donor kidney transplant recipients. Am J Transplant 2018;18(S4):674.

31. Pratt JR, Basheer SA, Sacks SH. Local synthesis of complement component C3 regulates acute renal transplant rejection. Nat Med 2002;8(6):582–7.

32. Strainic MG, Liu J, Huang D, et al. Locally produced complement fragments C5a and C3a provide both costimulatory and survival signals to naive CD4+ T cells. Immunity 2008;28(3):425–35.

33. Sheen JH, Strainic MG, Liu J, et al. TLR-induced murine dendritic cell (DC) activation requires DC-intrinsic complement. J Immunol 2017;199(1):278–91.

34. Cravedi P, Leventhal J, Lakhani P, et al. Immune cell-derived C3a and C5a costimulate human T cell alloimmunity. Am J Transplant 2013;13(10):2530–9.

35. Li K, Fazekasova H, Wang N, et al. Expression of complement components, receptors and regulators by human dendritic cells. Mol Immunol 2011;48(9–10):1121–7.
36. Liszewski MK, Kolev M, Le Friec G, et al. Intracellular complement activation sustains T cell homeostasis and mediates effector differentiation. Immunity 2013;39(6):1143–57.
37. Ghannam A, Fauquert JL, Thomas C, et al. Human complement C3 deficiency: Th1 induction requires T cell-derived complement C3a and CD46 activation. Mol Immunol 2014;58(1):98–107.
38. Strainic MG, Shevach EM, An F, et al. Absence of signaling into CD4(+) cells via C3aR and C5aR enables autoinductive TGF-beta1 signaling and induction of Foxp3(+) regulatory T cells. Nat Immunol 2013;14(2):162–71.
39. Okinaga S, Slattery D, Humbles A, et al. C5L2, a nonsignaling C5A binding protein. Biochemistry 2003;42(31):9406–15.
40. Verghese DA, Demir M, Chun N, et al. T cell expression of C5a receptor 2 augments murine regulatory T cell (TREG) generation and TREG-dependent cardiac allograft survival. J Immunol 2018;200(6):2186–98.
41. Stoermer KA, Morrison TE. Complement and viral pathogenesis. Virology 2011;411(2):362–73.
42. Ricklin D, Lambris JD. Complement in immune and inflammatory disorders: pathophysiological mechanisms. J Immunol 2013;190(8):3831–8.
43. Lublin DM, Atkinson JP. Decay-accelerating factor: biochemistry, molecular biology, and function. Annu Rev Immunol 1989;7:35–58.
44. Pavlov V, Raedler H, Yuan S, et al. Donor deficiency of decay-accelerating factor accelerates murine T cell-mediated cardiac allograft rejection. J Immunol 2008;181(7):4580–9.
45. Raedler H, Vieyra MB, Leisman S, et al. Anti-complement component C5 mAb synergizes with CTLA4Ig to inhibit alloreactive T cells and prolong cardiac allograft survival in mice. Am J Transplant 2011;11(7):1397–406.
46. Gueler F, Rong S, Gwinner W, et al. Complement 5a receptor inhibition improves renal allograft survival. J Am Soc Nephrol 2008;19(12):2302–12.
47. Horwitz J, Mathern D, Heeger P. C3a receptor regulates the CD8 T-cell alloresponse via intrinsic and extrinsic mechanisms. Am J Transplant 2018;18(S4):498.
48. Fang Y, Xu C, Fu YX, et al. Expression of complement receptors 1 and 2 on follicular dendritic cells is necessary for the generation of a strong antigen-specific IgG response. J Immunol 1998;160(11):5273–9.
49. Dempsey PW, Allison ME, Akkaraju S, et al. C3d of complement as a molecular adjuvant: bridging innate and acquired immunity. Science 1996;271(5247):348–50.
50. Marsh JE, Farmer CK, Jurcevic S, et al. The allogeneic T and B cell response is strongly dependent on complement components C3 and C4. Transplantation 2001;72(7):1310–8.
51. Wang H, Arp J, Liu W, et al. Inhibition of terminal complement components in presensitized transplant recipients prevents antibody-mediated rejection leading to long-term graft survival and accommodation. J Immunol 2007;179(7):4451–63.
52. Valenzuela NM, McNamara JT, Reed EF. Antibody-mediated graft injury: complement-dependent and complement-independent mechanisms. Curr Opin Organ Transplant 2014;19(1):33–40.
53. Stegall MD, Chedid MF, Cornell LD. The role of complement in antibody-mediated rejection in kidney transplantation. Nat Rev Nephrol 2012;8(11):670–8.

54. Jane-Wit D, Manes TD, Yi T, et al. Alloantibody and complement promote T cell-mediated cardiac allograft vasculopathy through noncanonical nuclear factor-kappaB signaling in endothelial cells. Circulation 2013;128(23): 2504–16.

55. Stegall MD, Diwan T, Raghavaiah S, et al. Terminal complement inhibition decreases antibody-mediated rejection in sensitized renal transplant recipients. Am J Transplant 2011;11(11):2405–13.

56. Locke JE, Magro CM, Singer AL, et al. The use of antibody to complement protein C5 for salvage treatment of severe antibody-mediated rejection. Am J Transplant 2009;9(1):231–5.

57. Burbach M, Suberbielle C, Brocheriou I, et al. Report of the inefficacy of eculizumab in two cases of severe antibody-mediated rejection of renal grafts. Transplantation 2014;98(10):1056–9.

58. Montgomery RA, Orandi BJ, Racusen L, et al. Plasma-derived C1 esterase inhibitor for acute antibody-mediated rejection following kidney transplantation: results of a randomized double-blind placebo-controlled pilot study. Am J Transplant 2016;16(12):3468–78.

59. Michielsen LA, van Zuilen AD, Muskens IS, et al. Complement polymorphisms in kidney transplantation: critical in graft rejection? Am J Transplant 2017;17(8): 2000–7.

60. Wang Z, Yang H, Guo M, et al. Impact of complement component 3/4/5 single nucleotide polymorphisms on renal transplant recipients with antibody-mediated rejection. Oncotarget 2017;8(55):94539–53.

61. Griesemer AD, Okumi M, Shimizu A, et al. Upregulation of CD59: potential mechanism of accommodation in a large animal model. Transplantation 2009;87(9): 1308–17.

62. Michielsen LA, van Zuilen AD, Kardol-Hoefnagel T, et al. Association between promoter polymorphisms in CD46 and CD59 in kidney donors and transplant outcome. Front Immunol 2018;9:972.

63. Budding K, van de Graaf EA, Kardol-Hoefnagel T, et al. A promoter polymorphism in the CD59 complement regulatory protein gene in donor lungs correlates with a higher risk for chronic rejection after lung transplantation. Am J Transplant 2016;16(3):987–98.

64. Loupy A, Lefaucheur C, Vernerey D, et al. Complement-binding anti-HLA antibodies and kidney-allograft survival. N Engl J Med 2013;369(13):1215–26.

65. Zeevi A, Lunz J, Feingold B, et al. Persistent strong anti-HLA antibody at high titer is complement binding and associated with increased risk of antibody-mediated rejection in heart transplant recipients. J Heart Lung Transplant 2013;32(1): 98–105.

66. Witt CA, Gaut JP, Yusen RD, et al. Acute antibody-mediated rejection after lung transplantation. J Heart Lung Transplant 2013;32(10):1034–40.

67. Wiebe C, Gareau AJ, Pochinco D, et al. Evaluation of C1q status and titer of de novo donor-specific antibodies as predictors of allograft survival. Am J Transplant 2017;17(3):703–11.

68. Vakeva A, Lehto T, Takala A, et al. Detection of a soluble form of the complement membrane attack complex inhibitor CD59 in plasma after acute myocardial infarction. Scand J Immunol 2000;52(4):411–4.

69. Budding K, van de Graaf EA, Kardol-Hoefnagel T, et al. Soluble CD59 is a novel biomarker for the prediction of obstructive chronic lung allograft dysfunction after lung transplantation. Sci Rep 2016;6:26274.

70. Tower CM, Reyes M, Nelson K, et al. Plasma C4d+ endothelial microvesicles increase in acute antibody-mediated rejection. Transplantation 2017;101(9): 2235–43.

71. Aibara N, Ohyama K, Hidaka M, et al. Immune complexome analysis of antigens in circulating immune complexes from patients with acute cellular rejection after living donor liver transplantation. Transpl Immunol 2018;48:60–4.

72. Thurman JM, Le Quintrec M. Targeting the complement cascade: novel treatments coming down the pike. Kidney Int 2016;90(4):746–52.

Donor-Specific HLA Antibodies as Biomarkers of Transplant Rejection

Olga A. Timofeeva, PhD, D(ABHI)

KEYWORDS

- Donor-specific antibody • Biomarker • Rejection • C1q • Titer • IgG subclass

KEY POINTS

- Anti- Human Leukocyte Antigen (Anti-HLA) donor specific antibodies (DSA) are increasingly recognized as biomarkers of antibody-mediated rejection and inferior graft survival in solid organ transplantation.
- Using Food and Drug Administration–National Institutes of Health Biomarkers, EndpointS, and other Tools (BEST) resource terms, DSAs can be classified as diagnostic, prognostic, risk, predictive, monitoring, and response-to-treatment biomarkers for graft rejection.
- Detection of DSAs must be interpreted within the context of assay limitations, including reactivity against denatured antigens, bead saturation, inhibitory factors, and reactivity against shared epitopes.
- DSA characteristics, including mean fluorescence intensity, titers, the ability to activate a complement cascade, and specific IgG subclasses, should be defined to further validate DSAs as actionable biomarkers.

INTRODUCTION

Currently, 114,362 US patients are waiting for an organ transplant (Organ Procurement and Transplantation Network data as of July 2018). In 2017, approximately 34,800 transplants were performed for all organs, but more than 50,000 patients were added to the wait list, of whom approximately 2500 were on the list due to failure of first transplant. One of the major reasons for allograft loss is immunologic damage. The incidence of hyperacute rejection caused by preformed anti-HLA donor-specific antibodies (DSAs) has been nearly eliminated by prospective antibody testing and crossmatching. Similarly, the incidence of acute T-cell–mediated injury has been significantly reduced with the effective multimodal application of immunosuppressive agents. Acute and chronic antibody-mediated rejections (ABMR), however, play a

Disclosure: The author has nothing to disclose.
Pathology and Laboratory Medicine, Temple University and Hospital, Lewis Katz School of Medicine, 3401 North Broad Street, Room A2-F388, Philadelphia, PA 19140, USA
E-mail address: olga.timofeeva@tuhs.temple.edu

critical role in allograft loss and are considered among the most important barriers that limit long-term outcomes.[1]

The mechanisms for ABMR injury involve binding of DSAs to antigenic targets on the allograft endothelium.[2] The clinical picture of ABMR has become progressively more complex and the multitude of promising biomarkers is currently being validated to improve the accuracy of diagnostic approaches and offer safe and effective tools for managing post-transplant patients.[3] DSAs have been increasingly recognized as a major cause for allograft rejection in acute, chronic, and subclinical/asymptomatic ABMR in kidney,[4] heart,[5,6] pancreas,[7–9] lung,[10,11] liver,[12] and small bowel[13,14] transplants. DSAs are viewed as markers of an ongoing antiallograft response and are currently under thorough evaluation as biomarkers in all solid organ transplants. Established technologies to detect and define DSAs can potentially provide an effective way of managing patients post-transplant. Many questions about the clinical application of DSA test results in the diagnosis, prognosis, prevention, and treatment of this disease, however, remain to be answered.

Biomarkers have the potential to significantly improve and accelerate the development of new therapies and form the basis for a precision approach to managing transplant recipients. The term, *biomarker*, and its various subgroupings, however, are commonly used imprecisely, which can slow their adoption, proper application, and significance. In 2016, the FDA and NIH published the first version of the glossary included in the Biomarkers, EndpointS, and other Tools (BEST) resource (Cagney, 2017; BEST, 2016) to harmonize and clarify terms used in translational science and medical product development and provide a common language for communication by those agencies.[15] This review evaluates which DSA characteristics may improve the validity of DSAs as a biomarker for diagnosis, prognosis, risk assessment, and prediction of response to therapy in solid organ recipients to improve long-term outcomes. (**Fig. 1**)

HLA DONOR-SPECIFIC ANTIBODIES AS A DIAGNOSTIC BIOMARKER FOR ANTIBODY-MEDIATED REJECTION

Accurate diagnosis is a prerequisite for successful treatment. A diagnostic biomarker is used to detect or confirm presence of a disease.[15]

ABMR became a distinct diagnostic entity after the Banff 2001 meeting, when roles of antibodies in causing rejection and the prognostic significance of C4d staining were

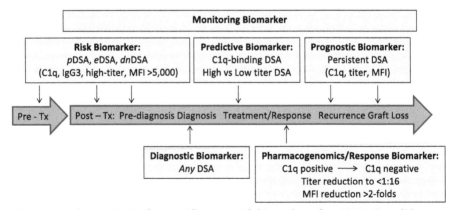

Fig. 1. DSA characteristics for specific types of biomarkers for ABMR in solid organ transplantation.

first recognized and DSA testing was introduced into clinical guidelines for the diagnosis of ABMR.[16] ABMR diagnostic criteria were first established for renal and heart allografts[16] and have subsequently been described for pancreas,[7] liver,[14] lung,[17] and intestine[18] allografts. Although diagnostic criteria for ABMR vary slightly across solid organs, endothelial cell injury, complement deposition using C4d staining, and mononuclear cell infiltration are recurrent manifestations in heart, lung, pancreas, and liver allografts. Because C4d staining has shown conflicting results in kidney,[19] heart,[20] lung,[21] and intestine,[14] the Banff 2013 working group defined criteria for diagnosing C4d-negative ABMR as a new diagnostic category in kidney allografts.[22] In addition, a new diagnostic entity was recognized, namely a subclinical or asymptomatic rejection, which happens without graft dysfunction.[23–25]

Although, DSAs are at the center of allograft injury, not all DSAs cause ABMR and/or graft loss.[26] One of the reasons for this phenomenon is that currently ABMR diagnosis requires evaluating only the presence of DSAs, which should be detected using a single-antigen bead assay (SAB). To define a pathogenic DSA, however, several parameters beyond simply DSA presence should be assessed, including DSA levels by mean fluorescence intensity (MFI) (when inhibition and bead saturation are addressed) and titer, subclass, target epitope, and complement binding (using C1q, C3d, or C4d binding assays).[27–29]

Recent insights in antibody-mediated molecular changes in kidney, heart, and lung allografts suggest that distinct DSA properties are associated with distinct allograft injury patterns.[30] DSAs can cause injury to the capillary endothelium by complement cascade activation.[27–29] This requires high-titer IgG3 or IgG1 DSAs.[31,32] DSAs can also activate Fc receptor–mediated recruitment of inflammatory cells, including macrophages and natural killer cells.[33] In addition, DSAs can trigger direct endothelial activation.[34] Detailed characterization of DSAs may help classify ABMR phenotypes not only in terms of timing and dynamics (early vs late and acute vs chronic) but also in terms of mechanisms of immunologic injury.

DONOR-SPECIFIC ANTIBODIES AS A PROGNOSTIC BIOMARKER

A prognostic biomarker is used to identify the likelihood of a clinical event, disease recurrence, or progression in patients who have the disease or medical condition of interest.[15]

It has been shown that untreated ABMR is associated with poor outcome in kidney, heart, and lung transplant recipients.[18,35–39] After successful treatment of the initial antibody-mediated injury, renal patients maintain stable graft function for years. Failure to reduce DSA levels in response to treatment is associated with a poor renal graft outcome.[40–42] This is a common law across various solid organ transplants. In renal transplant recipients, patients who achieved greater than 50% reduction in DSAs within 14 days experienced higher allograft survival,[43] whereas failure to lower DSA levels after the therapy predicted graft failure in patients with different ABMR phenotypes.[16] Among lung transplant recipients, those who developed DSAs but cleared them after treatment had outcomes similar to patients who did not develop DSAs. Furthermore, recipients in whom DSA depletion was successful were relatively more free of bronchiolitis obliterans syndrome and had better survival than those who had persistent DSAs.[44] Similarly, in heart transplantation, failure to eliminate DSAs after treatment led to poor survival after the diagnosis of ABMR.[45] Overall, several studies demonstrated that timely treatment of ABMR improves outcomes, whereas inability to clear DSAs leads to poor prognosis for graft survival.[16,41,46–48] Even in the case of slow progression of chronic ABMR, treatment of DSAs with a combination of rituximab and intravenous immunoglobulin (IVIG)[49] or with steroids/IVIG[50] shows improved kidney allograft function.

Patients with subclinical ABMR had the poorest kidney graft survival.[51] Subclinical ABMR often remains untreated, which leads to an increased risk of allograft loss because treatment guidelines are still not defined.[52] Several groups have demonstrated that increased DSA levels post-transplant correlate with a poor graft outcome regardless of whether or not the early graft function is stable.[53] Heart patients with asymptomatic ABMR had a greater risk of cardiac allograft vasculopathy.[24] Similarly, DSA-positive lung recipients without clinical ABMR had much worse prognosis compared with patients with ABMR who underwent treatment.[54] Based on these data, untreated or treatment-resistant DSAs may serve as biomarker of poor prognosis.

DONOR-SPECIFIC ANTIBODIES AS A RISK BIOMARKER FOR ANTIBODY-MEDIATED REJECTION AND GRAFT LOSS

A risk biomarker indicates the potential for developing a disease. It may also identify individuals for whom more vigilant surveillance is needed.[15] A risk biomarker is detected in individuals who seem healthy but are likely to get the disease, whereas a prognostic biomarker is detected in individuals who are diagnosed with the disease. Therefore, DSAs without signs of ABMR may serve as a risk biomarker for developing antibody-mediated rejection and eventually graft loss (**Fig. 1**).

Historically, DSAs were classified into preformed (preexisting) DSAs (pDSAs) and de novo DSAs (dnDSAs). pDSAs are detected in pretransplant serum and develop as a result of previous sensitizing events, such as blood transfusions, pregnancies, or prior transplants, and may cause ABMR early post-transplant. dnDSAs develop post-transplant as a result of the first encounter with donor HLA antigens and are responsible for late ABMR. Recently, a new term, early DSAs (eDSAs), was coined to describe a category of DSAs that were not detected prior to transplant but developed early post-transplant due to the activation of memory response.[39,55,56] eDSAs are associated with early ABMR.

Preformed Donor-specific Antibodies as a Risk Biomarker

Patients transplanted with pDSAs are at a higher risk of hyperacute/accelerated acute ABMR, chronic rejection, and allograft loss across all solid organs.[18,35–39] High-titer pDSAs that result in positive complement-dependent cytotoxicity (CDC) crossmatches and may cause hyperacute rejection can be effectively avoided or preemptively treated[57] based on immunologic risk defined in a center-specific manner.[58]

Kidney patients transplanted with pDSAs had a worse survival (61%) compared with both sensitized patients without HLA-DSAs (93%) and nonsensitized patients (84%).[59] Several studies showed that it is not simply presence or absence of DSAs but rather the quantity of DSAs assessed by MFI and/or complement binding that is associated with ABMR and acute allograft dysfunction.[60–63] Even though MFI values are not considered a precise quantitation of DSA levels, an increase in MFI is accompanied by decreased graft survival and increased relative risk for ABMR in both kidney and lung transplant patients. Kidney recipients with DSAs greater than 6000 MFI had greater than 100-fold higher risk for ABMR than patients with MFIs less than 465 (relative risk 113; 95% CI, 31–414).[59] Similarly lung recipients with DSAs greater than 5000 MFIs had 1-year survival of 33.3% compared with 71.4% for MFIs 2000 to 5000 and 62.5% for MFIs less than 2000 ($P = .0046$), suggesting DSAs greater than 5000 MFI as an independent predictor of poor patient survival within 1 year ($P = .0010$; hazard ratio

[HR] = 3.569).[64] In general, DSAs less than 3000 MFI had low rates of antibody-mediated rejection.[64–66] Recent observation by Gosset and colleagues[67] linked DSAs without ABMR to increased interstitial fibrosis and tubular atrophy. Similar to other studies, increased MFI values were associated with an increased interstitial fibrosis and tubular atrophy.[67] One of the conclusions from these reports is that pDSAs become progressively pathogenic with increase in MFI values. Therefore, it is critical to recognize the assay limitations and minimize the inherent issues when DSA specificities and levels are assessed and to incorporate quantitation of antibody levels to assess the risk of DSA burden.[51]

In addition to elevated MFI values, the presence of complement-fixing DSAs has emerged as an independent predictor of allograft loss. Capacity of HLA antibodies to activate complement has been suggested as a potential factor in directing their pathogenicity in the rejection process. In a seminal study published by Loupy and colleagues,[29] investigators differentiated DSAs by C1q binding (as a measure of the ability to activate a complement cascade), supporting the pathogenicity of DSAs as a predictor of graft failure. The 5-year graft survival rates for patients with no DSAs, non–C1q-binding DSAs, and C1q-binding DSAs were 94%, 93%, and 54%, respectively. Recent systematic review and meta-analysis showed that complement-fixing pDSAs carry the highest risk for adverse transplant outcomes in kidney, heart, lung, and liver recipients.[68]

Early Donor-specific Antibodies as a Risk Biomarker

Meanwhile, there are numerous reports that showed no correlation between pDSAs and ABMR development and transplant outcomes. Several recent studies shed light on this phenomenon. In a study of 22 heart transplant recipients with detectable pDSAs, but with negative T-cell and B-cell anti-human globulin CDC crossmatches, 3 different DSA dynamic patterns were identified after transplantation, including decreased, increased, and stable DSA levels.[69] Patients in whom DSAs-MFIs decreased during the first 2 weeks after surgery did not develop ABMR; 22% of patients with stable DSA levels and 85% of patients with increased DSA levels developed ABMR early after transplantation. In addition, 4 out of 39 sensitized patients (calculated panel-reactive antibodies >0%), who at the time of transplant did not have pDSAs, developed eDSAs within the first week post-transplant followed by ABMR in the first month. A similar observation was made in a study of 134 lung transplant recipients. DSAs with MFI greater than 3000 MFI at 1 month post-transplant but no pDSAs prior to transplant serve as an independent risk factor for mortality (HR 2.71; 95% CI, 1.34–5.47; $P<.01$).[70] In the case of eDSAs, even DSAs with MFIs 500 to 1000 and 1000 to 3000 strongly correlated with chronic lung allograft dysfunction (CLAD). Similarly, renal patients who cleared pDSAs 14 days post-transplant had excellent long-term outcomes.[71] Based on these studies, levels of eDSAs better correlate with long-term outcomes than levels of pDSAs. These studies warrant more frequent DSA testing early post-transplant in sensitized patients for better ABMR prediction.

De Novo Donor-specific Antibodies as a Risk Biomarker

Production of dnDSAs after any solid organ transplantation is a major risk factor for decreased long-term graft survival. Approximately 2% of low-risk renal transplant recipients develop dnDSAs each year, reaching 25% to 27% by 10 years post-transplant.[72–74] Within 5 years after the appearance of dnDSAs, 40% of patients lose their renal allografts.[74,75] The median 10-year graft survival for those with dnDSAs was lower than that of patients without DSAs (57% vs 96%; $P<.0001$).[76] Although at the time of initial dnDSA detection, many patients seem healthy, approximately

60% to 70% of them showed microvascular inflammation and evidence of antibody-mediated injury (intimal arteritis) on protocol biopsies at the time of initial DSA detection, suggesting that DSAs are present before allograft dysfunction.[76]

In cardiac transplantation, pediatric and adult heart transplant recipients develop dnDSAs with an incidence of approximately 30% to 40% by 10 years post-transplant.[77–80] Heart patients who developed dnDSAs 1 year after transplantation had the poorest survival.[78] dnDSAs are common after lung transplantation[17,81–83] and are associated with an increased risk of CLAD.[81,84–86] In pancreas,[7–9,87,88] liver,[12,89] and small bowel transplant recipients,[14,18,90–92] dnDSAs also result in inferior graft survival. Complement-activating dnDSAs, detected by C1q, C3d, or C4d binding assays, indicate the highest risk for ABMR and graft loss in kidney,[29,93] lung,[70] heart,[94] and liver.[95]

The utility of a risk biomarker depends on whether interventions are available to modify the risk of disease. Recent improvements in desensitization therapy have enabled the management of high-risk recipients, suggesting that the prevalence of early acute rejection can be significantly decreased with appropriate monitoring and preemptive DSA treatment.[96] In lung transplant patients, preemptive treatment of the eDSAs resulted in 4-year graft survival, which is similar to patients without antibodies.[55] In renal patients, high-dose IVIG with or without rituximab lowered DSA levels and stabilized graft function.[49,97] A recent study demonstrated that increased calcineurin inhibitor–based maintenance immunosuppression can improve outcomes in patients with dnDSAs in whom ABMR development has not yet begun.[98]

Previously, treating DSAs without ABMR was not justified; however, the latest research suggests that this concept needs to be revisited to improve long-term outcomes.[99] Clinical trials are warranted to establish how preemptive treatment of pDSAs, eDSAs, and dnDSAs may improve long-term graft survival and further establish DSAs as an actionable risk biomarker.

DONOR-SPECIFIC ANTIBODIES AS A MONITORING BIOMARKER

When any biomarker needs to be measured serially, it is placed in a category of monitoring biomarkers according to the BEST glossary definitions.[15]

The recommendations for post-transplant DSA monitoring have been summarized in a recent review[100] based on the consensus guidelines addressing technical issues of DSA testing.[101] Centers that perform DSA monitoring have demonstrated that despite technical limitations (**Fig. 1**),[102,103] the highly sensitive SAB assay seems a useful tool for post-transplant monitoring of HLA antibodies and for surveillance of ABMR when used appropriately.[46,47,74,104–110]

Recently, the HLA antibody assessment guidelines were expanded to include information regarding all major HLA loci (HLA-A, HLA-B, HLA-C, HLA-DRB1, HLA-DRB3/4/5, HLA-DQA1/DQB1, and HLA DPA1/DPB1), preferably at allele-specific level; to put in place measures to remove inhibition; to recognize potential epitope sharing; and to use a universal cutoff between 1000 MFIs and 1500 MFIs for comparing data between multiple centers.[56] Based on multicenter comprehensive assessment and standardization of SAB, a difference of less than 25% should not be considered clinically meaningful.[111]

Antibodies against denatured HLA antigens need to be recognized and studied separately.[101] It is known that some of the antibodies detected in SAB assays may be directed against cryptic epitopes on recombinant HLA proteins created by missing peptides and/or β2-macroglobulin.[112] This reactivity can be ruled out using screening/phenotype bead assays prepared with naturally expressed HLA antigens from transformed B cells.[113,114] The precise role of naturally occurring antibodies is not well understood yet,[115] but several studies suggest that such antibodies do not have clinical significance.[116–128] Several recent studies, including meta-analysis of 13 cohorts of lung recipients (total 3039 patients), showed that dnDSAs were associated with CLAD (HR = 2.02; 95% CI, 1.37–2.97; $P<.001$) only when combinations of screening assays and SAB were used. When SAB was used alone, dnDSAs were no longer associated with CLAD.[129] Despite the published estimates that approximately 20% of patients have antibodies against denatured antigens, numerous studies of post-transplant DSAs rely solely on SAB and, therefore, may detect clinically irrelevant antibodies. It may be beneficial to use the screening methods along with SAB for post-transplant monitoring to achieve a better correlation with other biomarkers. In addition, when the presence of DSAs is detected (and its reactivity with the native epitope is confirmed), it is recommended by Sensitization in Transplantation: Assessment of Risk 2017 guidelines to determine titers, C1q/C3d/C4d binding, and IgG subclass to define pathogenic DSA characteristics contributing to graft injury.[56]

DONOR-SPECIFIC ANTIBODIES AS PREDICTIVE AND PHARMACODYNAMICS/RESPONSE BIOMARKERS

A predictive biomarker is used to identify individuals who are more likely to respond to exposure to a particular medical product/therapy whereas pharmacodynamics/response biomarkers allow tracking a response to treatment.[15] Because all ABMR treatment therapies aim to remove or reduce DSA levels, DSA is a predictive biomarker in the sense that patients with ABMR (see **Fig. 1**) will undergo antibody reduction therapy, and also a pharmacodynamics/response biomarker, because it can be used to evaluate response to treatment.

There are different regimens for DSA removal/reduction, however, currently there are no guidelines for which therapy to use in the presence of DSAs of a specific type. Common approaches to DSA depletion include high doses of IVIG with or without rituximab, series of therapeutic plasma exchanges with or without low doses of IVIG, bortezomib or carfilzomib in combination with plasmapheresis/IVIG and rituximab, and eculizumab. More studies are needed to clarify which DSA characteristics can be used to decide on treatment regimen. For example, eculizumab is a monoclonal antibody that specifically binds to factor C5 and inhibits the terminal pathway of the complement cascade, preventing endothelial injury.[130] A review of eculizumab-treated ABMR cases concludes that cases of cd4-negative ABMR do not seem to improve with eculizumab treatment.[131] Because C4d is a marker of complement activation, eculizumab would be ineffective in this context of C4d-negative rejection. Whether complement-activating DSAs detected by C1q, C3d, or C4d assays could provide similar information remains to be investigated.

Another example of how DSA-specific characteristics can be used to guide selection of candidates is demonstrated by titers that can predict response to therapeutic plasma exchanges/IVIG treatment.[132] This study showed that antibodies with an initial titer greater than 1:512 could not be reduced despite a significant increase in the number of treatment cycles.[132] For patients with DSA titers greater than 1:512, it may be beneficial to add bortezomib, a proteasome inhibitor active against plasma cells, which was shown to effectively reduce high-titer DSAs in renal and heart transplant patients.[133–140] Therefore, knowledge regarding DSA titer can offer selecting the most effective treatment regimen in timely manner.

As for using DSAs as a pharmacodynamics/response biomarker, understanding the limitations of and information provided by SAB assays is critical. It has been shown that for strong DSAs, changes in MFI values do not correlate with the success of a treatment if the initial MFI values are greater than 10,000, which is most likely due to single-antigen bead saturation.[56,104,132,141] Antibody titration[46] or C1q-binding status[142] can serve as effective tool for monitoring efficacy of treatment (**Fig. 1**). For example, patients who became C1q negative post–ABMR treatment showed a significantly improved glomerular filtration rate with significantly reduced glomerulitis, peritubular capillaritis, interstitial inflammation, tubulitis, C4d deposition, and endarteritis compared with patients who remained C1q positive post-treatment.[142]

Overall, specific DSA characteristics, such as titers and C1q binding, can serve as both predictive biomarkers and biomarkers of response to treatment; however, more studies are needed to test this hypothesis.

SUMMARY

Introduction of DSA testing into clinical practice using SAB assays has led to the realization that DSAs may serve as biomarkers for ABMR and graft loss in solid organ transplant recipients. This has the potential for improving and accelerating the development of new therapies and precision-based approaches for the management of transplant recipients. The recently developed BEST glossary can help classify DSAs as biomarkers to improve their proper application. During the past decade, understanding of the limitations of DSA testing and defining clinically relevant DSA characteristics has improved. DSA characteristics, including MFI, titers, IgG subclass and complement activation, can serve as important biomarkers in the development of guidelines for immunologic risk assessments and clinical management of transplant recipients.

REFERENCES

1. Djamali A, Kaufman DB, Ellis TM, et al. Diagnosis and management of antibody-mediated rejection: current status and novel approaches. Am J Transplant 2014; 14(2):255–71.
2. Valenzuela NM, Reed EF. Antibodies in transplantation: the effects of HLA and non-HLA antibody binding and mechanisms of injury. Methods Mol Biol 2013; 1034:41–70.
3. Mengel M, Sis B, Haas M, et al. Banff 2011 meeting report: new concepts in antibody-mediated rejection. Am J Transplant 2012;12(3):563–70.
4. Davis S, Cooper JE. Acute antibody-mediated rejection in kidney transplant recipients. Transplant Rev (Orlando) 2017;31(1):47–54.
5. Vaughn GR, Jorgensen NW, Law YM, et al. Outcome of antibody-mediated rejection compared to acute cellular rejection after pediatric heart transplantation. Pediatr Transplant 2018;22(1).
6. Hammond ME, Kfoury AG. Antibody-mediated rejection in the cardiac allograft: diagnosis, treatment and future considerations. Curr Opin Cardiol 2017;32(3): 326–35.
7. Drachenberg CB, Torrealba JR, Nankivell BJ, et al. Guidelines for the diagnosis of antibody-mediated rejection in pancreas allografts-updated Banff grading schema. Am J Transplant 2011;11(9):1792–802.
8. de Kort H, Mallat MJ, van Kooten C, et al. Diagnosis of early pancreas graft failure via antibody-mediated rejection: single-center experience with 256 pancreas transplantations. Am J Transplant 2014;14(4):936–42.
9. Cantarovich D, De Amicis S, Akl A, et al. Posttransplant donor-specific anti-HLA antibodies negatively impact pancreas transplantation outcome. Am J Transplant 2011;11(12):2737–46.

10. Morrell MR, Pilewski JM, Gries CJ, et al. De novo donor-specific HLA antibodies are associated with early and high-grade bronchiolitis obliterans syndrome and death after lung transplantation. J Heart Lung Transplant 2014;33(12):1288–94.
11. Kulkarni HS, Bemiss BC, Hachem RR. Antibody-mediated rejection in lung transplantation. Curr Transplant Rep 2015;2(4):316–23.
12. Kaneku H, O'Leary JG, Banuelos N, et al. De novo donor-specific HLA antibodies decrease patient and graft survival in liver transplant recipients. Am J Transplant 2013;13(6):1541–8.
13. Cheng EY, Everly MJ, Kaneku H, et al. Prevalence and clinical impact of donor-specific alloantibody among intestinal transplant recipients. Transplantation 2017;101(4):873–82.
14. Wu GS. Updates on antibody-mediated rejection in intestinal transplantation. World J Transplant 2016;6(3):564–72.
15. FDA-NIH Biomarker Working Group. BEST (Biomarkers, EndpointS, and other Tools) Resource. Food and Drug Administration (US). Bethesda (MD): National Institute of Health; 2016.
16. Haas M, Mirocha J, Reinsmoen NL, et al. Differences in pathologic features and graft outcomes in antibody-mediated rejection of renal allografts due to persistent/recurrent versus de novo donor-specific antibodies. Kidney Int 2017;91(3): 729–37.
17. Levine DJ, Glanville AR, Aboyoun C, et al. Antibody-mediated rejection of the lung: a consensus report of the International Society for Heart and Lung Transplantation. J Heart Lung Transplant 2016;35(4):397–406.
18. Wu GS, Cruz RJ Jr, Cai JC. Acute antibody-mediated rejection after intestinal transplantation. World J Transplant 2016;6(4):719–28.
19. Cohen D, Colvin RB, Daha MR, et al. Pros and cons for C4d as a biomarker. Kidney Int 2012;81(7):628–39.
20. Kobashigawa J, Crespo-Leiro MG, Ensminger SM, et al. Report from a consensus conference on antibody-mediated rejection in heart transplantation. J Heart Lung Transplant 2011;30(3):252–69.
21. Roberts JA, Barrios R, Cagle PT, et al. The presence of anti-HLA donor-specific antibodies in lung allograft recipients does not correlate with C4d immunofluorescence in transbronchial biopsy specimens. Arch Pathol Lab Med 2014; 138(8):1053–8.
22. Haas M, Sis B, Racusen LC, et al. Banff 2013 meeting report: inclusion of c4d-negative antibody-mediated rejection and antibody-associated arterial lesions. Am J Transplant 2014;14(2):272–83.
23. Loupy A, Suberbielle-Boissel C, Hill GS, et al. Outcome of subclinical antibody-mediated rejection in kidney transplant recipients with preformed donor-specific antibodies. Am J Transplant 2009;9(11):2561–70.
24. Wu GW, Kobashigawa JA, Fishbein MC, et al. Asymptomatic antibody-mediated rejection after heart transplantation predicts poor outcomes. J Heart Lung Transplant 2009;28(5):417–22.
25. Kfoury AG, Hammond ME, Snow GL, et al. Cardiovascular mortality among heart transplant recipients with asymptomatic antibody-mediated or stable mixed cellular and antibody-mediated rejection. J Heart Lung Transplant 2009;28(8):781–4.
26. Valenzuela NM, Reed EF. Antibody-mediated rejection across solid organ transplants: manifestations, mechanisms, and therapies. J Clin Invest 2017;127(7): 2492–504.

27. Sicard A, Ducreux S, Rabeyrin M, et al. Detection of C3d-binding donor-specific anti-HLA antibodies at diagnosis of humoral rejection predicts renal graft loss. J Am Soc Nephrol 2015;26(2):457–67.

28. Smith JD, Hamour IM, Banner NR, et al. C4d fixing, luminex binding antibodies - a new tool for prediction of graft failure after heart transplantation. Am J Transplant 2007;7(12):2809–15.

29. Loupy A, Lefaucheur C, Vernerey D, et al. Complement-binding anti-HLA antibodies and kidney-allograft survival. N Engl J Med 2013;369(13):1215–26.

30. Halloran PF, Merino Lopez M, Barreto Pereira A. Identifying subphenotypes of antibody-mediated rejection in kidney transplants. Am J Transplant 2016; 16(3):908–20.

31. Everly MJ, Rebellato LM, Haisch CE, et al. Impact of IgM and IgG3 anti-HLA alloantibodies in primary renal allograft recipients. Transplantation 2014;97(5): 494–501.

32. O'Leary JG, Kaneku H, Banuelos N, et al. Impact of IgG3 subclass and C1q-fixing donor-specific HLA alloantibodies on rejection and survival in liver transplantation. Am J Transplant 2015;15(4):1003–13.

33. Dos Santos DC, Campos EF, Saraiva Camara NO, et al. Compartment-specific expression of natural killer cell markers in renal transplantation: immune profile in acute rejection. Transpl Int 2016;29(4):443–52.

34. Zhang X, Valenzuela NM, Reed EF. HLA class I antibody-mediated endothelial and smooth muscle cell activation. Curr Opin Organ Transplant 2012;17(4): 446–51.

35. O'Leary JG, Klintmalm GB. Impact of donor-specific antibodies on results of liver transplantation. Curr Opin Organ Transplant 2013;18(3):279–84.

36. O'Leary JG, Demetris AJ, Friedman LS, et al. The role of donor-specific HLA alloantibodies in liver transplantation. Am J Transplant 2014;14(4):779–87.

37. Lefaucheur C, Suberbielle-Boissel C, Hill GS, et al. Clinical relevance of preformed HLA donor-specific antibodies in kidney transplantation. Am J Transplant 2008;8(2):324–31.

38. Kim M, Townsend KR, Wood IG, et al. Impact of pretransplant anti-HLA antibodies on outcomes in lung transplant candidates. Am J Respir Crit Care Med 2014;189(10):1234–9.

39. Ius F, Sommer W, Tudorache I, et al. Early donor-specific antibodies in lung transplantation: risk factors and impact on survival. J Heart Lung Transplant 2014;33(12):1255–63.

40. Everly MJ, Everly JJ, Arend LJ, et al. Reducing de novo donor-specific antibody levels during acute rejection diminishes renal allograft loss. Am J Transplant 2009;9(5):1063–71.

41. Everly MJ, Rebellato LM, Ozawa M, et al. Beyond histology: lowering human leukocyte antigen antibody to improve renal allograft survival in acute rejection. Transplantation 2010;89(8):962–7.

42. Lefaucheur C, Nochy D, Andrade J, et al. Comparison of combination Plasmapheresis/IVIg/anti-CD20 versus high-dose IVIg in the treatment of antibody-mediated rejection. Am J Transplant 2009;9(5):1099–107.

43. Everly MJ, Terasaki PI. Monitoring and treating posttransplant human leukocyte antigen antibodies. Hum Immunol 2009;70(8):655–9.

44. Hachem RR, Yusen RD, Meyers BF, et al. Anti-human leukocyte antigen antibodies and preemptive antibody-directed therapy after lung transplantation. J Heart Lung Transplant 2010;29(9):973–80.

45. Hodges AM, Lyster H, McDermott A, et al. Late antibody-mediated rejection after heart transplantation following the development of de novo donor-specific human leukocyte antigen antibody. Transplantation 2012;93(6):650–6.

46. Gilbert A, Grafals M, Timofeeva O, et al. Pre-empting antibody-mediated rejection: a program of DSA monitoring and treatment can effectively prevent antibody mediated rejection. Clin Transplant 2016;32:93–101.

47. Rao S, Ghanta M, Lee IJ, et al. Impact of donor specific HLA antibody monitoring after kidney transplantation. Clin Transplant 2014;143–51.

48. Hachem RR, Kamoun M, Budev MM, et al. Human leukocyte antigens antibodies after lung transplantation: primary results of the HALT study. Am J Transplant 2018;18(9):2285–94.

49. Fehr T, Rusi B, Fischer A, et al. Rituximab and intravenous immunoglobulin treatment of chronic antibody-mediated kidney allograft rejection. Transplantation 2009;87(12):1837–41.

50. Redfield RR, Ellis TM, Zhong W, et al. Current outcomes of chronic active antibody mediated rejection - a large single center retrospective review using the updated BANFF 2013 criteria. Hum Immunol 2016;77(4):346–52.

51. Loupy A, Vernerey D, Tinel C, et al. Subclinical rejection phenotypes at 1 year post-transplant and outcome of kidney allografts. J Am Soc Nephrol 2015; 26(7):1721–31.

52. Orandi BJ, Chow EH, Hsu A, et al. Quantifying renal allograft loss following early antibody-mediated rejection. Am J Transplant 2015;15(2):489–98.

53. Kimball PM, Baker MA, Wagner MB, et al. Surveillance of alloantibodies after transplantation identifies the risk of chronic rejection. Kidney Int 2011;79(10): 1131–7.

54. Witt CA, Gaut JP, Yusen RD, et al. Acute antibody-mediated rejection after lung transplantation. J Heart Lung Transplant 2013;32(10):1034–40.

55. Ius F, Verboom M, Sommer W, et al. Preemptive treatment of early donor-specific antibodies with IgA- and IgM-enriched intravenous human immunoglobulins in lung transplantation. Am J Transplant 2018;18(9):2295–304.

56. Tambur AR, Campbell P, Claas FH, et al. Sensitization in transplantation: assessment of risk (STAR) 2017 working group meeting report. Am J Transplant 2018; 18(7):1604–14.

57. Tinckam KJ, Keshavjee S, Chaparro C, et al. Survival in sensitized lung transplant recipients with perioperative desensitization. Am J Transplant 2015; 15(2):417–26.

58. Zachary AA, Sholander JT, Houp JA, et al. Using real data for a virtual crossmatch. Hum Immunol 2009;70(8):574–9.

59. Lefaucheur C, Loupy A, Hill GS, et al. Preexisting donor-specific HLA antibodies predict outcome in kidney transplantation. J Am Soc Nephrol 2010;21(8): 1398–406.

60. Fine NM, Daly RC, Shankar N, et al. The role of donor-specific antibodies in acute cardiac allograft dysfunction in the absence of cellular rejection. Transplantation 2014;98(2):229–38.

61. Ware AL, Malmberg E, Delgado JC, et al. The use of circulating donor specific antibody to predict biopsy diagnosis of antibody-mediated rejection and to provide prognostic value after heart transplantation in children. J Heart Lung Transplant 2016;35(2):179–85.

62. Cicciarelli JC, Lemp NA, Chang Y, et al. Renal transplant patients biopsied for cause and tested for C4d, DSA, and IgG subclasses and C1q: which humoral markers improve diagnosis and outcomes? J Immunol Res 2017;2017:1652931.

63. Santos S, Malheiro J, Tafulo S, et al. Impact of preformed donor-specific antibodies against HLA class I on kidney graft outcomes: comparative analysis of exclusively anti-Cw vs anti-A and/or -B antibodies. World J Transplant 2016; 6(4):689–96.

64. Smith JD, Ibrahim MW, Newell H, et al. Pre-transplant donor HLA-specific antibodies: characteristics causing detrimental effects on survival after lung transplantation. J Heart Lung Transplant 2014;33(10):1074–82.

65. Caro-Oleas JL, Gonzalez-Escribano MF, Gonzalez-Roncero FM, et al. Clinical relevance of HLA donor-specific antibodies detected by single antigen assay in kidney transplantation. Nephrol Dial Transplant 2012;27(3):1231–8.

66. Yoo PS, Bonnel A, Kamoun M, et al. Clinical outcomes among renal transplant recipients with pre-transplant weakly reactive donor-specific antibodies. Clin Transplant 2014;28(1):127–33.

67. Gosset C, Viglietti D, Rabant M, et al. Circulating donor-specific anti-HLA antibodies are a major factor in premature and accelerated allograft fibrosis. Kidney Int 2017;92(3):729–42.

68. Bouquegneau A, Loheac C, Aubert O, et al. Complement-activating donor-specific anti-HLA antibodies and solid organ transplant survival: a systematic review and meta-analysis. PLoS Med 2018;15(5):e1002572.

69. de Castro MCR, Barbosa EA, Souza RP, et al. The kinetics of anti-HLA antibodies in the first year after kidney transplantation: in whom and when should they be monitored? J Transplant 2018;2018:8316860.

70. Le Pavec J, Suberbielle C, Lamrani L, et al. De-novo donor-specific anti-HLA antibodies 30 days after lung transplantation are associated with a worse outcome. J Heart Lung Transplant 2016;35(9):1067–77.

71. Zecher D, Bach C, Staudner C, et al. Characteristics of donor-specific anti-HLA antibodies and outcome in renal transplant patients treated with a standardized induction regimen. Nephrol Dial Transplant 2017;32(4):730–7.

72. Everly MJ, Rebellato LM, Haisch CE, et al. Incidence and impact of de novo donor-specific alloantibody in primary renal allografts. Transplantation 2013; 95(3):410–7.

73. Wiebe C, Nevins TE, Robiner WN, et al. The synergistic effect of class II HLA epitope-mismatch and nonadherence on acute rejection and graft survival. Am J Transplant 2015;15(8):2197–202.

74. Wiebe C, Nickerson P. Posttransplant monitoring of de novo human leukocyte antigen donor-specific antibodies in kidney transplantation. Curr Opin Organ Transplant 2013;18(4):470–7.

75. Wiebe C, Gibson IW, Blydt-Hansen TD, et al. Rates and determinants of progression to graft failure in kidney allograft recipients with de novo donor-specific antibody. Am J Transplant 2015;15(11):2921–30.

76. Wiebe C, Gibson IW, Blydt-Hansen TD, et al. Evolution and clinical pathologic correlations of de novo donor-specific HLA antibody post kidney transplant. Am J Transplant 2012;12(5):1157–67.

77. Chen CK, Manlhiot C, Conway J, et al. Development and impact of De Novo Anti-HLA antibodies in pediatric heart transplant recipients. Am J Transplant 2015;15(8):2215–22.

78. Smith JD, Banner NR, Hamour IM, et al. De novo donor HLA-specific antibodies after heart transplantation are an independent predictor of poor patient survival. Am J Transplant 2011;11(2):312–9.

79. Tran A, Fixler D, Huang R, et al. Donor-specific HLA alloantibodies: impact on cardiac allograft vasculopathy, rejection, and survival after pediatric heart transplantation. J Heart Lung Transplant 2016;35(1):87–91.

80. Omrani O, Alawwami M, Buraiki J, et al. Donor-specific HLA-DQ antibodies may contribute to poor graft outcome after heart transplantation. Ann Saudi Med 2018;38(2):97–104.

81. Tikkanen JM, Singer LG, Kim SJ, et al. De Novo DQ donor-specific antibodies are associated with chronic lung allograft dysfunction after lung transplantation. Am J Respir Crit Care Med 2016;194(5):596–606.

82. Hachem RR. Acute rejection and antibody-mediated rejection in lung transplantation. Clin Chest Med 2017;38(4):667–75.

83. Roux A, Bendib Le Lan I, Holifanjaniaina S, et al. Antibody-mediated rejection in lung transplantation: clinical outcomes and donor-specific antibody characteristics. Am J Transplant 2016;16(4):1216–28.

84. Roux A, Bendib Le Lan I, Holifanjaniaina S, et al. Characteristics of donor-specific antibodies associated with antibody-mediated rejection in lung transplantation. Front Med (Lausanne) 2017;4:155.

85. Verleden SE, Vanaudenaerde BM, Emonds MP, et al. Donor-specific and -nonspecific HLA antibodies and outcome post lung transplantation. Eur Respir J 2017;50(5).

86. Walton DC, Hiho SJ, Cantwell LS, et al. HLA matching at the eplet level protects against chronic lung allograft dysfunction. Am J Transplant 2016;16(9):2695–703.

87. Rudolph EN, Dunn TB, Mauer D, et al. HLA-A, -B, -C, -DR, and -DQ matching in pancreas transplantation: effect on graft rejection and survival. Am J Transplant 2016;16(8):2401–12.

88. Yadav K, Cotterell A, Kimball P, et al. Antibody mediated rejection due to de-novo DSA causing venous thrombosis of pancreas allograft - a case report. Transpl Immunol 2018;47:22–5.

89. Abu-Elmagd KM, Wu G, Costa G, et al. Preformed and de novo donor specific antibodies in visceral transplantation: long-term outcome with special reference to the liver. Am J Transplant 2012;12(11):3047–60.

90. Sindhi R, AshokKumar C, Mazariegos G, et al. Immune monitoring in small bowel transplantation. Curr Opin Organ Transplant 2010;15(3):349–56.

91. Berger M, Zeevi A, Farmer DG, et al. Immunologic challenges in small bowel transplantation. Am J Transplant 2012;12(Suppl 4):S2–8.

92. Rabant M, Racape M, Petit LM, et al. Antibody-mediated rejection in pediatric small bowel transplantation: capillaritis is a major determinant of C4d positivity in intestinal transplant biopsies. Am J Transplant 2018;18(9):2250–60.

93. Comoli P, Cioni M, Tagliamacco A, et al. Acquisition of C3d-binding activity by de novo donor-specific HLA antibodies correlates with graft loss in nonsensitized pediatric kidney recipients. Am J Transplant 2016;16(7):2106–16.

94. Chin C, Chen G, Sequeria F, et al. Clinical usefulness of a novel C1q assay to detect immunoglobulin G antibodies capable of fixing complement in sensitized pediatric heart transplant patients. J Heart Lung Transplant 2011;30(2):158–63.

95. Kozlowski T, Weimer ET, Andreoni K, et al. C1q test for identification of sensitized liver recipients at risk of early acute antibody-mediated rejection. Ann Transplant 2017;22:518–23.

96. Loupy A, Suberbielle-Boissel C, Zuber J, et al. Combined posttransplant prophylactic IVIg/anti-CD 20/plasmapheresis in kidney recipients with preformed donor-specific antibodies: a pilot study. Transplantation 2010;89(11):1403–10.

97. Billing H, Rieger S, Ovens J, et al. Successful treatment of chronic antibody-mediated rejection with IVIG and rituximab in pediatric renal transplant recipients. Transplantation 2008;86(9):1214–21.
98. Beland MA, Lapointe I, Noel R, et al. Higher calcineurin inhibitor levels predict better kidney graft survival in patients with de novo donor-specific anti-HLA antibodies: a cohort study. Transpl Int 2017;30(5):502–9.
99. Mengel M. Deconstructing interstitial fibrosis and tubular atrophy: a step toward precision medicine in renal transplantation. Kidney Int 2017;92(3):553–5.
100. Morath C, Opelz G, Zeier M, et al. Clinical relevance of HLA antibody monitoring after kidney transplantation. J Immunol Res 2014;2014:845040.
101. Tait BD, Susal C, Gebel HM, et al. Consensus guidelines on the testing and clinical management issues associated with HLA and non-HLA antibodies in transplantation. Transplantation 2013;95(1):19–47.
102. Liwski RS, Gebel HM. Of cells and microparticles: assets and liabilities of HLA antibody detection. Transplantation 2018;102(1S Suppl 1):S1–6.
103. Reed EF, Rao P, Zhang Z, et al. Comprehensive assessment and standardization of solid phase multiplex-bead arrays for the detection of antibodies to HLA. Am J Transplant 2013;13(7):1859–70.
104. Tambur AR, Wiebe C. HLA diagnostics: evaluating DSA strength by titration. Transplantation 2018;102(1S Suppl 1):S23–30.
105. Everly MJ. Using HLA antibody detection, monitoring, and treatment to improve long-term allograft survival. Clin Transplant 2010;317–22.
106. Everly MJ. Summarizing the use of donor specific anti-HLA antibody monitoring in transplant patients. Clin Transplant 2011;333–6.
107. Everly MJ. Donor-specific anti-HLA antibody monitoring and removal in solid organ transplant recipients. Clin Transplant 2011;319–25.
108. Mohamed MA, Muth B, Vidyasagar V, et al. Post-transplant DSA monitoring may predict antibody-mediated rejection in sensitized kidney transplant recipients. Clin Transplant 2011;389–94.
109. Ho J, Wiebe C, Gibson IW, et al. Immune monitoring of kidney allografts. Am J Kidney Dis 2012;60(4):629–40.
110. Viglietti D, Loupy A, Vernerey D, et al. Value of donor-specific anti-HLA antibody monitoring and characterization for risk stratification of kidney allograft loss. J Am Soc Nephrol 2017;28(2):702–15.
111. Reed EF, Rao P, Zhang Z, et al. Comprehensive assessment and standardization of solid phase multiplex-bead arrays for the detection of antibodies to HLA-drilling down on key sources of variation. Am J Transplant 2013;13(11):3050–1.
112. Jucaud V, Ravindranath MH, Terasaki PI. Conformational variants of the individual HLA-I antigens on luminex single antigen beads used in monitoring HLA antibodies: problems and solutions. Transplantation 2017;101(4):764–77.
113. Cao S, Courtwright AM, Lamattina AM, et al. The impact of screening method on HLA antibody detection before and after lung transplantation: a prospective pilot study. J Heart Lung Transplant 2018;37(4):531–3.
114. Gebel HM, Liwski RS, Bray RA. Technical aspects of HLA antibody testing. Curr Opin Organ Transplant 2013;18(4):455–62.
115. Zorn E, See SB. Polyreactive natural antibodies in transplantation. Curr Opin Organ Transplant 2017;22(1):8–13.
116. Sullivan HC, Gebel HM, Bray RA. Understanding solid-phase HLA antibody assays and the value of MFI. Hum Immunol 2017;78(7–8):471–80.

117. Bettinotti MP, Zachary AA, Leffell MS. Clinically relevant interpretation of solid phase assays for HLA antibody. Curr Opin Organ Transplant 2016;21(4):453–8.
118. Visentin J, Marroc M, Guidicelli G, et al. Clinical impact of preformed donor-specific denatured class I HLA antibodies after kidney transplantation. Clin Transplant 2015;29(5):393–402.
119. Visentin J, Guidicelli G, Nong T, et al. Evaluation of the iBeads assay as a tool for identifying class I HLA antibodies. Hum Immunol 2015;76(9):651–6.
120. Visentin J, Guidicelli G, Moreau JF, et al. Deciphering allogeneic antibody response against native and denatured HLA epitopes in organ transplantation. Eur J Immunol 2015;45(7):2111–21.
121. Oaks M, Michel K, Sulemanjee NZ, et al. Practical value of identifying antibodies to cryptic HLA epitopes in cardiac transplantation. J Heart Lung Transplant 2014;33(7):713–20.
122. Grenzi PC, de Marco R, Silva RZ, et al. Antibodies against denatured HLA class II molecules detected in luminex-single antigen assay. Hum Immunol 2013; 74(10):1300–3.
123. Kaneku H. 2012 annual literature review of donor-specific HLA antibodies after organ transplantation. Clin Transplant 2012;207–17.
124. Poli F, Benazzi E, Innocente A, et al. Heart transplantation with donor-specific antibodies directed toward denatured HLA-A*02:01: a case report. Hum Immunol 2011;72(11):1045–8.
125. Pereira S, Perkins S, Lee JH, et al. Donor-specific antibody against denatured HLA-A1: clinically nonsignificant? Hum Immunol 2011;72(6):492–8.
126. Visentin J, Guidicelli G, Taupin JL. Are complement-fixing antibodies against denatured HLA antigens clinically relevant? Exp Mol Pathol 2016;100(3):532–3.
127. Gao B, Rong C, Porcheray F, et al. Evidence to support a contribution of poly-reactive antibodies to HLA serum reactivity. Transplantation 2016;100(1): 217–26.
128. Cai J, Terasaki PI, Zhu D, et al. Complement-fixing antibodies against denatured HLA and MICA antigens are associated with antibody mediated rejection. Exp Mol Pathol 2016;100(1):45–50.
129. Courtwright A, Diamond JM, Wood I, et al. Detection and clinical impact of human leukocyte antigen antibodies in lung transplantation: a systematic review and meta-analysis. HLA 2018;91(2):102–11.
130. Touzot M, Couvrat-Desvergnes G, Castagnet S, et al. Differential modulation of donor-specific antibodies after B-cell depleting therapies to cure chronic antibody mediated rejection. Transplantation 2015;99(1):63–8.
131. Tran D, Boucher A, Collette S, et al. Eculizumab for the treatment of severe antibody-mediated rejection: a case report and review of the literature. Case Rep Transplant 2016;2016:9874261.
132. Pinelli DF, Zachary AA, Friedewald JJ, et al. Prognostic tools to assess candidacy for and efficacy of antibody removal therapy. Am J Transplant 2018. [Epub ahead of print].
133. Eskandary F, Bond G, Schwaiger E, et al. Bortezomib in late antibody-mediated kidney transplant rejection (BORTEJECT Study): study protocol for a randomized controlled trial. Trials 2014;15:107.
134. Krisl JC, Alloway RR, Shields AR, et al. Bortezomib-based antibody-mediated rejection therapy and simultaneous conversion to belatacept. Transplantation 2014;97(4):e30–2.
135. May LJ, Yeh J, Maeda K, et al. HLA desensitization with bortezomib in a highly sensitized pediatric patient. Pediatr Transplant 2014;18(8):E280–2.

136. Philogene MC, Sikorski P, Montgomery RA, et al. Differential effect of bortezomib on HLA class I and class II antibody. Transplantation 2014;98(6):660–5.

137. Yang KS, Jeon H, Park Y, et al. Use of bortezomib as anti-humoral therapy in kidney transplantation. J Korean Med Sci 2014;29(5):648–51.

138. Zinn MD, L'Ecuyer TJ, Fagoaga OR, et al. Bortezomib use in a pediatric cardiac transplant center. Pediatr Transplant 2014;18(5):469–76.

139. Ide K, Tanaka Y, Sasaki Y, et al. A phased desensitization protocol with rituximab and bortezomib for highly sensitized kidney transplant candidates. Transplant Direct 2015;1(5):e17.

140. Lee J, Kim BS, Park Y, et al. The effect of bortezomib on antibody-mediated rejection after kidney transplantation. Yonsei Med J 2015;56(6):1638–42.

141. Tambur AR, Herrera ND, Haarberg KM, et al. Assessing antibody strength: comparison of MFI, C1q, and titer information. Am J Transplant 2015;15(9):2421–30.

142. Viglietti D, Bouatou Y, Kheav VD, et al. Complement-binding anti-HLA antibodies are independent predictors of response to treatment in kidney recipients with antibody-mediated rejection. Kidney Int 2018;94(4):773–87.

Biomarkers for Early Complications After Hematopoietic Stem Cell Transplantation

Courtney M. Rowan, MD, MS[a],*, Sophie Paczesny, MD, PhD[b,c]

KEYWORDS

- Biomarkers - Hematopoietic stem cell transplantation - Proteomics
- Graft versus host disease

KEY POINTS

- Biomarkers should be categorized into diagnostic, prognostic, predictive, and response to treatment biomarkers based on the 2014 National Institutes of Health consensus report.
- Several proteomic biomarkers for acute graft-versus-host disease have been investigated by unbiased or hypothesis-driven approaches. Stimulation 2 has been the most validated and is a promising therapeutic target.
- Discovery of additional biomarkers for other posttransplant complications is ongoing and may improve diagnosis, prognosis, and the development of new therapeutic strategies.

INTRODUCTION

Hematopoietic stem cell transplantation (HSCT) is increasingly being used for a variety of malignant and nonmalignant conditions. With improvements in donor selection and conditional regimens, outcomes have improved. However, early posttransplant

C.M. Rowan has no conflict of interest.

C.M. Rowan is supported by a grant from the Showalter Research Trust Fund.

S. Paczesny has a patent on "Methods of detection of graft-versus-host disease" (US 20130115232A1, WO2013066369A3) licensed to Viracor-IBT Laboratories.

S. Paczesny is supported by grants from the National Cancer Institute (R01CA168814), National Institute of Child Health and Human Development (R01HD074587, U54HD090215), and the Leukemia & Lymphoma Society (1293-15).

[a] Department of Pediatrics, Division of Critical Care, Indiana University School of Medicine, 705 Riley Hospital Drive, Room 4900, Indianapolis, IN 46202, USA; [b] Department of Pediatrics, Melvin and Bren Simon Cancer Center, Indiana University School of Medicine, 1044 West Walnut Street, Room R4-425, Indianapolis, IN 46202, USA; [c] Department of Microbiology Immunology, Melvin and Bren Simon Cancer Center, Indiana University School of Medicine, 1044 West Walnut Street, Room R4-425, Indianapolis, IN 46202, USA

* Corresponding author.

E-mail address: coujohns@iu.edu

complications remain a barrier for overall success and survival. Issues such as acute graft-versus-host disease (aGVHD), sinusoidal obstructive syndrome (SOS), and idiopathic pneumonia syndrome (IPS) can dramatically increase morbidity and mortality. For example, up to one-half of patients who have undergone allogeneic HSCT can be affected by aGVHD[1] and are at increased risk for mortality.

Biomarkers can offer an effective method for early identification of complications related to HSCT and potentially guide treatments. Biomarkers have gained popularity over the years as a way to provide objective, unbiased information. As technology has advanced, there has been an explosion in the development and applications of biomarkers in an array of specialties. These markers can be obtained from a variety of medical samples, such as blood and urine, but can also be thought of in the broader sense to include data such as radiographic images obtained from use of other technologies. An ideal biomarker would be obtained from a readily available, noninvasive sample that could be easily collected at multiple time points. Currently, plasma and serum remain the most common sources for biomarkers and effectively provide information on systemic disorders that often affect the transplant recipient, such as aGVHD.

In a National Institutes of Health–sponsored working group, biomarkers were categorized into 4 types: diagnostic, prognostic, predictive, and response to treatment[2] (**Table 1**). A diagnostic biomarker helps a clinician identify a disease rapidly or differentiate between diseases with similar presentations. A prognostic biomarker should aid a clinician in the anticipated course of a disease or the development of a particular complication. A predictive biomarker gives information about how a patient or disease progression will likely respond to a specific treatment, therapy, or intervention when measured before the treatment. Finally, a response to treatment marker can be used to monitor the treatment response and could substitute for a clinical response

Table 1
Categories of biomarkers as defined by the National Institutes of Health working group

Category	Definition	Example
Diagnostic	• Can help a clinician identify a disease rapidly so that treatment can be initiated • Can help to differentiate diseases with similar clinical presentations	REG3α can help to differentiate GI GVHD from other causes of non-GVHD diarrhea[28]
Prognostic	• Can aid the clinician in the anticipated course of disease • Can also help determine the likelihood of developing a particular complication	A panel of HA, VCAM, and L-ficolin drawn on day 0 of HSCT can serve as a prognostic panel for the future development of SOS[34]
Predictive	• Measured before therapy is initiated • Helps to determine how a disease will progress following therapy • Can give information on how a patient will respond to a particular treatment of intervention	ST2 can serve as a predictive marker for response to therapy for GVHD[14]
Response to treatment	• Measured after therapy is initiated • Can help monitor therapeutic response • Could potentially be used as a substitute for a clinical response	MAGIC biomarkers (ST2 and Reg3α) measured at 1 wk after initiation of steroids can predict steroids resistant disease and nonrelapsed mortality[16]

endpoint. Unlike a predictive marker, it is measured after treatment is initiated to monitor therapeutic response.

OMICS TECHNOLOGIC ADVANCES AND THE DEVELOPMENT OF BIOMARKERS

The recent technologic advances combined with their decreasing cost have led to a rapid increase in the application of omics in translational research and then in clinic. There are many different types of omics, but the most popular remain genomics, transcriptomics, and proteomics. The foundation of the omics field was built on genomics, which is the study of how genetic variants are associated with disease development or prognosis. In addition, it is being increasingly applied to stratify patients at risk for adverse events to certain drugs (ie, pharmacogenomics). Transcriptomics measure gene activity by investigating the messenger RNA that codes for different proteins. Proteomics investigates protein quantity and function. It is important because it measures both gene function and the host environment, but is complicated due to the sheer volume of proteins. These omics all carry different importance. For this review, the authors focus on the most relevant and recent biomarkers that have been validated in different cohorts.

The development of a biomarker is complicated and involves many steps from discovery to implementation in the routine clinical care of patients. **Fig. 1** highlights the important steps of development. These steps must all be followed to ensure the validity and clinical utility of newly discovered biomarkers.

BIOMARKERS FOR EARLY COMPLICATIONS AFTER HEMATOPOIETIC STEM CELL TRANSPLANTATION
Acute Graft-Versus-Host Disease

aGVHD is one of the best studied post-HSCT complications because it remains a major barrier to the overall success of this procedure. Because the presentation is diverse and the diagnosis relies entirely on clinical symptoms, there has been a quest to develop and validate biomarkers to aid in early diagnosis and prognosis. Furthermore, many of these biomarkers are being developed as potential novel therapeutic targets. **Table 2** features an overview of the most recent and validated biomarkers for aGVHD.

Genomic markers for the development and severity of aGVHD following HSCT have been investigated. In addition to the well-known risk of major histocompatibility complex disparity,[3] single nucleotide polymorphisms (SNPs) for mismatches in minor histocompatibility antigens have also been found to be risk factors for the occurrence of aGVHD, and increasing genome-wide recipient mismatching results in a substantial increased risk for grades III–IV GVHD.[4] Genomic markers remain complicated to investigate because of the need to understand the genome of the donor and the recipient pre-HSCT and after HSCT, and the small effect of each SNP requires large cohorts of thousands of HSCT patients to get meaningful and reproducible data.[5]

Recent transcriptomics analysis in the nonhuman primate have found that blocking OX40L using the blocking antibody KY1005 helped to control Th1 cells while preserving the reconstitution of regulatory T cells (Tregs) and prolonged GVHD-free survival. There was an additional benefit when combined with sirolimus.[6] This antibody is currently being tested in a clinical trial through the Pediatric Blood and Marrow Transplant Consortium.

A variety of proteomic markers have been studied, and the most validated and recent ones are presented in **Table 2**. Several of the interleukins and their receptors (IL-2, IL-2Rα, IL-6, IL-8, IL-12, and IL-18) have been investigated, and IL-2Rα and IL-6 have emerged as the most useful markers for aGVHD.[7–9] Using a screen of patient

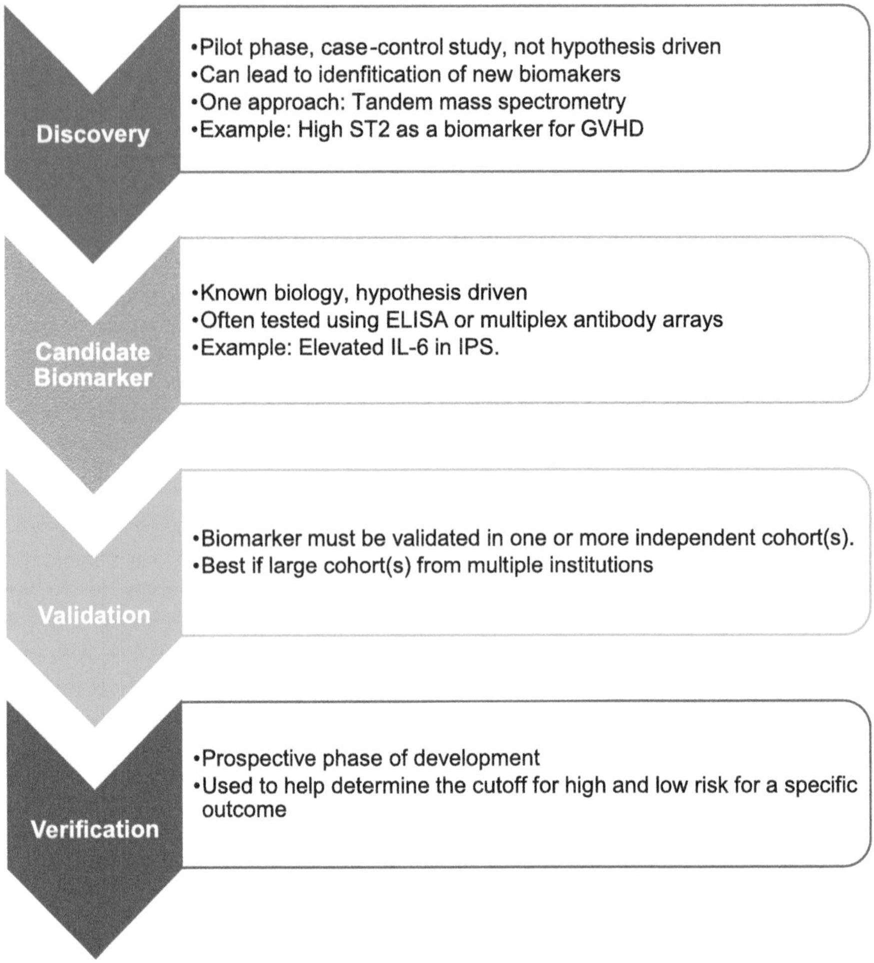

Discovery
- Pilot phase, case-control study, not hypothesis driven
- Can lead to idenfitication of new biomakers
- One approach: Tandem mass spectrometry
- Example: High ST2 as a biomarker for GVHD

Candidate Biomarker
- Known biology, hypothesis driven
- Often tested using ELISA or multiplex antibody arrays
- Example: Elevated IL-6 in IPS.

Validation
- Biomarker must be validated in one or more independent cohort(s).
- Best if large cohort(s) from multiple institutions

Verification
- Prospective phase of development
- Used to help determine the cutoff for high and low risk for a specific outcome

Fig. 1. There are several steps involved in the development of a biomarker for clinical use. The first step is a discovery phase that usually compares 20 to 40 cases and controls. This is often done with mass spectrometry. Candidate biomarkers are biomarkers that are often chosen based on biologic plausibility. Studies of candidate biomarkers are hypothesis driven. These markers often are in the early phases of study and lack extensive validation. Once a newly discovered biomarker demonstrates promising statistical association, validation must be performed. This is usually done using high-throughput immunoassay. The cohorts should be independent, and the validation is stronger if the cohort is large and from multiple institutions. Finally, the biomarker should be verified. This is often done in large prospective studies that can help to determine cutoffs for high or low risk for a specific outcome.

plasma samples by competitive hybridization to arrays of antibodies specific for diverse proteins, the first biomarker panel for aGVHD, including 4 different proteins IL-2Rα, tumor necrosis factor receptor 1 (TNFR1), IL-8, and hepatocyte growth factor (HGF), was identified and validated in a training and validation set of hundreds of patients.[9] Although Denileukin Diftitox, an anti-IL-2Rα antibody, did not show benefit for the treatment of aGVHD,[10] IL-6 has been more promising for prophylaxis against

Table 2
Biomarkers for acute graft-versus-host disease

Name	Study	(n)	Biomarker Type	Associations and Time Points in aGVHD
Plasma markers				
4 biomarker panel: IL-2-receptor-α, HGF, IL-8, TNFR1	Paczesny et al,[9] 2009	424	• Diagnosis • Prognostic	• Can discriminate patients with GVHD at onset of clinical symptoms • Prognostic abilities for severity of GVHD
Interleukin-6 (IL-6)	Kennedy et al,[7] 2014	48 patients: phase 1/2 clinical trial	• Therapeutic target	• Prophylactic tocilizumab given to adults undergoing allogeneic HSCT had decreased incidence of aGVHD
	McDonald et al,[8] 2015	74 training cohort 76 validation cohort	• Diagnostic • Prognostic	• Increased at onset of aGVHD • Associated with severity of GVHD and NRM
ST2	Vander Lugt et al,[14] 2013	673 in total from 3 independent sets	• Predictive	• Increased level at 14 d after HSCT predicts response to aGVHD treatment and 6-mo mortality
	McDonald et al,[8] 2015	74 training cohort 76 validation cohort 167 patients without GVHD	• Diagnostic • Prognostic	• Increased at onset of aGVHD • Associated with severity of GVHD and NRM
	Levine et al,[46] 2015	328 training set 164 test set 300 validation set	• Predictive	• Increased levels predictive of NRM from aGVHD
	Abu Zaid et al,[15] 2017	211 patients (independent cohort of previously identified biomarkers)	• Predictive	• Increased levels on day 28 after HSCT were associated with NRM
	Hartwell et al,[18] 2017	620 training set 667 validation set	• Prognostic	• Increased day 7 were prognostic for development of aGVHD and NRM
	McDonald et al,[17] 2017	165 patients with aGVHD	• Response to treatment	• ST2 combined with TIM3 measured on day 14 of steroid therapy can predict response to treatment
	Major-Monfried et al,[16] 2018	236 test set 142 validation set 129 validation set	• Response to treatment	• ST2 combined with REG3α (MAGIC biomarkers) measured at 1 wk after initiation of steroids can predict steroid refractory disease and NRM

(continued on next page)

Table 2
(continued)

Name	Study	(n)	Biomarker Type	Associations and Time Points in aGVHD
TIM3	McDonald et al,[8] 2015	74 training set 76 validation set 167 patients without GVHD	• Diagnostic • Prognostic	• Increased at onset of aGVHD • Associated with severity of GVHD and NRM
	Abu Zaid et al,[15] 2017	211 patients (independent cohort of previously identified biomarkers)	• Predictive	• Increased levels on day 28 after HSCT were associated with NRM
Amphiregulin	Holtan et al,[29] 2018	251 patients with aGVHD	• Prognostic risk score	• High levels (>33 pg/mL) could refine risk categories within the Minnesota aGVHD clinical risk score • Associated with NRM and response to steroids
Skin specific				
Elafin	Paczesny et al,[25] 2010	522: discovery 492: validation	• Diagnostic • Prognostic	• Diagnostic ability for skin GVHD • Associated with severity of disease and NRM
	Bruggen et al,[47] 2015	59	• Prognostic	• Elevated levels in skin are associated with poor prognosis of skin GVHD
GI specific				
REG3α	Ferrara et al,[28] 2011	20 discovery 1014 validation set	• Diagnostic • Predictive • Prognostic	• Elevated at onset of GI aGVHD • Level at onset predicts response to aGVHD treatment and NRM
	Harris et al,[27] 2012	954 patients, 3 centers	• Diagnostic	• Best biomarker to discern GI GVHD from non-GVHD diarrhea
TIM3	Hansen et al,[26] 2013	20: discovery set 127: validation set 22: validation set	• Diagnostic • Prognostic	• Levels elevated in those with GI aGVHD prior onset of clinical symptoms • Increased levels associated with severity of gut GVHD

Liver specific				
REG3α, HGF, and KRT18	Harris et al,[27] 2012	954 patients, 3 centers	• Diagnostic	• Elevated in patients with liver GVHD, not validated due to low incidence
Cellular markers				
Regulatory T cells	Magenau et al,[21] 2010	215	• Diagnostic • Predictive	• Lower Tregs in peripheral blood are associated with aGVHD • Tregs frequency at GVHD onset were predictive on response to therapy
CD146+ T cells	Li et al,[22] 2016	20 discovery set 214 validation set	• Prognostic	• Increased T cells expressing CD146 at day +14 after HSCT was associated with increased risk for GI GVHD
CD30	Chen et al,[23] 2012	53	• Diagnostic	• Elevated CD30 levels at the time of clinical presentation of aGVHD
	Chen et al,[24] 2017	34	• Clinical trial	• Phase 1 trial of brentuximab vedotin, antibody drug for CD30, found to have 38% response rate in steroid-refractory GI aGVHD
Invariant natural killer T cells	Chaidos et al,[20] 2012	57	• Prognostic	• High levels in donor graft was associated with a decrease in the development of GVHD

Abbreviation: NRM, nonrelapsed mortality.

aGVHD. The use of tocilizumab in a phase 1/2 trial demonstrated a decrease in occurrence of aGVHD but no overall survival advantage.[7] Stimulation 2 (ST2), the IL-33 receptor, is a marker that has been discovered through an unbiased tandem mass spectrometry approach and has been validated in several cohorts as a diagnostic, prognostic, predictive, and response to treatment biomarker.[8,11–17] It has been tested in a variety of patients with different conditioning, transplant donor source, and degrees of match.[11,12] As early as day 7 or 14 after HSCT, it can serve as a prognostic marker for aGVHD and nonrelapsed mortality.[8,14,18] Furthermore, it may be a promising therapeutic target. ST2 blockade in murine models has demonstrated the ability to decrease the severity of GVHD and associated mortality.[19]

Cellular markers have also been studied, including Tregs, CD146T cells, CD30, and invariant natural killer T cells.[20–23] CD146-expressing T cells and upregulation of CCR5 (a chemokine receptor) were found to be prognostic for gastrointestinal (GI) GVHD as early as day 14 after HSCT.[22] A phase 1 clinical trial for brentuximab vedotin, an antibody-drug targeting CD30, has been tested for steroid-refractory aGVHD. In this trial, there was almost a 40% response rate with 15% achieving complete remission.[24]

Organ-specific markers have also been discovered. Elafin, which is overexpressed in inflammatory skin disorders, was found to be associated with the diagnosis of skin GVHD.[25] GI and liver GVHD markers include HGF, cytokeratine-18 fragments (KRT18), T-cell immunoglobulin domain and mucin domain (TIM-3), and regenerating islet-derived 3-α (REG3α), with REG3α emerging as the most validated biomarker specifically for GI GVHD with prognostic ability.[26–28] Recently, hypothesis-driven markers such as amphiregulin have emerged. Amphiregulin, an epidermal growth factor receptor ligand, was found to accurately define patients with a high-risk Minnesota aGVHD risk score, and to predict steroid responsiveness and nonrelapsed mortality (NRM).[29]

Sinusoidal Obstruction Syndrome

SOS, previously known as veno-occlusive disease, is a serious post-HSCT complication that affects the sinusoidal endothelial cells of the liver. It has been reported to occur in up to 13% of HSCT recipients, and when severe, is associated with multiorgan failure and significant mortality.[30] The diagnosis of SOS remains challenging because it is dependent mostly on clinical presentation and supported with blood work showing elevated bilirubin and ultrasound results of the liver demonstrating reversal of the hepatic flow.

Although many markers of coagulation, such as antithrombin, thrombomodulin, protein C, von Willebrand factor, and plasminogen activator inhibitor-1, have been found to be associated with SOS in early studies,[31–33] these markers are nonspecific and have not been well validated in current HSCT populations. Given the endothelial involvement, markers of endothelial dysfunction have been investigated. Using state-of-the art proteomics, a panel of 5 proteins (angiopoietin 2 [Ang2], hyaluronic acid [HA], vascular adhesion molecule-1 [VCAM-1], ST2, and L-ficolin) has been identified and validated with diagnostic value. All biomarkers were found to be elevated with the exception of L-ficolin, which was reduced.[34] HA and VCAM-1, combined with L-ficolin on day 0 of HSCT, is an early prognostic panel of markers for SOS[34] (**Table 3**).

Pulmonary Complications

Pulmonary complications remain a significant source of early transplant-related mortality. Part of the difficulty in treating post-HSCT pulmonary disease is the diverse infectious and noninfectious causes that are difficult to understand, diagnose, and treat. Complications, such as IPS, require ruling out infectious causes before the institution of more specific IPS therapy. To that end, diagnostic markers for IPS have recently

Table 3
Biomarkers for sinusoidal obstructive syndrome after HSCT

Name	Study	(n)	Biomarker Type	Associations and Time Points in SOS
Ang2, HA, L-ficolin, ST2, VCAM	Akil et al,[34] 2015	40 discovery 45 training set 35 validation	Diagnostic	• Composite panel for the diagnosis of SOS • All markers increased except L-ficolin, which is decreased
HA, L-ficolin, VCAM	Akil et al,[34] 2015	Derived from cohort above	Prognostic	• Prognostic panel at day 0 of HSCT for the development of SOS • All markers increased except L-ficolin, which is decreased
L-ficolin	Abu Zaid et al,[15] 2017	211	Prognostic	• Low level on day 28 was associated with the development of SOS

been identified. IL-6 and ST2 are good diagnostic markers for IPS, and TNFR1 is able to distinguish IPS from underlying viral causes.[35] This same group of biomarkers has been investigated for general respiratory failure, which carries up to a 60% mortality in this population.[36] ST2 and IL-6 on day 7 after HSCT were found to be great prognostic markers for the future development of respiratory failure in an adult and pediatric cohort.[37] However, these findings need to be validated in an independent cohort. Biomarkers for pulmonary complication offer the benefit of not only early prognosis but also a method to understand potential underlying biology of the disease process and offer new therapeutic targets.

Other Early Transplant Complications

Biomarkers for other early post-HSCT complications have also been investigated. Posttransplant diabetes mellitus (PTDM) has been reported in both pediatric and adult patients who have undergone allogeneic HSCT.[38] There is an association with hyperglycemia in adults after HSCT and the occurrence of GVHD and overall mortality.[39,40] As such, early identification and institution of therapy are important for this population. A large adult cohort revealed that elevated ST2 was associated with PTDM.[41] This association held when investigated in an isolated pediatric cohort.[42]

Thrombotic microangiopathy (TMA) is a post-HSCT complication associated with endothelial injury and complement activation that can lead to increased mortality and morbidity.[43] Many organs can be affected leading to multiorgan dysfunction and death. Diagnosis of this disease is challenging because of lack of uniformed acceptance of diagnostic criteria.[44] Discovery of specific biomarkers may lead to improved therapeutic decisions. Recently, ST2 on day 14 after HSCT has been found elevated in patients with TMA.[45]

SUMMARY

The advancement in technology, particularly in the field of omics, has led to numerous discoveries of biomarkers for early post-HSCT complications. Future research must include the testing of newly discovered biomarkers against existing, validated biomarkers. Work also needs to be done to implement the promising, validated biomarkers into clinical practice in a time-efficient and cost-effective manner. The prognostic biomarkers should be incorporated into clinical trials so that the effect of early recognition on the outcomes of HSCT recipients can be assessed. Diagnostic biomarkers can help to differentiate the complex variety of diseases that can be present in this population. Finally, biomarkers that can serve as therapeutic targets should be further studied. Many of these post-HSCT complications have limited or nonspecific therapeutic options. For example, corticosteroids are the first-line therapy for aGVHD. Using biomarkers to help identify underlying biologic pathways may open new therapeutic avenues that deserve investigation. This major advancement in technology allows for early diagnosis of complications, risk stratification for complications, and potential new therapeutic targets. All of these strides can improve the utilization of life-saving allogeneic HSCT while minimizing complications and mortality.

REFERENCES

1. Zeiser R, Blazar BR. Acute graft-versus-host disease - biologic process, prevention, and therapy. N Engl J Med 2017;377(22):2167–79.
2. Paczesny S, Hakim FT, Pidala J, et al. National Institutes of Health consensus development project on criteria for clinical trials in chronic Graft-versus-host disease: III. The 2014 Biomarker Working Group report. Biol Blood Marrow Transplant 2015;21(5):780–92.
3. Flomenberg N, Baxter-Lowe LA, Confer D, et al. Impact of HLA class I and class II high-resolution matching on outcomes of unrelated donor bone marrow transplantation: HLA-C mismatching is associated with a strong adverse effect on transplantation outcome. Blood 2004;104(7):1923–30.
4. Martin PJ, Levine DM, Storer BE, et al. Genome-wide minor histocompatibility matching as related to the risk of graft-versus-host disease. Blood 2017;129(6): 791–8.
5. Karaesmen E, Rizvi AA, Preus LM, et al. Replication and validation of genetic polymorphisms associated with survival after allogeneic blood or marrow transplant. Blood 2017;130(13):1585–96.
6. Tkachev V, Furlan SN, Watkins B, et al. Combined OX40L and mTOR blockade controls effector T cell activation while preserving Treg reconstitution after transplant. Sci Transl Med 2017;9(408) [pii:eaan3085].
7. Kennedy GA, Varelias A, Vuckovic S, et al. Addition of interleukin-6 inhibition with tocilizumab to standard graft-versus-host disease prophylaxis after allogeneic stem-cell transplantation: a phase 1/2 trial. Lancet Oncol 2014;15(13):1451–9.
8. McDonald GB, Tabellini L, Storer BE, et al. Plasma biomarkers of acute GVHD and nonrelapse mortality: predictive value of measurements before GVHD onset and treatment. Blood 2015;126(1):113–20.
9. Paczesny S, Krijanovski OI, Braun TM, et al. A biomarker panel for acute graft-versus-host disease. Blood 2009;113(2):273–8.
10. Alousi AM, Weisdorf DJ, Logan BR, et al. Etanercept, mycophenolate, denileukin, or pentostatin plus corticosteroids for acute graft-versus-host disease: a randomized phase 2 trial from the Blood and Marrow Transplant Clinical Trials Network. Blood 2009;114(3):511–7.
11. Ponce DM, Hilden P, Mumaw C, et al. High day 28 ST2 levels predict for acute graft-versus-host disease and transplant-related mortality after cord blood transplantation. Blood 2015;125(1):199–205.

12. Kanakry CG, Bakoyannis G, Perkins SM, et al. Plasma-derived proteomic biomarkers in human leukocyte antigen-haploidentical or human leukocyte antigen-matched bone marrow transplantation using post-transplantation cyclophosphamide. Haematologica 2017;102(5):932–40.
13. Nelson RP Jr, Khawaja MR, Perkins SM, et al. Prognostic biomarkers for acute graft-versus-host disease risk after cyclophosphamide-fludarabine nonmyeloablative allotransplantation. Biol Blood Marrow Transplant 2014;20(11):1861–4.
14. Vander Lugt MT, Braun TM, Hanash S, et al. ST2 as a marker for risk of therapy-resistant graft-versus-host disease and death. N Engl J Med 2013;369(6):529–39.
15. Abu Zaid M, Wu J, Wu C, et al. Plasma biomarkers of risk for death in a multicenter phase 3 trial with uniform transplant characteristics post-allogeneic HCT. Blood 2017;129(2):162–70.
16. Major-Monfried H, Renteria AS, Pawarode A, et al. MAGIC biomarkers predict long-term outcomes for steroid-resistant acute GVHD. Blood 2018;131(25):2846–55.
17. McDonald GB, Tabellini L, Storer BE, et al. Predictive value of clinical findings and plasma biomarkers after fourteen days of prednisone treatment for acute graft-versus-host disease. Biol Blood Marrow Transplant 2017;23(8):1257–63.
18. Hartwell MJ, Ozbek U, Holler E, et al. An early-biomarker algorithm predicts lethal graft-versus-host disease and survival. JCI Insight 2017;2(3):e89798.
19. Zhang J, Ramadan AM, Griesenauer B, et al. ST2 blockade reduces sST2-producing T cells while maintaining protective mST2-expressing T cells during graft-versus-host disease. Sci Transl Med 2015;7(308):308ra160.
20. Chaidos A, Patterson S, Szydlo R, et al. Graft invariant natural killer T-cell dose predicts risk of acute graft-versus-host disease in allogeneic hematopoietic stem cell transplantation. Blood 2012;119(21):5030–6.
21. Magenau JM, Qin X, Tawara I, et al. Frequency of CD4(+)CD25(hi)FOXP3(+) regulatory T cells has diagnostic and prognostic value as a biomarker for acute graft-versus-host-disease. Biol Blood Marrow Transplant 2010;16(7):907–14.
22. Li W, Liu L, Gomez A, et al. Proteomics analysis reveals a Th17-prone cell population in presymptomatic graft-versus-host disease. JCI insight 2016;1(6) [pii:e86660].
23. Chen YB, McDonough S, Hasserjian R, et al. Expression of CD30 in patients with acute graft-versus-host disease. Blood 2012;120(3):691–6.
24. Chen YB, Perales MA, Li S, et al. Phase 1 multicenter trial of brentuximab vedotin for steroid-refractory acute graft-versus-host disease. Blood 2017;129(24):3256–61.
25. Paczesny S, Braun TM, Levine JE, et al. Elafin is a biomarker of graft-versus-host disease of the skin. Sci Transl Med 2010;2(13):13ra12.
26. Hansen JA, Hanash SM, Tabellini L, et al. A novel soluble form of Tim-3 associated with severe graft-versus-host disease. Biol Blood Marrow Transplant 2013;19(9):1323–30.
27. Harris AC, Ferrara JL, Braun TM, et al. Plasma biomarkers of lower gastrointestinal and liver acute GVHD. Blood 2012;119(12):2960–3.
28. Ferrara JL, Harris AC, Greenson JK, et al. Regenerating islet-derived 3-alpha is a biomarker of gastrointestinal graft-versus-host disease. Blood 2011;118(25):6702–8.
29. Holtan SG, DeFor TE, Panoskaltsis-Mortari A, et al. Amphiregulin modifies the Minnesota acute graft-versus-host disease risk score: results from BMT CTN 0302/0802. Blood Adv 2018;2(15):1882–8.
30. Coppell JA, Richardson PG, Soiffer R, et al. Hepatic veno-occlusive disease following stem cell transplantation: incidence, clinical course, and outcome. Biol Blood Marrow Transplant 2010;16(2):157–68.

31. Lee JH, Lee KH, Kim S, et al. Relevance of proteins C and S, antithrombin III, von Willebrand factor, and factor VIII for the development of hepatic veno-occlusive disease in patients undergoing allogeneic bone marrow transplantation: a prospective study. Bone Marrow Transplant 1998;22(9):883–8.

32. Lee JH, Lee KH, Lee JH, et al. Plasminogen activator inhibitor-1 is an independent diagnostic marker as well as severity predictor of hepatic veno-occlusive disease after allogeneic bone marrow transplantation in adults conditioned with busulphan and cyclophosphamide. Br J Haematol 2002;118(4):1087–94.

33. Cutler C, Kim HT, Ayanian S, et al. Prediction of veno-occlusive disease using biomarkers of endothelial injury. Biol Blood Marrow Transplant 2010;16(8):1180–5.

34. Akil A, Zhang Q, Mumaw CL, et al. Biomarkers for diagnosis and prognosis of sinusoidal obstruction syndrome after hematopoietic cell transplantation. Biol Blood Marrow Transplant 2015;21(10):1739–45.

35. Seo S, Yu J, Jenkins IC, et al. Diagnostic and prognostic plasma biomarkers for idiopathic pneumonia syndrome after hematopoietic cell transplantation. Biol Blood Marrow Transplant 2018;24(4):678–86.

36. Rowan CM, Gertz SJ, McArthur J, et al. Invasive mechanical ventilation and mortality in pediatric hematopoietic stem cell transplantation: a multicenter study. Pediatr Crit Care Med 2016;17(4):294–302.

37. Rowan CM, Moser EAS, Bakoyannis G, et al. Prognostic and predictive biomarkers for respiratory failure and related mortality post allogeneic hematopoietic cell transplantation. Biol Blood Marrow Transplant 2018;24(3):S301.

38. Majhail NS, Challa TR, Mulrooney DA, et al. Hypertension and diabetes mellitus in adult and pediatric survivors of allogeneic hematopoietic cell transplantation. Biol Blood Marrow Transplant 2009;15(9):1100–7.

39. Gebremedhin E, Behrendt CE, Nakamura R, et al. Severe hyperglycemia immediately after allogeneic hematopoietic stem-cell transplantation is predictive of acute graft-versus-host disease. Inflammation 2013;36(1):177–85.

40. Fuji S, Kim SW, Mori S, et al. Hyperglycemia during the neutropenic period is associated with a poor outcome in patients undergoing myeloablative allogeneic hematopoietic stem cell transplantation. Transplantation 2007;84(7):814–20.

41. Johnpulle RA, Paczesny S, Jung DK, et al. Metabolic complications precede alloreactivity and are characterized by changes in suppression of tumorigenicity 2 signaling. Biol Blood Marrow Transplant 2017;23(3):529–32.

42. Teagarden AM, Moser E, Rowan CM, et al. Early ST2 levels are associated with the diagnosis of post-transplant diabetes mellitus. Paper presented at: Pediatric Academic Society 2018; Toronto, Canda.

43. Jodele S, Davies SM, Lane A, et al. Diagnostic and risk criteria for HSCT-associated thrombotic microangiopathy: a study in children and young adults. Blood 2014;124(4):645–53.

44. Rosenthal J. Hematopoietic cell transplantation-associated thrombotic microangiopathy: a review of pathophysiology, diagnosis, and treatment. J Blood Med 2016;7:181–6.

45. Rotz SJ, Dandoy CE, Davies SM. ST2 and endothelial injury as a link between GVHD and microangiopathy. N Engl J Med 2017;376(12):1189–90.

46. Levine JE, Braun TM, Harris AC, et al. A prognostic score for acute graft-versus-host disease based on biomarkers: a multicentre study. Lancet Haematol 2015;2(1):e21–9.

47. Bruggen MC, Petzelbauer P, Greinix H, et al. Epidermal elafin expression is an indicator of poor prognosis in cutaneous graft-versus-host disease. J Invest Dermatol 2015;135(4):999–1006.

Biomarkers in Solid Organ Transplantation

John Choi, MD, Albana Bano, MD, Jamil Azzi, MD*

KEYWORDS

- Transplant • Biomarker • Allograft • Rejection • Transplant immunology

KEY POINTS

- Biomarkers in solid organ transplantation are critical tools in assessing immunologic risks and preventing graft rejection.
- A paucity of sensitive and specific biomarkers hinders outcome of both the graft and the recipient.
- Number of novel biomarkers are being introduced; understanding the biological concept and methods can guide effective application of these powerful tools.

INTRODUCTION

Since the first human kidney transplant in 1954,[1] transplantation has expanded to various organs including heart, lung, liver, pancreas, and even vascularized composites (limbs and face). The outcome for each organ clearly supports the transplantation to be the best management option. Transplantation improves quality of life and is cost effective when compared with other supportive options in end organ diseases[2–12]; more important, it is a life-saving event.

A number of challenges remain, despite the promising data and achievements in organ transplantation. One of the most striking facts is the lack of advancement in long-term graft survival.[13] Although the 1-year survival in kidney transplant recipient has significantly improved between 1989 and 2008, the long-term graft survival did not show much improvement. Although this finding may be attributable to an increased number of higher risk profile donors and recipients in the pool, it underscores the lack of biological and clinical knowledge in long-term graft management. Another concern is the aggravating organ shortage to accommodate increased demand. Based on Organ Procurement and Transplantation Network data as of January 2018, number of patients awaiting organ transplantation has exceeded 110,000 in

Disclosure Statement: Funding support was provided by NIH grants to the authors Dr.Choi T32DK007527 and Dr. Azzi R01AI134842 and the author Dr. Bano have no disclosure.
Transplantation Research Center, Renal Division, Brigham and Women's Hospital, Harvard Medical School, 221 Longwood Avenue, Boston, MA 02115, USA
* Corresponding author.
E-mail address: jazzi@rics.bwh.harvard.edu

the United States. Last but not least, the number of therapeutic agents used in transplantation, mainly the immunosuppressive regimen, has been relatively stagnant over past decades.[14] To overcome such challenges, there has been increasing interest in developing novel biomarkers that can guide risk assessment, prognostication, and management.

Recapitulating specific aims in transplantation can help with the systematic categorization of biomarkers. Some of the main goals of transplantation include (1) optimizing allograft and living donor assessment, (2) advancing matching algorithm and immunologic risks evaluation, (3) improving allograft survival, and (4) minimizing unintended side effects from the immunosuppressive regimen. Although certain biomarkers may reveal useful information in multiple domains, a judicious combination of tests is crucial for successful outcomes. In this review, we explore the laboratory process and clinical application of selective biomarkers. Finally, we introduce novel biomarkers that were recently discovered and are undergoing validation.

INTRODUCTION OF BIOMARKERS IN SOLID ORGAN TRANSPLANTATION

A biomarker is defined as "a characteristic that is, objectively measured and evaluated as an indicator of normal biological processes, pathogenic processes, or pharmacologic responses to a therapeutic intervention."[15] An ideal biomarker should provide an accurate assessment of the disease status and provide predictive and prognostic value. It should be easy to collect, simple to run the assay, and provide results efficiently and cost effectively.

There is an interesting story behind the first biomarker tested in solid organ transplantation. Before laboratory tests were available to measure alloimmunity in preparation for kidney transplants, full-thickness skin grafts were exchanged between the donor and the recipient to test tissue compatibility.[1] After confirming that there was no evidence of skin graft rejection, Murray and colleagues[16] proceeded with the transplant, and validated the successful graft acceptance. A few years after the first kidney transplant, Patel and colleagues[17] discovered the risk of allograft hyperacute rejection associated with the cytotoxicity of recipient serum (containing antidonor antibody) on donor cells. This revolutionary method is now called a microcytotoxicity test and is the basis for different tests performed in the laboratory. Since then, a number of powerful assays have been introduced for donor–recipient matching and posttransplant management.

TISSUE TYPING AND CROSS-MATCH

During the pretransplantation evaluation, a series of critical tests are performed at the tissue typing laboratory. The assessment begins with the HLA typing of both the donor and the recipient. Luminex reverse polymerase chain reaction sequence-specific oligonucleotide has been a popular method for HLA typing. The Luminex system is based on internally color-coded beads that are in turn coated with various sequence-specific oligonucleotide probes that bind target HLA alleles. When DNA binds, it is subsequently labeled with streptavidin conjugated with R-phycoerythin. Flow cytometry can identify the bead and the presence of amplicon of specific allele as a final read out based on the intensity and characteristics of the signal. Although the resolution for typing is generally lower than that with other techniques such as the sequence-specific primers method or sequence-based typing, polymerase chain reaction sequence specific oligonucleotide is widely accepted as standard practice owing to its simplicity and reproducibility. HLA typing by real-time polymerase chain reaction is more recently becoming a method of choice in several tissue typing laboratories as well.

The more powerful application of the Luminex bead platform is the detection of antibodies circulating in the recipient. The presence of donor-specific antibodies (DSA) correlates with allograft rejection and failure.[18–20] In this US Food and Drug Administration–approved test, the color-coded bead is coated with HLA molecules and incubated with the subject's serum. Anti-IgG antibody conjugated with phycoerythin is then used as a secondary antibody for read out. The Luminex-based solid phase antibody screen has revolutionized the field, because the information can be registered in United Nation of Organ Sharing's online database system, UNet, for virtual cross-matching. Virtual cross-matching, compared with manual wet cross-matching, drastically decreases the time taken and increases the chance of identifying the best match of candidates with available donors. Virtual matching is essentially an assessment of compatibility of donor and recipient based on a paper report on antigens of the donor and antibodies of the potential recipient. This approach is useful in case of import donors, when the time to perform a wet cross-match is usually not there. Solid phase antibody assay is also performed posttransplantation for de novo DSA surveillance. There are caveats to this assay, because not all antibodies exercise cytotoxicity.

Microcytotoxicity, as discussed elsewhere in this article, is an example of a screening tool for clinically relevant DSA. This discovery has been used for many decades in a format of complement-dependent cytotoxicity, which uses rabbit complement to target donor cell-bound antibodies. However, owing to its technical complexity as well as its suboptimal sensitivity and specificity, series of modifications were made on the Luminex-based solid phase assays. Currently, the C1q assay is a popular assay of choice for detecting complement binding anti-HLA antibodies in patient serum.[21] This flow cytometry-based assay quantifies the recipient's C1q bound to antibodies linked to the donor cell to infer the ability of initiating the classical pathway. Complement-binding antibodies as detected by C1q assay or by other means show higher correlation for acute rejection, antibody-mediated rejection, transplant glomerulopathy, and graft failure when compared with C1q nonbinding DSA.[22,23] In general, it has been shown that high titered antibodies are usually complement binding; this is due to the fact that a high molar amount of antibody is required to recruit complement to mediate cytotoxicity. Not only donor-specific-IgG antibodies, but also donor cell-binding IgM antibodies can be detected with this assay. Although this may be viewed as suboptimal specificity, DSA IgG-negative/IgM-positive patients were found to have antibody-mediated rejection with future development of DSA IgG, suggesting the clinical significance of IgM binding.[24]

ADDITIONAL RISK ASSESSMENT TOOLS

Advances in technology and accumulating data enabled the matching of donors and recipients at the level of epitopes for each of the HLA molecules. Using 3-dimensional modeling, a computer program from the database (HLAMatchmaker) can identify alloantigenic eplets when the high-resolution (4-digit) HLA genotype is provided. Studies have shown an association between degree of epitope mismatch to corresponding risk of antibody-mediated rejection.[25–28] With a dramatic decrease in sequencing cost, epitope matching may become a standard practice in the near future.

Increasing evidence is reported on critical role of non-HLA antibodies in transplantation.[29,30] A number of non-HLA molecules expressed on the allograft display polymorphisms thereby priming the recipient's B cells for alloantibody production in a stressed environment.[30,31] In addition to these non-HLA molecules from the allograft, previously unexposed self-antigens may be uncovered in the setting of inflammation and increase the probability of development of autoantibodies. These antibodies are clinically associated with a higher risk for hyperacute rejection, short-term graft survival, and antibody-mediated rejection.[32–38] Since the report of antiendothelial cell antibodies,[32] multiple important non-HLA antibodies have been identified. Major histocompatibility class 1–related chain A antigens that share the major histocompatibility locus have been well-described as being related to an increased risk for kidney allograft failure.[39] The presence of anti-major histocompatibility class 1–related chain A antigen antibodies can be tested on a Luminex-based platform. The antiangiotensin type II receptor, which is also associated with an increased risk of recurrent focal segmental glomerulosclerosis,[40–42] can be tested with an enzyme-linked immunosorbent assay. Although these panels are not routinely tested at this time, assays are available at selective transplant centers.

BIOMARKERS FOR ALLOGRAFT MONITORING

Currently available noninvasive tests are generally not able to detect early allograft dysfunction and discriminate rejection from other types of allograft injury. For example, a change in the serum creatinine level is the prototypical alarm for kidney allograft injury to prompt further investigation. Unfortunately, creatinine remains relatively stable until significant damage occurs (not sensitive), and can be increased owing to multiple possible etiologies (not specific).[43,44] In most cases, when clinicians cannot rule out rejection, only a few options are available: an antibody panel to check DSA and a biopsy for histopathology.[45,46] Biopsies have been the gold standard for diagnosing rejection, although the paradigm has been focused on developing accurate noninvasive biomarkers. The approach for identifying a noninvasive biomarker is appealing, because it will minimize the risk and resources associated with biopsying an organ in case of a suspected rejection.[47–51] In addition, novel biomarkers may help to classify different forms of rejection on a molecular basis that will assist in formulating the most effective treatment.[52] In the following paragraphs, we introduce some of the biomarkers that have passed various stages of validation phases. In addition, we briefly discuss potential preclinical studies that may have implications for future biomarker development.

Urine is an attractive source for biomarker mining owing to its ability to be collected conveniently. Urinary biomarkers have high potentials for translation through a longitudinal monitoring method. In addition, the composition is directly affected by graft function in kidney transplantation. One of the most well-validated, noninvasive rejection markers is the urine messenger RNA study by Suthanthiran and Muthukumar.[53] The group isolated RNA from urine cell pellets and tested messenger RNA level of CD3ε and IP-10 with 18S rRNA, markers that distinguished acute cellular rejection from antibody-mediated rejection and borderline rejection. In addition, the signature urinary messenger RNA were elevated before the detection of biopsy-proven rejection, which showed that these markers were predictive. This was a multicenter study through clinical trials in organ transplantation (CTOT-04) consortium, which strengthens the reproducibility.

Urinary proteins were also tested as potential biomarkers. Because chemokines are essential in recruiting inflammatory cells,[54] CXCR3-binding protein CXCL9, and CXCL10 were identified as correlated with allograft rejection.[55,56] Bead-based techniques can be applied again for urinary protein detection, by coating them with antibodies for proteins of interest. Follow-up studies further confirmed the role of CXCL9 in discriminating acute T-cell–mediated rejection and CXCL10 in antibody-mediated rejection.[57-60] The limitation with urinary chemokines was their inability to distinguish between allograft rejection and BK nephropathy.[57]

The microarray is another attractive platform for testing multiple signature transcriptions and has been mainly used with biopsy samples. A few years ago the molecular diagnostic system was introduced to evaluate the allograft biopsy samples at a gene expression level.[61] This assay interrogated the current limitation with morphology-based diagnosis of acute cellular rejection and antibody-mediated rejection. The group further tested microarray system in a multicenter, large cohort and showed correlations between the selected pathogenesis-based transcript sets and their associated diagnosis showing its superior diagnostic resolution and predictive power compared with the current histopathologic diagnosis.[62,63] The Genomics of Chronic Allograft Rejection (GoCAR) study[64] is another example of a microarray based biomarker discovery, where authors from multiple centers extracted RNA from frozen biopsy samples and tested the differential expression of 13 different genes, and showed a correlation with kidney fibrosis development. The main goals of microarray-based systems are to identify subclinical, at-risk groups and prevent the progression of allograft failure and fibrosis.

A donor-derived cell-free DNA kit (CareDx, Inc., Brisbane, CA) is another ground-breaking technique that has been introduced to the biomedical field. Previously, cell-free DNA has been well-described in fetomaternal genetics and lately in oncology as a novel tool for monitoring circulating tumor signal. The introduction of next-generation sequencing was key to the momentum of this platform,[65] because the cost and time necessary for the assay has now become clinically relevant. In this assay, the donor-derived cell-free DNA detects the frequency of donor single nucleotide polymorphisms and this has been shown to be an effective assay to discriminate rejection in multiple systems. such as the kidney, pancreas, liver, heart, and lung.[66-71] It also showed a predictive value as the level was elevated months before a biopsy-proven rejection event.[71]

Finally, our group developed a platform, an integrated kidney exosomes analysis to rapidly detect kidney allograft rejection with high accuracy using urine sample.[72] Extracellular vesicles facilitate intercellular communication and play a critical role in transplant immunology. As T cells infiltrate kidney tubules during acute cellular rejection, exosomes are shed into tubular lumen with signature membrane protein from parent T cell (CD3 in our study). T-cell extracellular vesicles in urine samples are enriched with magnetic beads coated with anti-CD3 antibody. Captured extracellular vesicles are then labeled with horseradish peroxidase conjugated anti-CD63 antibody, which is a marker used to identify exosomes. For read out, the complex is mixed with a chromogenic electron mediator to generate measurable electronic current. Currently, a multicenter prospective study is being conducted to test the predictive value of this assay in a large cohort of patients.

BIOMARKERS FOR IMMUNE MONITORING

Transplant recipients suffer from infection and malignancy, which stems from the toxicity of long-term immunosuppressive regimens.[73] Clinical trials were conducted to test the safety of immunosuppression withdrawal in hope of minimizing the burden of potent medications; so far, withdrawal was shown to be associated with increased risk of rejection and allograft failure.[74,75] One's immunosuppression regimen is currently managed according to each center's protocol in an effort to reflect immunologic risks specific to each institution's patient population. In particular, the calcineurin inhibitor, the central component of an immunosuppressive regimen, is titrated based on the serum trough level.[76] However, the target level does not reflect the individual's immune system leading to overimmunosuppression or underimmunosuppression. There are limited methods with which to test immune cell function; therefore, there is an increasing demand for the development of a novel immune monitoring platform.

Interferon (IFN)-γ enzyme-linked immunosorbent spot (ELISPOT) is tested to infer the donor memory T-cell activity. The assay quantifies IFN-γ production by mixing isolated recipient memory T cells to donor cells.[77] Elevated IFN-γ production correlates with an increased risk of developing acute cellular rejection and having progressive allograft failure.[78–80] The limitation has been intercenter variation, partly owing to the variation in induction therapy[81] and the technical complexity for standardization.[78] Further optimization with a panel of reactive T cells in place of donor cells, which is often inaccessible after transplantation, and may enhance the usefulness of the ELISPOT assay.

When overimmunosuppression is suspected, a US Food and Drug Administration-approved (ViraCor-IBT, Immuknow, Lee's Summit) assay can provide insight on the recipient's immune function.[82] The Immuknow assay exploits the T-cell production of ATP by antigen presentation. CD4$^+$ T cells isolated from the recipient's peripheral blood mononuclear cells are stimulated with mitogen. The induced intracellular ATP level is then measured in a luminometer after adding luciferin/luciferase mixture. A low level of ATP correlates with overimmunosuppression and infections.[83–86] In addition, a single-center, randomized, controlled trial on a liver transplant recipient showed improved allograft survival rate with Immuknow-assisted titration of immunosuppressive regimen.[87] However, different studies failed to prevent rejection based on Immuknow, suggesting technical difficulties with standardizing the test.[84–86,88]

Although current immune monitoring assays stem from T-cell biology, increasing attention has been focused on B-cell function, which is directly linked with acute and chronic antibody-mediated injury.[89] Quantifying DSA generating B-cell function, especially memory B-cell function, may be a sensitive method to predict future antibody production and chronic graft failure.[90] HLA-specific B-cell clones can be detected by HLA tetramer staining, and these B-cell clone frequencies correlated with future DSA detection.[91–93] It is worth mentioning that ELISPOT, which is currently used for memory T-cell function, was initially introduced for B-cell clone detection.[94] Studies have shown the feasibility of detecting DSA-producing B-cell clone with ELISPOT.[95,96] Although limitations with clinical translation are expected owing to the rarity and bias in the circulating memory B-cell population,[97–99] functional B-cell monitoring will become an essential biomarker in the near future in conjunction with advancement in B-cell biology.

DONOR CANDIDATE AND ALLOGRAFT QUALITY ASSESSMENT

The accurate assessment of allograft quality during organ procurement and the living donor candidate assessment are essential steps that can affect the expanding donor pool and safety of living donors. At present, assessment is heavily based on crude clinical data, including demographics, medical conditions, cause of death (for deceased donor), candidate allograft function, ischemia time, and postprocurement biopsy on high-risk allografts. However, novel molecular tests are also available to assist risk assessments.

Concern among the transplant community has increased because an increased risk of end-stage renal disease and hypertension was detected in black donors.[100,101] The APOL1 gene variant has been on spotlight as a causal polymorphism for the high frequency of chronic renal failure among African Americans.[102] The presence of 2 high-risk APOL1 alleles has been associated with increased risk of focal segmental glomerulosclerosis and end-stage renal disease.[103,104] Allografts from APOL1 high-risk donors showed a higher frequency of collapsing focal segmental glomerulosclerosis,[105] and young African American donors carrying 2 high-risk APOL1 alleles were identified as the highest risk group for developing chronic kidney disease.[106] Recently, a study was conducted to stratify the donor outcome among black living kidney donors with varying number of high-risk alleles.[107] The study revealed the association of high-risk APOL1 genotype and accelerated estimated glomerular filtration rate loss in donors and is expected to be followed by a large cohort prospective study (APOLLO study). Although there is no current guideline regarding whether or not the APOL1 genotype should be tested routinely, our center counsels on the potential implication of high-risk variation to at-risk group donor candidates while making decision on proceeding with a genetic test. Further study results will guide generating consensus among the transplant society.[108]

SUMMARY

Owing to the complex medical conditions in patients with end-organ disease and the convoluted nature of alloimmunity, biomarkers serve a critical role in transplant medicine. Perhaps we are witnessing the most exciting time in transplant biomarkers—a number of promising biomarkers are being examined at different validation phases and are being introduced in everyday practice, awaiting wide implementation. The discovery of candidate biomarkers has accelerated as a result of advances in science and technology. Examples shared in this review include the donor-derived cell-free DNA test and the APOL1 gene test that would have been impossible without the innovation in sequencing. High-throughput analysis such as single cell analysis[109] and the -omics approach[110] opened a door to discover biomarkers through a hypothesis-generating fashion that complements traditional hypothesis-based experiments. It is imperative for researchers, clinicians, industrial, and administrative bodies to continue to work hand in hand to design an efficient pipeline of biomarkers to address unmet needs for patients.

REFERENCES

1. Merrill JP, Murray JE, Harrison JH, et al. Successful homotransplantation of the human kidney between identical twins. JAMA 1956;160(4):277–82.
2. Wood RP, Ozaki CF, Katz SM, et al. Liver transplantation. The last ten years. Surg Clin North Am 1994;74(5):1133–54.
3. Annual data report of the US Organ Procurement and Transplantation Network (OPTN) and the scientific registry of transplant recipients (SRTR). Introduction. Am J Transplant 2013;13(Suppl 1):8–10.
4. Large SR, English TA, Wallwork J. Heart and heart-lung transplantation, Papworth Hospital, 1979-1989. Clin Transpl 1989;73–8.
5. O'Brien BJ, Buxton MJ, Ferguson BA. Measuring the effectiveness of heart transplant programmes: quality of life data and their relationship to survival analysis. J Chronic Dis 1987;40(Suppl 1):137S–58S.
6. Lough ME, Lindsey AM, Shinn JA, et al. Life satisfaction following heart transplantation. J Heart Transplant 1985;4(4):446–9.
7. Bunzel B, Grundbock A, Laczkovics A, et al. Quality of life after orthotopic heart transplantation. J Heart Lung Transplant 1991;10(3):455–9.
8. Russell JD, Beecroft ML, Ludwin D, et al. The quality of life in renal transplantation–a prospective study. Transplantation 1992;54(4):656–60.

9. Witzke O, Becker G, Franke G, et al. Kidney transplantation improves quality of life. Transplant Proc 1997;29(1–2):1569–70.

10. Starzl TE, Koep LJ, Schroter GP, et al. The quality of life after liver transplantation. Transplant Proc 1979;11(1):252–6.

11. Colonna JO 2nd, Brems JJ, Hiatt JR, et al. The quality of survival after liver transplantation. Transplant Proc 1988;20(1 Suppl 1):594–7.

12. Bravata DM, Olkin I, Barnato AE, et al. Health-related quality of life after liver transplantation: a meta-analysis. Liver Transpl Surg 1999;5(4):318–31.

13. Lamb KE, Lodhi S, Meier-Kriesche HU. Long-term renal allograft survival in the United States: a critical reappraisal. Am J Transplant 2011;11(3):450–62.

14. Stegall MD, Morris RE, Alloway RR, et al. Developing new immunosuppression for the next generation of transplant recipients: the path forward. Am J Transplant 2016;16(4):1094–101.

15. Biomarkers Definitions Working Group. Biomarkers and surrogate endpoints: preferred definitions and conceptual framework. Clin Pharmacol Ther 2001; 69(3):89–95.

16. Murray JE, Hills W. The first successful organ transplants in man. JACS 2005; 200(1):5–9.

17. Patel R, Terasaki PI. Significance of the positive crossmatch test in kidney transplantation. N Engl J Med 1969;280(14):735–9.

18. Lefaucheur C, Loupy A, Hill GS, et al. Preexisting donor-specific HLA antibodies predict outcome in kidney transplantation. J Am Soc Nephrol 2010;21(8): 1398–406.

19. Mao Q, Terasaki PI, Cai J, et al. Extremely high association between appearance of HLA antibodies and failure of kidney grafts in a five-year longitudinal study. Am J Transplant 2007;7(4):864–71.

20. Wiebe C, Gibson IW, Blydt-Hansen TD, et al. Evolution and clinical pathologic correlations of de novo donor-specific HLA antibody post kidney transplant. Am J Transplant 2012;12(5):1157–67.

21. Chen G, Tyan DB. C1q assay for the detection of complement fixing antibody to HLA antigens. Methods Mol Biol 2013;1034:305–11.

22. Chin C, Chen G, Sequeria F, et al. Clinical usefulness of a novel C1q assay to detect immunoglobulin G antibodies capable of fixing complement in sensitized pediatric heart transplant patients. J Heart Lung Transplant 2011;30(2):158–63.

23. Yabu JM, Higgins JP, Chen G, et al. C1q-fixing human leukocyte antigen antibodies are specific for predicting transplant glomerulopathy and late graft failure after kidney transplantation. Transplantation 2011;91(3):342–7.

24. Chen G, Sequeira F, Tyan DB. Novel C1q assay reveals a clinically relevant subset of human leukocyte antigen antibodies independent of immunoglobulin G strength on single antigen beads. Hum Immunol 2011;72(10):849–58.

25. Duquesnoy RJ, Takemoto S, de Lange P, et al. HLAmatchmaker: a molecularly based algorithm for histocompatibility determination. III. Effect of matching at the HLA-A,B amino acid triplet level on kidney transplant survival. Transplantation 2003;75(6):884–9.

26. Lim WH, Wong G, Heidt S, et al. Novel aspects of epitope matching and practical application in kidney transplantation. Kidney Int 2018;93(2):314–24.

27. Sypek M, Kausman J, Holt S, et al. HLA epitope matching in kidney transplantation: an overview for the general nephrologist. Am J Kidney Dis 2018;71(5): 720–31.

28. Wiebe C, Pochinco D, Blydt-Hansen TD, et al. Class II HLA epitope matching-A strategy to minimize de novo donor-specific antibody development and improve outcomes. Am J Transplant 2013;13(12):3114–22.
29. Li L, Wadia P, Chen R, et al. Identifying compartment-specific non-HLA targets after renal transplantation by integrating transcriptome and "antibodyome" measures. Proc Natl Acad Sci U S A 2009;106(11):4148–53.
30. Opelz G, Collaborative Transplant Study. Non-HLA transplantation immunity revealed by lymphocytotoxic antibodies. Lancet 2005;365(9470):1570–6.
31. Terasaki PI. Deduction of the fraction of immunologic and non-immunologic failure in cadaver donor transplants. Clin Transpl 2003;449–52.
32. Brasile L, Rodman E, Shield CF 3rd, et al. The association of antivascular endothelial cell antibody with hyperacute rejection: a case report. Surgery 1986; 99(5):637–40.
33. Harmer AW, Haskard D, Koffman CG, et al. Novel antibodies associated with unexplained loss of renal allografts. Transpl Int 1990;3(2):66–9.
34. Jackson AM, Kuperman MB, Montgomery RA. Multiple hyperacute rejections in the absence of detectable complement activation in a patient with endothelial cell reactive antibody. Am J Transplant 2012;12(6):1643–9.
35. Jordan SC, Yap HK, Sakai RS, et al. Hyperacute allograft rejection mediated by anti-vascular endothelial cell antibodies with a negative monocyte crossmatch. Transplantation 1988;46(4):585–7.
36. Niikura T, Yamamoto I, Nakada Y, et al. Probable C4d-negative accelerated acute antibody-mediated rejection due to non-HLA antibodies. Nephrology (Carlton) 2015;20(Suppl 2):75–8.
37. Sumitran-Karuppan S, Tyden G, Reinholt F, et al. Hyperacute rejections of two consecutive renal allografts and early loss of the third transplant caused by non-HLA antibodies specific for endothelial cells. Transpl Immunol 1997;5(4): 321–7.
38. Perrey C, Brenchley PE, Johnson RW, et al. An association between antibodies specific for endothelial cells and renal transplant failure. Transpl Immunol 1998; 6(2):101–6.
39. Zou Y, Stastny P, Susal C, et al. Antibodies against MICA antigens and kidney-transplant rejection. N Engl J Med 2007;357(13):1293–300.
40. Alachkar N, Gupta G, Montgomery RA. Angiotensin antibodies and focal segmental glomerulosclerosis. N Engl J Med 2013;368(10):971–3.
41. Mujtaba MA, Sharfuddin AA, Book BL, et al. Pre-transplant angiotensin receptor II type 1 antibodies and risk of post-transplant focal segmental glomerulosclerosis recurrence. Clin Transplant 2015;29(7):606–11.
42. Delville M, Sigdel TK, Wei C, et al. A circulating antibody panel for pretransplant prediction of FSGS recurrence after kidney transplantation. Sci Transl Med 2014;6(256):256ra136.
43. Waikar SS, Betensky RA, Emerson SC, et al. Imperfect gold standards for kidney injury biomarker evaluation. J Am Soc Nephrol 2012;23(1):13–21.
44. Nankivell BJ, Alexander SI. Rejection of the kidney allograft. N Engl J Med 2010; 363(15):1451–62.
45. Halawa A. The early diagnosis of acute renal graft dysfunction: a challenge we face. The role of novel biomarkers. Ann Transplant 2011;16(1):90–8.
46. Williams WW, Taheri D, Tolkoff-Rubin N, et al. Clinical role of the renal transplant biopsy. Nat Rev Nephrol 2012;8(2):110–21.
47. Diaz-Buxo JA, Donadio JV Jr. Complications of percutaneous renal biopsy: an analysis of 1,000 consecutive biopsies. Clin Nephrol 1975;4(6):223–7.

48. Stiles KP, Yuan CM, Chung EM, et al. Renal biopsy in high-risk patients with medical diseases of the kidney. Am J Kidney Dis 2000;36(2):419–33.
49. Kersnik Levart T, Kenig A, Buturovic Ponikvar J, et al. Real-time ultrasound-guided renal biopsy with a biopsy gun in children: safety and efficacy. Acta Paediatr 2001;90(12):1394–7.
50. Chesney DS, Brouhard BH, Cunningham RJ. Safety and cost effectiveness of pediatric percutaneous renal biopsy. Pediatr Nephrol 1996;10(4):493–5.
51. Mahoney MC, Racadio JM, Merhar GL, et al. Safety and efficacy of kidney transplant biopsy: Tru-Cut needle vs sonographically guided biopsy gun. AJR Am J Roentgenol 1993;160(2):325–6.
52. Sarwal M, Chua MS, Kambham N, et al. Molecular heterogeneity in acute renal allograft rejection identified by DNA microarray profiling. N Engl J Med 2003; 349(2):125–38.
53. Suthanthiran M, Muthukumar T. Urinary-cell mRNA and acute kidney-transplant rejection. N Engl J Med 2013;369(19):1860–1.
54. Nelson PJ, Krensky AM. Chemokines, chemokine receptors, and allograft rejection. Immunity 2001;14(4):377–86.
55. Segerer S, Cui Y, Eitner F, et al. Expression of chemokines and chemokine receptors during human renal transplant rejection. Am J Kidney Dis 2001;37(3): 518–31.
56. Hu H, Aizenstein BD, Puchalski A, et al. Elevation of CXCR3-binding chemokines in urine indicates acute renal-allograft dysfunction. Am J Transplant 2004;4(3):432–7.
57. Jackson JA, Kim EJ, Begley B, et al. Urinary chemokines CXCL9 and CXCL10 are noninvasive markers of renal allograft rejection and BK viral infection. Am J Transplant 2011;11(10):2228–34.
58. Hricik DE, Nickerson P, Formica RN, et al. Multicenter validation of urinary CXCL9 as a risk-stratifying biomarker for kidney transplant injury. Am J Transplant 2013;13(10):2634–44.
59. Schaub S, Nickerson P, Rush D, et al. Urinary CXCL9 and CXCL10 levels correlate with the extent of subclinical tubulitis. Am J Transplant 2009;9(6):1347–53.
60. Rabant M, Amrouche L, Lebreton X, et al. Urinary C-X-C motif chemokine 10 independently improves the noninvasive diagnosis of antibody-mediated kidney allograft rejection. J Am Soc Nephrol 2015;26(11):2840–51.
61. Halloran PF, Reeve JP, Pereira AB, et al. Antibody-mediated rejection, T cell-mediated rejection, and the injury-repair response: new insights from the Genome Canada studies of kidney transplant biopsies. Kidney Int 2014;85(2): 258–64.
62. Halloran PF, Famulski KS, Reeve J. Molecular assessment of disease states in kidney transplant biopsy samples. Nat Rev Nephrol 2016;12(9):534–48.
63. Halloran PF, Reeve J, Akalin E, et al. Real time central assessment of kidney transplant indication biopsies by microarrays: the INTERCOMEX Study. Am J Transplant 2017;17(11):2851–62.
64. O'Connell PJ, Zhang W, Menon MC, et al. Biopsy transcriptome expression profiling to identify kidney transplants at risk of chronic injury: a multicentre, prospective study. Lancet 2016;388(10048):983–93.
65. Voelkerding KV, Dames SA, Durtschi JD. Next-generation sequencing: from basic research to diagnostics. Clin Chem 2009;55(4):641–58.
66. Knight SR, Thorne A, Faro MLL. Donor-specific Cell-Free DNA as a biomarker in solid organ transplantation. A systematic review. Transplantation 2018. https://doi.org/10.1097/TP.0000000000002482.

67. Agbor-Enoh S, Tunc I, De Vlaminck I, et al. Applying rigor and reproducibility standards to assay donor-derived cell-free DNA as a non-invasive method for detection of acute rejection and graft injury after heart transplantation. J Heart Lung Transplant 2017;36(9):1004–12.

68. Schutz E, Fischer A, Beck J, et al. Graft-derived cell-free DNA, a noninvasive early rejection and graft damage marker in liver transplantation: a prospective, observational, multicenter cohort study. PLoS Med 2017;14(4):e1002286.

69. Zou J, Duffy B, Slade M, et al. Rapid detection of donor cell free DNA in lung transplant recipients with rejections using donor-recipient HLA mismatch. Hum Immunol 2017;78(4):342–9.

70. Gordon PM, Khan A, Sajid U, et al. An Algorithm measuring donor cell-free DNA in plasma of cellular and solid organ transplant recipients that does not require donor or recipient genotyping. Front Cardiovasc Med 2016;3:33.

71. Beck J, Oellerich M, Schulz U, et al. Donor-derived cell-free DNA is a novel universal biomarker for allograft rejection in solid organ transplantation. Transplant Proc 2015;47(8):2400–3.

72. Park J, Lin HY, Assaker JP, et al. Integrated kidney exosome analysis for the detection of kidney transplant rejection. ACS Nano 2017;11(11):11041–6.

73. Fishman JA. Infection in solid-organ transplant recipients. N Engl J Med 2007; 357(25):2601–14.

74. Hricik DE, Formica RN, Nickerson P, et al. Adverse outcomes of tacrolimus withdrawal in immune-quiescent kidney transplant recipients. J Am Soc Nephrol 2015;26(12):3114–22.

75. Kasiske BL, Chakkera HA, Louis TA, et al. A meta-analysis of immunosuppression withdrawal trials in renal transplantation. J Am Soc Nephrol 2000;11(10): 1910–7.

76. Schiff J, Cole E, Cantarovich M. Therapeutic monitoring of calcineurin inhibitors for the nephrologist. Clin J Am Soc Nephrol 2007;2(2):374–84.

77. Hricik DE, Rodriguez V, Riley J, et al. Enzyme linked immunosorbent spot (ELISPOT) assay for interferon-gamma independently predicts renal function in kidney transplant recipients. Am J Transplant 2003;3(7):878–84.

78. Ashoor I, Najafian N, Korin Y, et al. Standardization and cross validation of alloreactive IFNgamma ELISPOT assays within the clinical trials in organ transplantation consortium. Am J Transplant 2013;13(7):1871–9.

79. Nather BJ, Nickel P, Bold G, et al. Modified ELISPOT technique–highly significant inverse correlation of post-Tx donor-reactive IFNgamma-producing cell frequencies with 6 and 12 months graft function in kidney transplant recipients. Transpl Immunol 2006;16(3–4):232–7.

80. Nickel P, Presber F, Bold G, et al. Enzyme-linked immunosorbent spot assay for donor-reactive interferon-gamma-producing cells identifies T-cell presensitization and correlates with graft function at 6 and 12 months in renal-transplant recipients. Transplantation 2004;78(11):1640–6.

81. Hricik DE, Augustine J, Nickerson P, et al. Interferon gamma ELISPOT testing as a risk-stratifying biomarker for kidney transplant injury: results from the CTOT-01 multicenter study. Am J Transplant 2015;15(12):3166–73.

82. Sottong PR, Rosebrock JA, Britz JA, et al. Measurement of T-lymphocyte responses in whole-blood cultures using newly synthesized DNA and ATP. Clin Diagn Lab Immunol 2000;7(2):307–11.

83. Kowalski RJ, Post DR, Mannon RB, et al. Assessing relative risks of infection and rejection: a meta-analysis using an immune function assay. Transplantation 2006;82(5):663–8.

84. Huskey J, Gralla J, Wiseman AC. Single time point immune function assay (ImmuKnow) testing does not aid in the prediction of future opportunistic infections or acute rejection. Clin J Am Soc Nephrol 2011;6(2):423–9.

85. Wang Z, Liu X, Lu P, et al. Performance of the ImmuKnow assay in differentiating infection and acute rejection after kidney transplantation: a meta-analysis. Transplant Proc 2014;46(10):3343–51.

86. Moon HH, Kim TS, Lee S, et al. Serial ImmuKnow assay in stable kidney transplant recipients. Cent Eur J Immunol 2014;39(1):96–9.

87. Ravaioli M, Neri F, Lazzarotto T, et al. Immunosuppression modifications based on an immune response assay: results of a randomized, controlled trial. Transplantation 2015;99(8):1625–32.

88. He J, Li Y, Zhang H, et al. Immune function assay (ImmuKnow) as a predictor of allograft rejection and infection in kidney transplantation. Clin Transplant 2013; 27(4):E351–8.

89. Kwun J, Bulut P, Kim E, et al. The role of B cells in solid organ transplantation. Semin Immunol 2012;24(2):96–108.

90. Valujskikh A, Bromberg JS. Literature watch: implications for transplantation. Am J Transplant 2013;13(5):1117.

91. Zachary AA, Kopchaliiska D, Montgomery RA, et al. HLA-specific B cells: I. A method for their detection, quantification, and isolation using HLA tetramers. Transplantation 2007;83(7):982–8.

92. Zachary AA, Kopchaliiska D, Montgomery RA, et al. HLA-specific B cells: II. Application to transplantation. Transplantation 2007;83(7):989–94.

93. Zachary AA, Lucas DP, Montgomery RA, et al. Rituximab prevents an anamnestic response in patients with cryptic sensitization to HLA. Transplantation 2013;95(5):701–4.

94. Czerkinsky CC, Nilsson LA, Nygren H, et al. A solid-phase enzyme-linked immunospot (ELISPOT) assay for enumeration of specific antibody-secreting cells. J Immunol Methods 1983;65(1–2):109–21.

95. Heidt S, Roelen DL, de Vaal YJ, et al. A NOVel ELISPOT assay to quantify HLA-specific B cells in HLA-immunized individuals. Am J Transplant 2012;12(6): 1469–78.

96. Karahan GE, de Vaal YJ, Roelen DL, et al. Quantification of HLA class II-specific memory B cells in HLA-sensitized individuals. Hum Immunol 2015;76(2–3): 129–36.

97. Thaunat O, Patey N, Caligiuri G, et al. Chronic rejection triggers the development of an aggressive intragraft immune response through recapitulation of lymphoid organogenesis. J Immunol 2010;185(1):717–28.

98. Thaunat O, Field AC, Dai J, et al. Lymphoid neogenesis in chronic rejection: evidence for a local humoral alloimmune response. Proc Natl Acad Sci U S A 2005; 102(41):14723–8.

99. Bachelet T, Couzi L, Lepreux S, et al. Kidney intragraft donor-specific antibodies as determinant of antibody-mediated lesions and poor graft outcome. Am J Transplant 2013;13(11):2855–64.

100. Doshi MD, Goggins MO, Li L, et al. Medical outcomes in African American live kidney donors: a matched cohort study. Am J Transplant 2013;13(1):111–8.

101. Muzaale AD, Massie AB, Wang MC, et al. Risk of end-stage renal disease following live kidney donation. JAMA 2014;311(6):579–86.

102. Genovese G, Friedman DJ, Ross MD, et al. Association of trypanolytic ApoL1 variants with kidney disease in African Americans. Science 2010;329(5993): 841–5.

103. Kopp JB, Smith MW, Nelson GW, et al. MYH9 is a major-effect risk gene for focal segmental glomerulosclerosis. Nat Genet 2008;40(10):1175–84.
104. Ma L, Langefeld CD, Comeau ME, et al. APOL1 renal-risk genotypes associate with longer hemodialysis survival in prevalent nondiabetic African American patients with end-stage renal disease. Kidney Int 2016;90(2):389–95.
105. Kalil RS, Smith RJ, Rastogi P, et al. Late reoccurrence of collapsing FSGS after transplantation of a living-related kidney bearing APOL 1 risk variants without disease evident in donor supports the second hit hypothesis. Transplant Direct 2017;3(8):e185.
106. Locke JE, Sawinski D, Reed RD, et al. Apolipoprotein L1 and chronic kidney disease risk in young potential living kidney donors. Ann Surg 2018;267(6):1161–8.
107. Doshi MD, Ortigosa-Goggins M, Garg AX, et al. APOL1 genotype and renal function of black living donors. J Am Soc Nephrol 2018;29(4):1309–16.
108. Young BA, Fullerton SM, Wilson JG, et al. Clinical genetic testing for APOL1: are we there yet? Semin Nephrol 2017;37(6):552–7.
109. Wu H, Malone AF, Donnelly EL, et al. Single-cell transcriptomics of a human kidney allograft biopsy specimen defines a diverse inflammatory response. J Am Soc Nephrol 2018;29(8):2069–80.
110. Sarwal MM, Benjamin J, Butte AJ, et al. Transplantomics and biomarkers in organ transplantation: a report from the first international conference. Transplantation 2011;91(4):379–82.

The Role of Costimulatory Pathways in Transplant Tolerance

Mayuko Uehara, MD, PhD, Martina M. McGrath, MD, MB, BCh*

KEYWORDS

- T-cell costimulation • Regulatory T cell • Tolerance • CD28 • CTLA-4 • CD40
- CD154 • LFA-1

KEY POINTS

- Costimulatory signals delivered to T cells at the time of antigen presentation are critical to T-cell activation.
- CD28:CD80/CD86 is the most important T-cell costimulatory pathway involved in transplant rejection.
- Cytotoxic T-lymphocyte-associated protein 4 (CTLA-4) immunoglobulin blocks CD28-mediated costimulation but also has an impact on the suppressive function of regulatory T cells.
- CD40:CD154 blockade has shown impressive results in animal models, and efforts to translate these findings into humans are ongoing.
- Attempts to develop novel agents to block costimulation for clinical use have been hampered by increased risk of infection and other off-target effects.

INTRODUCTION

More than 37,000 patients underwent solid organ transplantation in the United States in 2017. A life-saving procedure, transplantation carries with it the need for lifelong immunosuppression to prevent rejection. The most common cause of late allograft loss remains chronic rejection.[1,2] Also, immunosuppressive drugs, such as tacrolimus, mycophenolic acid, and steroids, have significant side effects, which contribute to morbidity and mortality post-transplantation.[3,4] Thus, success in the field of transplantation is limited by the suboptimal efficacy and significant toxicity of present-day

Disclosures: The authors have no nothing to disclose.
This work is supported by the American Heart Association, under award number 14FTF19620001 to Martina M. McGrath.
Transplantation Research Center, Renal Division, Brigham and Women's Hospital, Harvard Medical School, 221 Longwood Avenue, Boston, MA, 02115, USA
* Corresponding author.
E-mail address: mmcgrath8@bwh.harvard.edu

immunosuppressive therapies. Furthermore, despite significant advances in understanding of immune recognition and activation that take place during transplantation, few novel immunosuppressive drugs have received Food and Drug Administration (FDA) approval in recent years.

One of the major breakthroughs in transplantation immunology was the discovery of T-cell costimulation as a critical step in T-cell activation.[5–7] Over the past 3 decades, understanding of these complex pathways and how multiple molecules interact to direct and control the immune response has grown exponentially. Recognition of the central role of T-cell costimulation in alloimmune activation has raised hopes for more targeted immunotherapy that may prevent chronic rejection without many of the metabolic side effects of current treatments.

This article reviews the role of T-cell costimulation in transplant rejection and tolerance and outlines its effect on the function of effector and regulatory T cells (Tregs). Several of the most important T-cell costimulatory pathways implicated in transplant rejection are focused on and their clinical relevance in the care of transplant recipients discussed, with emphasis on therapeutic agents undergoing or approaching clinical trials.

TRANSPLANT REJECTION, T-CELL COSTIMULATION, AND TOLERANCE

After transplantation, donor antigen derived from the allograft is carried by dendritic cells (DCs) to the allograft draining lymph nodes.[8] There, DCs encounter naïve T cells and present donor antigen, initiating T-cell priming. Antigens is presented by DCs to T cells which leads to T-cell activation in a few different ways, including direct allorecognition, where donor-derived DCs bearing donor major histocompatibility (MHC) molecules are recognized by T cells, and indirect allorecognition, where recipient DCs, having trafficked to the graft and picked up and processed donor antigen, present it on their own MHC molecules.[8,9] A third form of T-cell activation, semidirect allorecognition, occurs when DCs become cross-dressed with donor-derived MHC molecules carrying donor peptides, which are then presented to T cells in the draining lymph node, initiating T-cell activation and proliferation.[10,11]

T-cell receptor (TCR) recognition of a peptide presented on MHC provides what is known as signal 1 for T-cell activation. At the same time, for full activation, T cells also require signal 2, a costimulatory signal. Signal 3, which promotes T-cell differentiation into different subsets (such as helper T cell [T_H] 1, T_H2, or T_H17), is provided by the surrounding cytokine milieu. When antigen is presented in the absence of signal 2, T cells become anergic and are unable to proliferate, differentiate into effector T cells, or produce cytokines.[12,13] There exists a large array of cosignaling molecules, which can either increase (costimulatory) or decrease (coinhibitory) T-cell activation.[7] These molecules differ in their expression across cell populations and can have multiple ligands or binding partners, generating a complex network of signals. The ultimate fate of a naïve T-cell–encountering antigen is determined by the balance of costimulatory and coinhibitory signals it receives at the time of antigen recognition.[14] Memory T cells, which can rapidly proliferate and produce large amount of cytokines in response to antigen re-exposure, have lower costimulatory requirements than naïve T cells,[15] rendering them more challenging to control clinically.

Transplantation tolerance is generally defined as lack of immune activity against the allograft in the absence of maintenance immunosuppression, and occurring in the presence of intact immune system.[16] This is an active process and occurs where effector immunity is either suppressed or deleted in an antigen-specific manner. Tregs are central to the maintenance of transplant tolerance, but other regulatory cells of innate and adaptive origin (including B cells, DCs, natural killer [NK] cells, and other T cells) are increasingly recognized to play important roles.[16]

The goal of achieving durable transplantation tolerance in the clinic remains elusive. Several academic centers have clinical protocols that combine bone marrow and kidney transplantation. These protocols have been successful in inducing tolerance in carefully selected patients.[17–19] This approach, however, is not feasible for the vast majority of patients awaiting solid organ transplantation. Therefore, other mechanisms of inducing tolerance, including costimulatory blockade, remain active areas of investigation. Targeting individual costimulatory pathways has shown success in mouse models, but in more complex systems, in particular those involving memory T-cell responses, targeting several pathways using combination therapies will likely be required to induce and maintain robust tolerance.

CD28/CTLA-4/B7 T-LYMPHOCYTE–ASSOCIATED ANTIGEN 4/B7
CD28/B7 Costimulation

The CD28 pathway is the most important and best-studied costimulatory pathway in transplantation. CD28 is a transmembrane cell surface glycoprotein and belongs to the immunoglobulin (Ig) superfamily.[20] It has extracellular variable Ig-like, transmembrane, and cytoplasmic domains.[21] CD28 is constitutively expressed on naïve as well as activated and memory T cells, on all $CD4^+$ and $CD8^+$ T cells in mice, and approximately 80% of $CD4^+$ and half of $CD8^+$ T cells in humans.[22,23] This pattern of expression indicates that CD28 contributes to early antigen recognition and activation of T cells. The extracellular domain of CD28 interacts with its ligands, CD80 (B7-1) or CD86 (B7-2) expressed on antigen-presenting cells (APCs).[22] CD80 and CD86 seem to have overlapping functions. CD86 is expressed later, however, than CD80 after DC activation,[24] which suggests they may have distinct roles.[25–27] CD80 is the major initial ligand of cytotoxic T-lymphocyte associated protein-4 (CTLA-4) in the maintenance of immune tolerance. This inhibitory function can be modulated by up-regulation of CD86, which is the main ligand for CD28.[28]

Interaction of CD28, either with its ligands (CD80 or CD86) or with monoclonal antibodies, triggers phosphorylation of tyrosine residues on the cytoplasmic domain (Tyr^{189} in the YMNM motif)[29,30] of CD28 and results in the recruitment of Src homology 2 (SH2)-domain of the p85 subunit of phosphatidyl inositol 3-kinase (PI3K)[31–33] and the growth factor receptor bound protein 2 (Grb2),[30,34] which has approximately 10-fold to 100-fold less affinity than the p85 SH2-domain.[35] Through these intracellular signaling pathways, CD28 stimulation modulates T-cell proliferation, differentiation, and effector functions. These pathways regulate gene transcription via nuclear factor κB (NF-κB),[36,37] cell-cycle progression and survival via mitochondria associated Bcl-2 and Bcl-xL,[38–42] secretion of cytokines and chemokines via the guanine nucleotide exchange factor Vav1,[43] and metabolism via mTOR.[44,45]

Despite the critical role of the CD28/B7 costimulatory pathway in T-cell activation, mice with deficiencies in this pathway do not consistently show defective alloimmune responses against a transplanted graft. In murine models of graft-versus-host disease (GVHD), although CD28-deficient donor T cells fail to induce GVHD, CD28-deficient host mice develop systemic sclerosis, consistent with chronic GVHD, suggesting that T cells can be activated and alloreactive, even when part of the CD28/B7 pathway is absent.[46,47] In experimental models for solid organ transplantation, the authors have observed that CD28 knockout mice reject fully MHC-mismatched heart allografts, albeit slightly more slowly than wild-type controls (mean survival time: 12 days compared with approximately 8 days for control mice). Furthermore, other investigators have similarly shown that CD28 knockout mice reject MHC-mismatched transplants, regardless of the graft type.[48,49] Also, the absence of the ligands, CD80 and CD86, has an impact on allograft rejection. In studies using recipient mice lacking both CD80 and CD86 (CD80/CD86$^{-/-}$ mice), wild-type heart allografts were not rejected. Wild-type recipients, however, can effectively reject CD80/CD86$^{-/-}$ heart allografts, indicating that the site of expression of costimulatory molecules and their ligands have a great impact on their effect.[50] These data reflect the complexity of function of costimulatory pathways and the significant redundancy within the overall network of costimulatory molecules. They also speak to the challenges in targeting these molecules therapeutically.

Regulatory T Cells: CD28 and CTLA-4

Tregs are characterized by the expression of the transcription factor Foxp3. They play a crucial role in immune homeostasis by controlling the activities of activated T cells. In transplantation, the balance between Treg and T effector activity is a critical determinant of graft outcome. CD28 plays an important role in Treg development and homeostasis. Thymic development and peripheral homeostasis of Tregs is dependent on CD28-mediated production of interleukin (IL)-2[51,52] and mice deficient in CD28 or its ligands, CD80/CD86, have a markedly reduced number of natural Tregs and increased susceptibility to autoimmunity.[53,54] Much of the work examining the role of CD28 in Tregs has been done using CD28 knockout mice or blocking anti-B7 antibodies and has confirmed the requirement for CD28 in Treg development.[55,56] Turka and colleagues[57] demonstrated the importance of CD28 in Treg function postmaturation using mice with conditional knockout of CD28 on Tregs, the CD28-ΔTreg mice. Despite normal numbers of Tregs, proliferation and survival of Tregs in CD28-ΔTreg mice were markedly impaired.[57] Mice with Tregs lacking CD28 also had a markedly increased susceptibility to autoimmune disease, demonstrating the importance of CD28 in the function and survival of Tregs.[57] Furthermore, blockade of CD28 in vivo using CTLA-4 Ig (discussed later) seems to have variable effects on Treg function, as discussed in detail by Bluestone and colleagues.[58]

CTLA-4 is also a member of the Ig superfamily of cosignaling molecules and shares approximately 30% homology with CD28. CTLA-4 is localized in intracellular vesicles in resting T cells and is expressed on the cell surface after TCR ligation/CD28 costimulation.[59,60] CTLA-4 competes with CD28 for binding to CD80 and CD86; it binds the B7 ligands with much greater affinity and, in contrast to CD28, delivers a coinhibitory signal to the T cell on ligation.[61–63] Tregs express high levels of CTLA-4, which is their primary mechanism of T-cell suppression.[64] The importance of CTLA-4 in immune regulation is emphasized by the severity of disease states occurring in its absence. Mice genetically deficient in CTLA-4 die within 3 weeks of birth from severe lymphoproliferative disorder and autoimmune disease.[65] Blockade or deletion of CD28 or its ligands CD80 and CD86 prevents the development of autoimmunity, suggesting that excessive CD28-mediated costimulation drives the pathology observed in the absence of CTLA-4.[66]

Ligation with CTLA-4 and B7 negatively regulates T cells through several important mechanisms. Aside from competitively inhibiting T-cell costimulation via CD28, it inhibits T-cell activation, cell-cycle progression[67,68] and CD28-dependent IL-2 production.[67] CTLA-4 also increases T-cell motility, limiting the contact time between T cells and APCs, thereby decreasing T-cell activation.[69] Finally, it has been reported that CTLA-4 also binds surface CD80 and CD86 and internalizes them for degradation, a process that is up-regulated after Treg activation.[70,71]

Targeting CD28 Costimulation in Transplantation

CTLA-4 Ig is a fusion protein, developed more than 2 decades ago as an immunosuppressive agent targeted at CD28-mediated costimulation.[62] Exploiting the much greater affinity of B7 molecules for CTLA-4 than CD28, CTLA-4 Ig competitively inhibits the interaction between CD28 and B7, thereby blocking the costimulatory signal. Numerous preclinical studies have demonstrated that CTLA-4 Ig prolongs allograft and xenograft survival in rodent models, such as islet, heart, and kidney transplantation,[72–74] and has synergistic effect on transplant survival when given with additional agents.[75,76] The CTLA-4 Ig, Abatacept (Orencia, Bristol-Myers Squibb, USA), was first approved by the FDA for the treatment of rheumatoid arthritis.[77] It was found ineffective in nonhuman primate (NHP) studies in transplantation due to its lower affinity binding to CD86 compared with CD80.[78] The molecule was reengineered with 2 amino acid substitutions to increase its binding affinity to both CD80 and CD86 and its now known as belatacept (Nulojix, Bristol-Myers Squibb, USA). Belatacept is the only FDA-approved costimulatory blockade agent for clinical use in transplantation.[79,80] Phase III trials in kidney transplant recipients (Belatacept Evaluation of Nephroprotection and Efficacy as First-line Immunosuppression Trial [BENEFIT]) have shown that treatment with belatacept leads to graft survival similar to that observed with traditional immunosuppression using cyclosporin. Initial studies demonstrated increased early rates of acute cellular rejection with belatacept treatment.[80] Longerterm follow-up studies have also shown similar rates of overall graft survival in belatacept-treated and cyclosporine-treated patients. Those treated with belatacept, however, showed better kidney function (higher glomerular filtration rate) at long-term follow-up.[80]

In addition, belatacept-treated patients showed lower frequency of de novo donorspecific anti-HLA antibody (dnDSA) formation at 3 years post-transplant.[81] It has been proposed that decreased dnDSA formation is as a result of blockade of CD28 signaling by lymph node–resident follicular helper T cells (T_{FH}), which provide critical B-cell help to produce mature, affinity-switched humoral responses. Studies using murine transplant models also have demonstrated that blockade of CD28 cosignaling using either CTLA-4 Ig or an anti-CD28 antibody leads to better control of the humoral alloimmune response, and reductions in dnDSA.[81,82]

One potential disadvantage of CD28 blockade using CTLA-4 Ig is its concomitant blockade of CTLA-4–mediated coinhibitory signaling and its effect on Treg function. As described previously, the absence of CD28 slightly delays the rejection of fully mismatched cardiac transplants. Treating CD28 knockout transplant recipients, however, with CTLA-4 Ig leads to accelerated rejection, underscoring the inhibitory role of CTLA-4, even in the absence of CD28.[83] The proinflammatory T_H17 cells, which are involved in autoimmune disease and implicated in some models of transplant rejection, express high levels of CTLA-4, and it has been suggested that CTLA-4 plays a role in the suppression also of T_H17 cells.[84] CD28 blockade using CTLA-4 Ig has been shown, however, to be relatively ineffective in controlling T_H17 responses, because the blockade also impairs coinhibitory signaling.[85]

Furthermore, as outlined previously, CD28 signaling is critical for Treg development, proliferation, and survival and blockade of this pathway could have negative effects on Treg function. CTLA-4 Ig was shown to lead to accelerated rejection in a Tregdependent mouse model of transplantation.[86] The data on its effect on Treg induction are, however, conflicting. Early studies showed that CTLA-4 Ig impaired the induction of Tregs in vitro.[87] But more recently, ex vivo costimulatory blockade of peripheral blood mononuclear cells using CTLA-4 Ig has been used to generate allospecific

Tregs in vitro with the aim of producing Tregs for clinical use.[83] Although the ex vivo work is an initial proof of concept, further investigation is necessary to assess the stability, in vivo function, and survival of Tregs generated under CD28 blockade.

CTLA-4 Ig in Tolerance Induction

Although current clinical protocols to induce transplant tolerance do not include CTLA-4 Ig, there have been studies NHPs to evaluate its utility in tolerance induction protocols. Kawai and colleagues[86] successfully induced tolerance in a small number of NHP transplant recipients using a protocol of total body irradiation, thymic irradiation, and T-cell depletion with thymoglobulin prior to kidney and bone marrow transplant, followed by treatment with belatacept and the calcineurin inhibitor, cyclosporine. Three of 5 NHP recipients had long-term allograft survival without immunosuppression, suggesting that belatacept could be clinically useful. Despite good allograft outcomes, Treg numbers failed to increase substantially in these recipients, a finding that contrasts with other tolerance inducing protocols, namely, using anti-CD154, again indicating that belatacept may impair Treg induction and/or survival in vivo.[88]

The same group recently reported on an NHP study aimed at inducing tolerance through delayed bone marrow transplantation. This approach could be applicable to recipients of deceased donor transplants. In this study, NHP renal transplant recipients were treated with conventional immunosuppression for 4 months, who then underwent bone marrow transplantation after treatment with thymoglobin and belatacept. Despite achieving long-term transplant survival and donor-specific T-cell tolerance without maintenance immunosuppression, late donor-specific anti-HLA antibodies were identified, suggesting that using short-term belatacept at the time of bone marrow transplant fails to control the humoral alloimmune response in the longer term.[89]

CD28-Negative T Cells and Costimulatory Blockade

As humans ages, they accumulate an increasing number of CD28⁻ T cells. These are terminally differentiated, antigen-experienced T cells with lower replicative capacity and shorter life span than CD28⁺ T cells. Most commonly, increasing accumulation of CD8⁺ CD28⁻ T cells is associated with immune senescence; impaired responses to infection and vaccination; and neoplasia and is most commonly observed in older adults.[90] Because belatacept has become clinically available, there is increasing interest in the role of these cells in transplantation, particularly in the setting of costimulatory blockade.

As shown in BENEFIT, a sizable minority of kidney transplant patients develop rejection despite treatment with belatacept in what is known as costimulatory blockade-resistant rejection (CoBRR).[79,91] Belatacept has less activity against CD28⁻ T cells[92] and transplanted patients with CoBRR showed greater accumulation of CD28⁻ T cells.[93] A subset of CD28⁻ T cells has a proinflammatory phenotype with increased expression of proinflammatory cytokines (interferon [IFN]-γ, tumor necrosis factor [TNF]-α, and Interleukin [IL]-2)[94] and cytotoxic effector molecules (CD107a and granzyme B).[95] Other CD28⁻ T cells express the prototypic Treg transcription factor, Foxp3, and exhibit immunoregulatory functions.[90] Several small observational studies have reported increased circulating levels of CD8⁺ CD28⁻ T cells in stable allograft recipients.[96–98] Therefore, the significance of CD28⁻ T cells in transplantation is unclear. It seems that their costimulation requirements differ substantially from CD28⁺ T cells. Studies are ongoing to assess how they can be therapeutically manipulated.

Future Agents to Target CD28

Given the concerns that the efficacy of CD28 blockade with CTLA-4 Ig is limited by concurrent blockade of CTLA-4 coinhibition, there have been ongoing efforts to develop an antibody with specificity for CD28. An initial phase I trial of one novel anti-CD28 antibody resulted in life-threatening cytokine storm in 6 participants, requiring prolonged ICU-level care.[99] This antibody was subsequently found to cross-link CD28 and act as a superagonist in humans, a phenomenon not observed in preclinical studies. Advances in antibody generation, however, have produced anti–CD28-specific antibodies that are incapable of cross-linking. In preclinical studies, novel anti-CD28 antibodies have demonstrated significant inhibition of alloreactive CD8$^+$ T-cell responses and prolongation of graft survival.[100,101] It seems that among other mechanisms, intact CTLA-4 coinhibition in the absence of CD28 costimulation leads to enhanced Treg function and improved outcomes.[102] A CD28 domain-specific antibody, lulizumab pegol, has now moved to a phase II trial study in lupus.[103] Another anti-CD28 antibody, FR104, licensed by Janssen Biotech, USA, has produced prolongation of renal allograft survival and prevention of xenoGVHD in NHP, with superior efficacy to belatacept in both models.[104,105] FR104 was recently studied in a phase I study of healthy human volunteers and may have the potential for future applications in transplantation.[106]

CD40:CD154 (CD40 LIGAND)

CD40:CD154 is an important costimulatory pathway that impacts the function of many immune cells critical to the adaptive immune response and targeting this pathway has shown considerable promise in animal models of transplantation. Both CD40 and CD154 are type II transmembrane proteins and members of the TNF superfamily.[107] Murine and human CD40 share 62% homology in amino acid sequence and 78% of their cytoplasmic domains are identical.[108] CD40 is expressed on APCs, B cells, DCs, macrophages and multiple nonhematopoietic cells such as fibroblasts and endothelial cells. CD154 is 83% identical in mice and humans at the nucleotide level[109] and is up-regulated on CD4$^+$ T cells and endothelial cells after activation.

This pathway has been extensively studied in transplantation and plays a critical role in T-cell:B-cell interaction to generate high-affinity antibodies.[110] In addition, the interaction between CD40 expressed on T cells and CD154 expressed on APCs leads to maturation of DCs, with enhanced cytokine production and costimulatory molecule expression and increased ability to promote T effector differentiation.[111] Blockade of CD40:CD154 on DCs promotes a tolerogenic DC phenotype and leads to increased Treg induction.[112,113] CD40:CD154 is also a central pathway in T:T-cell interactions, where CD40 expressed by CD8$^+$ T cells serves as an important switch factor promoting CD8$^+$ T effector responses and inhibiting Treg differentiation.[112] This process can be inhibited with CD40 blockade, leading to increased Treg induction.

Blockade of CD40:CD154 in Transplantation

Blockade of the CD40:CD154 pathway has shown a striking effect on the alloimmune response. Anti-CD154 antibody blockade led to prolonged graft survival in murine models of skin and heart transplant,[114,115] and, in an NHP model, CD154 blockade led to long-term renal allograft survival with loss of donor-specific reactivity.[116] Antibodies inhibiting CD40 and CD154 have shown efficacy in disrupting germinal center formation and preventing alloantibody formation.[117,118] Blockade of this pathway, using either anti-CD154 or anti-CD40, has also been shown in multiple models to increase Tregs in vivo, predominantly through induction of Tregs from naïve T cells.[115,119]

Blockade of CD40:CD154 has shown significant synergistic effects when combined with CTLA-4 Ig, producing long-term graft survival in skin and cardiac allografts.[120,121] Mechanistic studies of combination therapy showed that although CTLA-4 Ig had detrimental effects on natural Tregs, anti-CD154 promoted conversion of induced Tregs, thereby promoting an overall tolerogenic milieu.[115] Furthermore, coadministration of CD40:CD154 blockade with donor-specific transfusion or bone marrow transplantation is a highly effective method of tolerance induction in skin, heart, and islet transplantation.[111]

The clinical translation of anti-CD154 antibodies was abandoned, however, due to a significant incidence of thromboembolic complications, initially observed in NHP models.[122,123] CD154 is expressed on activated platelets, and several anti-CD154 antibodies (hu5C8, IDEC-131, and ABI793) were associated with platelet activation, promoting large vessel thromboses.[124–126] Therefore, current approaches to targeting this pathway have focused on the development of CD40-blocking antibodies and comparable efficacy has been reported.

Future Agents to Target CD40:CD154

ASKP1240 is a fully humanized anti-CD40 antibody that blocks CD40:CD154 interactions and suppresses both cell-mediated and antibody immune responses without immunogenic and thromboembolic events.[127] ASKP1240 has been tested in NHP models as an alternative to anti-CD154 monoclonal antibody. It was found to be well tolerated, without thrombotic complications, and led to significant increases in kidney, liver, and islet transplant survival.[128–130] ASKP1240 was tested in a phase Ib trial, where it was given to kidney transplant recipients at the time of transplant in addition to standard immunosuppression and was well tolerated without complications.[131] This study was followed by an open-label, noninferiority study of 138 renal transplant recipients, comparing treatment with ASKP1240 in combination with mycophenolate mofetil or tacrolimus. Reported only in abstract form to date, combination therapy with ASKP1240 and mycophenolate mofetil was ineffective. Patients experienced increased rates of acute rejection compared with standard treatment. The combination of tacrolimus and ASKP1240 resulted in rates of rejection similar to control but was associated with increased rates of viral infection.[132] This agent was also tested recently as immunotherapy for psoriasis but showed no improvement in outcomes over placebo.[133] Currently, there are multiple ongoing studies to assess the effect of CD40 blockade with ASKP1240 in transplantation, and more data are forthcoming in the future.

Concurrently, other anti-CD40 antibodies are under investigation, including 4D11, 2C10R4, and HCD122. These agents have also demonstrated prolonged allograft survival of cardiac and kidney transplant in NHP models. These antibodies are associated with varying degrees of B-cell depletion, leading to a delay or inhibition of alloantibody production.[134,135] To assess if the observed improvements in transplant survival were due to blockade of CD40 or B-cell depletion, a novel Fc silent anti-CD40 antibody, CFZ533, was investigated in an NHP model of renal transplantation.[136] Transplant outcomes were excellent, and, despite a lack of B-cell depletion, CFZ533 prevented the formation of germinal centers, a key site of alloantibody generation. This agent is currently under investigation in a phase II clinical trial in renal transplant recipients.

LFA-1: ICAM-1

Antigen-experienced effector memory T (Tem) cells decrease their expression of CD28 and are, therefore, relatively resistant to the effects of CD28 blockade with CTLA-4 Ig. Memory T cells have reduced costimulatory requirements and enhanced proliferative capacity and can rapidly orchestrate an effector response against the allograft. Controlling the memory response to transplantation is a challenging issue, with few therapeutic options at present.

Tem cells are characterized by increased expression of adhesion molecules, including lymphocyte function–associated antigen 1 (LFA-1).[137,138] Recruitment of activated T cells to the transplanted organ is critical to the process of rejection. LFA-1 expressed on Tem cells binds to intercellular adhesion molecule-1 (ICAM-1) expressed on endothelial cells, promoting T-cell migration to the allograft in transplantation.[139] LFA-1/ICAM-1 binding also provides a costimulatory signal, enhances activation and proliferation of naïve CD8[+] T cells, and increases the adhesion between DCs and T cells.[140,141]

Murine studies have shown that blockade of the interaction between LFA-1 and ICAM-1 prolongs the survival of skin, cardiac, and islet allografts due to the inhibition of priming of naïve alloreactive T cells.[142–144] Antagonizing LFA-1 also inhibits the trafficking, proliferation, and effector functions of donor-reactive Tem cells in murine and NHP models.[139,145] Given the lack of efficacy of CD28 blockade in controlling Tem responses, LFA-1 antagonism was an attractive option for combined therapy. When combined with CTLA-4 Ig, anti–LFA-1 led to prolonged allograft survival and increased Treg numbers in a sensitized murine model of skin transplantation[146] and in an NHP islet transplant model, this combination therapy effectively controlled memory T-cell responses and decreased the rate of development of donor-specific antibodies.[137,145] Attempts to replicate this effect in an NHP renal transplant model, however, using 2 different anti–LFA-1 antibodies, showed no improvement in allograft survival over CTLA-4 Ig alone and increased rates of viral infections, reflecting differences in immune activation that occur in different transplant models.[146–148]

Based on the promising NHP findings, an anti–LFA-1 monoclonal antibody efalizumab was tested in clinical trials for allogeneic islet transplantation[149] and kidney transplantation.[150] Similar to NHP model, the patients treated with efalizumab and rapamycin showed marked increase of Treg in peripheral blood.[149] Both studies showed benefit in terms of improved allograft survival, and the therapy was well tolerated. In 2008, however, there were several reports of patients on long-term treatment with efalizumab developing fatal progressive multifocal leukoencephalopathy, secondary to reactivation of JC virus within the central nervous system.[151] The drug was voluntarily withdrawn from the market by its manufacturers in 2009. The future role of LFA-1 antagonism in transplantation is unclear.

OTHER PATHWAYS UNDER PRECLINICAL INVESTIGATION IN TRANSPLANTATION
ICOS: ICOSL

Inducible T-cell costimulatory (ICOS [CD278]) molecule also belongs to the Ig superfamily and shares significant structural similarity to CD28 and CTLA-4 in humans.[152] Despite this similarity, ICOS does not interact with CD80 or CD86 but interacts with ICOS ligand (ICOSL [B7h]).[153,154] ICOS is expressed on activated T cells, and some NK, NK T cells, and Treg populations and expression are increased in acutely and chronically rejecting allografts. ICOS:ICOSL interaction is critical for the generation of T_{FH} cells, which differentiate from naïve CD4+ T cells.[155,156] T_{FH} cells migrate from the T:B-cell border into the B-cell follicle and germinal center within the lymph node, where they provide critical help for B-cell proliferation, plasma cell formation, and isotype switching.[155,157] Antibody blockade of ICOS signaling, administered with either cyclosporin or anti-CD40, produced long-term allograft survival in several mouse models.[158-160] In an NHP model, however, ICOS blockade failed to prolong kidney or cardiac allograft survival, when added to belatacept or anti-CD40 antibody treatment.[159,161] This negative finding may reflect the fact that T-cell responses were well controlled in these NHP models, and ICOS blockade may be more relevant in situations where germinal center formation and humoral responses are more prominent. In keeping with this hypothesis, a phase 1b clinical trial using a human anti-ICOSL monoclonal antibody (ICOSL Ig [AMG557]) showed benefit in patients with active lupus arthritis.[162] Future studies are needed to identify if targeting ICOS is beneficial in transplantation, particularly in control of humoral rejection.

OX40:OX40 Ligand

OX40, a member of the TNF receptor superfamily, is expressed on activated T cells on TCR/CD28 stimulation.[163] Its ligand, OX40L, is expressed on activated APC, endothelium, and T cells.[164-166] The expression patterns of OX40 and OX40L suggest that OX40 promotes the differentiation and maintenance of activated T cells. This is highlighted by a study showing that after activation, OX40$^{-/-}$ T cells initially have normal proliferation and cytokine production but fail to maintain these responses and undergo apoptosis at approximately 4 days to 8 days after activation.[167] Furthermore, OX40 costimulation impairs the expression of Foxp3, blocks the induction of Tregs from naïve CD4+ T cells, and significantly impairs the suppressive function of existing Tregs.[168-170]

The effect of blockade of OX40:OX40L in murine models of transplantation reflects these findings. Although OX40 blockade did not have an impact on T-cell proliferation, it led to significantly decreased accumulation of T cells in lymph nodes and reduced survival, resulting in improved allograft outcomes.[171-174] Treg survival and suppressive functions were also considerably enhanced by OX40 blockade. This combination of effects makes OX40:OX40L pathway an attractive target for future studies in transplantation.[174]

SUMMARY

A substantial number of costimulatory and coinhibitory pathways are activated after transplantation, and the net effect of these signals shapes the T-cell response to the allograft. CD28:B7 is the dominant costimulatory pathway but important roles are played by other molecules, in particular CTLA-4 and the CD40:CD154 pathway. The first-in-class costimulatory agent, belatacept, has shown significant improvements in renal transplant function in long-term follow-up, but widespread use has been tempered by concerns about increased risk of early acute rejection and its effect on Treg populations.

Given the complex network of costimulatory molecules and significant overlap between their functions, a combinatorial strategy targeting multiple pathways will likely be required to produce transplant tolerance. As outlined in this article, multiple novel agents are in the early phases of clinical development, raising optimism that, in the future, a more tailored approach to costimulatory blockade may be possible based on the needs of individual patients.

REFERENCES

1. Ojo AO, Hanson JA, Wolfe RA, et al. Long-term survival in renal transplant recipients with graft function. Kidney Int 2000;57:307–13.
2. Prakash J, Ghosh B, Singh S, et al. Causes of death in renal transplant recipients with functioning allograft. Indian J Nephrol 2012;22:264–8.
3. Bamoulid J, Staeck O, Halleck F, et al. The need for minimization strategies: current problems of immunosuppression. Transpl Int 2015;28:891–900.
4. Silva HT Jr, Yang HC, Meier-Kriesche HU, et al. Long-term follow-up of a phase III clinical trial comparing tacrolimus extended-release/MMF, tacrolimus/MMF, and cyclosporine/MMF in de novo kidney transplant recipients. Transplantation 2014;97:636–41.
5. Li XC, Rothstein DM, Sayegh MH. Costimulatory pathways in transplantation: challenges and new developments. Immunol Rev 2009;229:271–93.
6. June CH, Ledbetter JA, Linsley PS, et al. Role of the CD28 receptor in T-cell activation. Immunol Today 1990;11:211–6.
7. McGrath MM, Najafian N. The role of coinhibitory signaling pathways in transplantation and tolerance. Front Immunol 2012;3:47.
8. Martin-Fontecha A, Lanzavecchia A, Sallusto F. Dendritic cell migration to peripheral lymph nodes. Handb Exp Pharmacol 2009;(188):31–49.
9. Benichou G, Tocco G. The road to transplant tolerance is paved with good dendritic cells. Eur J Immunol 2013;43:584–8.
10. Marino J, Babiker-Mohamed MH, Crosby-Bertorini P, et al. Donor exosomes rather than passenger leukocytes initiate alloreactive T cell responses after transplantation. Sci Immunol 2016;1:aaf8759.
11. Campana S, De Pasquale C, Carrega P, et al. Cross-dressing: an alternative mechanism for antigen presentation. Immunol Lett 2015;168:349–54.
12. Jenkins MK, Schwartz RH. Antigen presentation by chemically modified splenocytes induces antigen-specific T cell unresponsiveness in vitro and in vivo. J Exp Med 1987;165:302–19.
13. Adams AB, Ford ML, Larsen CP. Costimulation blockade in autoimmunity and transplantation: the CD28 pathway. J Immunol 2016;197:2045–50.
14. Marchingo JM, Kan A, Sutherland RM, et al. T cell signaling. Antigen affinity, costimulation, and cytokine inputs sum linearly to amplify T cell expansion. Science 2014;346:1123–7.
15. Sprent J, Surh CD. T cell memory. Annu Rev Immunol 2002;20:551–79.
16. Robinson KA, Orent W, Madsen JC, et al. Maintaining T cell tolerance of alloantigens: lessons from animal studies. Am J Transplant 2018;18:1843–56.
17. Kawai T, Cosimi AB, Spitzer TR, et al. HLA-mismatched renal transplantation without maintenance immunosuppression. N Engl J Med 2008;358:353–61.
18. Leventhal J, Abecassis M, Miller J, et al. Chimerism and tolerance without GVHD or engraftment syndrome in HLA-mismatched combined kidney and hematopoietic stem cell transplantation. Sci Transl Med 2012;4:124ra28.
19. Scandling JD, Busque S, Shizuru JA, et al. Chimerism, graft survival, and withdrawal of immunosuppressive drugs in HLA matched and mismatched patients after living donor kidney and hematopoietic cell transplantation. Am J Transplant 2015;15:695–704.
20. Sharpe AH, Freeman GJ. The B7-CD28 superfamily. Nat Rev Immunol 2002;2:116–26.

21. Buonavista N, Balzano C, Pontarotti P, et al. Molecular linkage of the human CTLA4 and CD28 Ig-superfamily genes in yeast artificial chromosomes. Genomics 1992;13:856–61.

22. Harper K, Balzano C, Rouvier E, et al. CTLA-4 and CD28 activated lymphocyte molecules are closely related in both mouse and human as to sequence, message expression, gene structure, and chromosomal location. J Immunol 1991; 147:1037–44.

23. Gross JA, St John T, Allison JP. The murine homologue of the T lymphocyte antigen CD28. Molecular cloning and cell surface expression. J Immunol 1990; 144:3201–10.

24. Hathcock KS, Laszlo G, Pucillo C, et al. Comparative analysis of B7-1 and B7-2 costimulatory ligands: expression and function. J Exp Med 1994;180:631–40.

25. Pentcheva-Hoang T, Egen JG, Wojnoonski K, et al. B7-1 and B7-2 selectively recruit CTLA-4 and CD28 to the immunological synapse. Immunity 2004;21: 401–13.

26. Collins AV, Brodie DW, Gilbert RJ, et al. The interaction properties of costimulatory molecules revisited. Immunity 2002;17:201–10.

27. Linsley PS, Greene JL, Brady W, et al. Human B7-1 (CD80) and B7-2 (CD86) bind with similar avidities but distinct kinetics to CD28 and CTLA-4 receptors. Immunity 1994;1:793–801.

28. Sansom DM, Manzotti CN, Zheng Y. What's the difference between CD80 and CD86? Trends Immunol 2003;24:314–9.

29. Michel F, Attal-Bonnefoy G, Mangino G, et al. CD28 as a molecular amplifier extending TCR ligation and signaling capabilities. Immunity 2001;15:935–45.

30. Schneider H, Cai YC, Cefai D, et al. Mechanisms of CD28 signalling. Res Immunol 1995;146:149–54.

31. Pages F, Ragueneau M, Rottapel R, et al. Binding of phosphatidylinositol-3-OH kinase to CD28 is required for T-cell signalling. Nature 1994;369:327–9.

32. Harada Y, Tanabe E, Watanabe R, et al. Novel role of phosphatidylinositol 3-kinase in CD28-mediated costimulation. J Biol Chem 2001;276:9003–8.

33. Bjorgo E, Solheim SA, Abrahamsen H, et al. Cross talk between phosphatidylinositol 3-kinase and cyclic AMP (cAMP)-protein kinase a signaling pathways at the level of a protein kinase B/beta-arrestin/cAMP phosphodiesterase 4 complex. Mol Cell Biol 2010;30:1660–72.

34. Higo K, Oda M, Morii H, et al. Quantitative analysis by surface plasmon resonance of CD28 interaction with cytoplasmic adaptor molecules Grb2, Gads and p85 PI3K. Immunol Invest 2014;43:278–91.

35. Schneider H, Cai YC, Prasad KV, et al. T cell antigen CD28 binds to the GRB-2/SOS complex, regulators of p21ras. Eur J Immunol 1995;25:1044–50.

36. Thaker YR, Schneider H, Rudd CE. TCR and CD28 activate the transcription factor NF-kappaB in T-cells via distinct adaptor signaling complexes. Immunol Lett 2015;163:113–9.

37. Tuosto L. NF-kappaB family of transcription factors: biochemical players of CD28 co-stimulation. Immunol Lett 2011;135:1–9.

38. Wei MC, Zong WX, Cheng EH, et al. Proapoptotic BAX and BAK: a requisite gateway to mitochondrial dysfunction and death. Science 2001;292:727–30.

39. Lindsten T, Ross AJ, King A, et al. The combined functions of proapoptotic Bcl-2 family members bak and bax are essential for normal development of multiple tissues. Mol Cell 2000;6:1389–99.

40. Hoff H, Knieke K, Cabail Z, et al. Surface CD152 (CTLA-4) expression and signaling dictates longevity of CD28null T cells. J Immunol 2009;182:5342–51.

41. Boise LH, Minn AJ, Noel PJ, et al. CD28 costimulation can promote T cell survival by enhancing the expression of Bcl-xL. Immunity. 1995. 3: 87-98. J Immunol 2010;185:3788–99.
42. Boise LH, Noel PJ, Thompson CB. CD28 and apoptosis. Curr Opin Immunol 1995;7:620–5.
43. David R, Ma L, Ivetic A, et al. T-cell receptor- and CD28-induced Vav1 activity is required for the accumulation of primed T cells into antigenic tissue. Blood 2009; 113:3696–705.
44. Arnold CR, Pritz T, Brunner S, et al. T cell receptor-mediated activation is a potent inducer of macroautophagy in human CD8(+)CD28(+) T cells but not in CD8(+)CD28(-) T cells. Exp Gerontol 2014;54:75–83.
45. Hamilton KS, Phong B, Corey C, et al. T cell receptor-dependent activation of mTOR signaling in T cells is mediated by Carma1 and MALT1, but not Bcl10. Sci Signal 2014;7:ra55.
46. Harada Y, Tokushima M, Matsumoto Y, et al. Critical requirement for the membrane-proximal cytosolic tyrosine residue for CD28-mediated costimulation in vivo. J Immunol 2001;166:3797–803.
47. Akieda Y, Wakamatsu E, Nakamura T, et al. Defects in regulatory T cells due to CD28 deficiency induce a qualitative change of allogeneic immune response in chronic graft-versus-host disease. J Immunol 2015;194:4162–74.
48. Yamada A, Kishimoto K, Dong VM, et al. CD28-independent costimulation of T cells in alloimmune responses. J Immunol 2001;167:140–6.
49. Maier S, Tertilt C, Chambron N, et al. Inhibition of natural killer cells results in acceptance of cardiac allografts in CD28-/- mice. Nat Med 2001;7:557–62.
50. Mandelbrot DA, Furukawa Y, McAdam AJ, et al. Expression of B7 molecules in recipient, not donor, mice determines the survival of cardiac allografts. J Immunol 1999;163:3753–7.
51. Bour-Jordan H, Bluestone JA. Regulating the regulators: costimulatory signals control the homeostasis and function of regulatory T cells. Immunol Rev 2009; 229:41–66.
52. Tang Q, Henriksen KJ, Boden EK, et al. Cutting edge: CD28 controls peripheral homeostasis of CD4+CD25+ regulatory T cells. J Immunol 2003;171:3348–52.
53. Salomon B, Lenschow DJ, Rhee L, et al. B7/CD28 costimulation is essential for the homeostasis of the CD4+CD25+ immunoregulatory T cells that control autoimmune diabetes. Immunity 2000;12:431–40.
54. Tai X, Cowan M, Feigenbaum L, et al. CD28 costimulation of developing thymocytes induces Foxp3 expression and regulatory T cell differentiation independently of interleukin 2. Nat Immunol 2005;6:152–62.
55. Sempowski GD, Cross SJ, Heinly CS, et al. CD7 and CD28 are required for murine CD4+CD25+ regulatory T cell homeostasis and prevention of thyroiditis. J Immunol 2004;172:787–94.
56. Heinly CS, Sempowski GD, Lee DM, et al. Comparison of thymocyte development and cytokine production in CD7-deficient, CD28-deficient and CD7/CD28 double-deficient mice. Int Immunol 2001;13:157–66.
57. Zhang R, Huynh A, Whitcher G, et al. An obligate cell-intrinsic function for CD28 in tregs. J Clin Invest 2013;123:580–93.
58. Esensten JH, Helou YA, Chopra G, et al. CD28 Costimulation: from mechanism to therapy. Immunity 2016;44:973–88.
59. Mead KI, Zheng Y, Manzotti CN, et al. Exocytosis of CTLA-4 is dependent on phospholipase D and ADP ribosylation factor-1 and stimulated during activation of regulatory T cells. J Immunol 2005;174:4803–11.

60. Alegre ML, Noel PJ, Eisfelder BJ, et al. Regulation of surface and intracellular expression of CTLA4 on mouse T cells. J Immunol 1996;157:4762–70.
61. Guinan EC, Gribben JG, Boussiotis VA, et al. Pivotal role of the B7:CD28 pathway in transplantation tolerance and tumor immunity. Blood 1994;84:3261–82.
62. Linsley PS, Brady W, Urnes M, et al. CTLA-4 is a second receptor for the B cell activation antigen B7. J Exp Med 1991;174:561–9.
63. Crepeau RL, Ford ML. Challenges and opportunities in targeting the CD28/CTLA-4 pathway in transplantation and autoimmunity. Expert Opin Biol Ther 2017;17:1001–12.
64. Read S, Malmstrom V, Powrie F. Cytotoxic T lymphocyte-associated antigen 4 plays an essential role in the function of CD25(+)CD4(+) regulatory cells that control intestinal inflammation. J Exp Med 2000;192:295–302.
65. Waterhouse P, Penninger JM, Timms E, et al. Lymphoproliferative disorders with early lethality in mice deficient in Ctla-4. Science 1995;270:985–8.
66. Tai X, Van Laethem F, Sharpe AH, et al. Induction of autoimmune disease in CTLA-4-/- mice depends on a specific CD28 motif that is required for in vivo costimulation. Proc Natl Acad Sci U S A 2007;104:13756–61.
67. Walunas TL, Bakker CY, Bluestone JA. CTLA-4 ligation blocks CD28-dependent T cell activation. J Exp Med 1996;183:2541–50.
68. Schneider H, Smith X, Liu H, et al. CTLA-4 disrupts ZAP70 microcluster formation with reduced T cell/APC dwell times and calcium mobilization. Eur J Immunol 2008;38:40–7.
69. Walker LS, Sansom DM. Confusing signals: recent progress in CTLA-4 biology. Trends Immunol 2015;36:63–70.
70. Misra N, Bayry J, Lacroix-Desmazes S, et al. Cutting edge: human CD4+CD25+ T cells restrain the maturation and antigen-presenting function of dendritic cells. J Immunol 2004;172:4676–80.
71. Qureshi OS, Zheng Y, Nakamura K, et al. Trans-endocytosis of CD80 and CD86: a molecular basis for the cell-extrinsic function of CTLA-4. Science 2011;332:600–3.
72. Lenschow DJ, Zeng Y, Thistlethwaite JR, et al. Long-term survival of xenogeneic pancreatic islet grafts induced by CTLA4Ig. Science 1992;257:789–92.
73. Pearson TC, Alexander DZ, Winn KJ, et al. Transplantation tolerance induced by CTLA4-Ig. Transplantation 1994;57:1701–6.
74. Azuma H, Chandraker A, Nadeau K, et al. Blockade of T-cell costimulation prevents development of experimental chronic renal allograft rejection. Proc Natl Acad Sci U S A 1996;93:12439–44.
75. Yamada A, Murakami M, Ijima K, et al. Long-term acceptance of major histocompatibility complex-mismatched cardiac allograft induced by a low dose of CTLA4IgM plus FK506. Microbiol Immunol 1996;40:513–8.
76. Uehara M, Solhjou Z, Banouni N, et al. Ischemia augments alloimmune injury through IL-6-driven CD4(+) alloreactivity. Sci Rep 2018;8:2461.
77. Kremer JM, Westhovens R, Leon M, et al. Treatment of rheumatoid arthritis by selective inhibition of T-cell activation with fusion protein CTLA4Ig. N Engl J Med 2003;349:1907–15.
78. Levisetti MG, Padrid PA, Szot GL, et al. Immunosuppressive effects of human CTLA4Ig in a non-human primate model of allogeneic pancreatic islet transplantation. J Immunol 1997;159:5187–91.

79. Vincenti F, Charpentier B, Vanrenterghem Y, et al. A phase III study of belatacept-based immunosuppression regimens versus cyclosporine in renal transplant recipients (BENEFIT study). Am J Transplant 2010;10:535–46.

80. Vincenti F, Larsen CP, Alberu J, et al. Three-year outcomes from BENEFIT, a randomized, active-controlled, parallel-group study in adult kidney transplant recipients. Am J Transplant 2012;12:210–7.

81. Badell IR, La Muraglia GM 2nd, Liu D, et al. Selective CD28 blockade results in superior inhibition of donor-specific T follicular helper cell and antibody responses relative to CTLA4-Ig. Am J Transplant 2018;18:89–101.

82. Leibler C, Thiolat A, Henique C, et al. Control of humoral response in renal transplantation by belatacept depends on a direct effect on B cells and impaired T follicular helper-B cell crosstalk. J Am Soc Nephrol 2018;29:1049–62.

83. Lin H, Rathmell JC, Gray GS, et al. Cytotoxic T lymphocyte antigen 4 (CTLA4) blockade accelerates the acute rejection of cardiac allografts in CD28-deficient mice: CTLA4 can function independently of CD28. J Exp Med 1998; 188:199–204.

84. Krummey SM, Floyd TL, Liu D, et al. Candida-elicited murine Th17 cells express high Ctla-4 compared with Th1 cells and are resistant to costimulation blockade. J Immunol 2014;192:2495–504.

85. Ying H, Yang L, Qiao G, et al. Cutting edge: CTLA-4-B7 interaction suppresses Th17 cell differentiation. J Immunol 2010;185:1375–8.

86. Riella LV, Liu T, Yang J, et al. Deleterious effect of CTLA4-Ig on a Treg-dependent transplant model. Am J Transplant 2012;12:846–55.

87. Levitsky J, Miller J, Huang X, et al. Inhibitory effects of belatacept on allospecific regulatory T-cell generation in humans. Transplantation 2013;96:689–96.

88. Yamada Y, Boskovic S, Aoyama A, et al. Overcoming memory T-cell responses for induction of delayed tolerance in nonhuman primates. Am J Transplant 2012; 12:330–40.

89. Hotta K, Oura T, Dehnadi A, et al. Long-term nonhuman primate renal allograft survival without ongoing immunosuppression in recipients of delayed donor bone marrow transplantation. Transplantation 2018;102:e128–36.

90. Mou D, Espinosa J, Lo DJ, et al. CD28 negative T cells: is their loss our gain? Am J Transplant 2014;14:2460–6.

91. Durrbach A, Pestana JM, Pearson T, et al. A phase III study of belatacept versus cyclosporine in kidney transplants from extended criteria donors (BENEFIT-EXT study). Am J Transplant 2010;10:547–57.

92. Xu H, Perez SD, Cheeseman J, et al. The allo- and viral-specific immunosuppressive effect of belatacept, but not tacrolimus, attenuates with progressive T cell maturation. Am J Transplant 2014;14:319–32.

93. Espinosa J, Herr F, Tharp G, et al. CD57(+) CD4 T cells underlie belatacept-resistant allograft rejection. Am J Transplant 2016;16:1102–12.

94. Lo DJ, Weaver TA, Stempora L, et al. Selective targeting of human alloresponsive CD8+ effector memory T cells based on CD2 expression. Am J Transplant 2011;11:22–33.

95. Strioga M, Pasukoniene V, Characiejus D. CD8+ CD28- and CD8+ CD57+ T cells and their role in health and disease. Immunology 2011;134:17–32.

96. Trzonkowski P, Zilvetti M, Chapman S, et al. Homeostatic repopulation by CD28-CD8+ T cells in alemtuzumab-depleted kidney transplant recipients treated with reduced immunosuppression. Am J Transplant 2008;8:338–47.

97. Lin YX, Yan LN, Li B, et al. A significant expansion of CD8+ CD28- T-suppressor cells in adult-to-adult living donor liver transplant recipients. Transplant Proc 2009;41:4229–31.

98. Colovai AI, Mirza M, Vlad G, et al. Regulatory CD8+CD28- T cells in heart transplant recipients. Hum Immunol 2003;64:31–7.

99. Suntharalingam G, Perry MR, Ward S. Cytokine storm in a phase 1 trial of the anti-CD28 monoclonal antibody TGN1412. N Engl J Med 2006;355:1018–28.

100. Liu D, Krummey SM, Badell IR, et al. 2B4 (CD244) induced by selective CD28 blockade functionally regulates allograft-specific CD8+ T cell responses. J Exp Med 2014;211:297–311.

101. Liu D, Suchard SJ, Nadler SG, et al. Inhibition of donor-reactive CD8+ T cell responses by selective CD28 blockade is independent of reduced ICOS expression. PLoS One 2015;10:e0130490.

102. Poirier N, Azimzadeh AM, Zhang T, et al. Inducing CTLA-4-dependent immune regulation by selective CD28 blockade promotes regulatory T cells in organ transplantation. Sci Transl Med 2010;2:17ra10.

103. Shi R, Honczarenko M, Zhang S, et al. Pharmacokinetic, pharmacodynamic, and safety profile of a novel Anti-CD28 domain antibody antagonist in healthy subjects. J Clin Pharmacol 2017;57:161–72.

104. Poirier N, Dilek N, Mary C, et al. FR104, an antagonist anti-CD28 monovalent fab' antibody, prevents alloimmunization and allows calcineurin inhibitor minimization in nonhuman primate renal allograft. Am J Transplant 2015;15:88–100.

105. Hippen KL, Watkins B, Tkachev V, et al. Preclinical testing of antihuman CD28 Fab' antibody in a novel nonhuman primate small animal rodent model of xenogenic graft-versus-host disease. Transplantation 2016;100:2630–9.

106. Poirier N, Blancho G, Hiance M, et al. First-in-human study in healthy subjects with FR104, a pegylated monoclonal antibody fragment antagonist of CD28. J Immunol 2016;197:4593–602.

107. Vogel LA, Noelle RJ. CD40 and its crucial role as a member of the TNFR family. Semin Immunol 1998;10:435–42.

108. Torres RM, Clark EA. Differential increase of an alternatively polyadenylated mRNA species of murine CD40 upon B lymphocyte activation. J Immunol 1992;148:620–6.

109. Armitage RJ, Fanslow WC, Strockbine L, et al. Molecular and biological characterization of a murine ligand for CD40. Nature 1992;357:80–2.

110. Kean LS, Turka LA, Blazar BR. Advances in targeting co-inhibitory and co-stimulatory pathways in transplantation settings: the Yin to the Yang of cancer immunotherapy. Immunol Rev 2017;276:192–212.

111. Pinelli DF, Ford ML. Novel insights into anti-CD40/CD154 immunotherapy in transplant tolerance. Immunotherapy 2015;7:399–410.

112. Liu D, Ferrer IR, Konomos M, et al. Inhibition of CD8+ T cell-derived CD40 signals is necessary but not sufficient for Foxp3+ induced regulatory T cell generation in vivo. J Immunol 2013;191:1957–64.

113. Ochando JC, Homma C, Yang Y, et al. Alloantigen-presenting plasmacytoid dendritic cells mediate tolerance to vascularized grafts. Nat Immunol 2006;7:652–62.

114. Hancock WW, Sayegh MH, Zheng XG, et al. Costimulatory function and expression of CD40 ligand, CD80, and CD86 in vascularized murine cardiac allograft rejection. Proc Natl Acad Sci U S A 1996;93:13967–72.

115. Pinelli DF, Wagener ME, Liu D, et al. An anti-CD154 domain antibody prolongs graft survival and induces Foxp3(+) iTreg in the absence and presence of CTLA-4 Ig. Am J Transplant 2013;13:3021–30.
116. Kirk AD, Burkly LC, Batty DS, et al. Treatment with humanized monoclonal antibody against CD154 prevents acute renal allograft rejection in nonhuman primates. Nat Med 1999;5:686–93.
117. Chen J, Yin H, Xu J, et al. Reversing endogenous alloreactive B cell GC responses with anti-CD154 or CTLA-4Ig. Am J Transplant 2013;13:2280–92.
118. Kim EJ, Kwun J, Gibby AC, et al. Costimulation blockade alters germinal center responses and prevents antibody-mediated rejection. Am J Transplant 2014;14: 59–69.
119. Ferrer IR, Wagener ME, Song M, et al. Antigen-specific induced Foxp3+ regulatory T cells are generated following CD40/CD154 blockade. Proc Natl Acad Sci U S A 2011;108:20701–6.
120. Zhu P, Chen YF, Chen XP, et al. Mechanisms of survival prolongation of murine cardiac allografts using the treatment of CTLA4-Ig and MR1. Transplant Proc 2008;40:1618–24.
121. Larsen CP, Elwood ET, Alexander DZ, et al. Long-term acceptance of skin and cardiac allografts after blocking CD40 and CD28 pathways. Nature 1996;381: 434–8.
122. Kawai T, Andrews D, Colvin RB, et al. Thromboembolic complications after treatment with monoclonal antibody against CD40 ligand. Nat Med 2000;6:114.
123. Koyama I, Kawai T, Andrews D, et al. Thrombophilia associated with anti-CD154 monoclonal antibody treatment and its prophylaxis in nonhuman primates. Transplantation 2004;77:460–2.
124. Henn V, Slupsky JR, Grafe M, et al. CD40 ligand on activated platelets triggers an inflammatory reaction of endothelial cells. Nature 1998;391:591–4.
125. Charafeddine AH, Kim EJ, Maynard DM, et al. Platelet-derived CD154: ultrastructural localization and clinical correlation in organ transplantation. Am J Transplant 2012;12:3143–51.
126. Vincenti F. What's in the pipeline? New immunosuppressive drugs in transplantation. Am J Transplant 2002;2:898–903.
127. Okimura K, Maeta K, Kobayashi N, et al. Characterization of ASKP1240, a fully human antibody targeting human CD40 with potent immunosuppressive effects. Am J Transplant 2014;14:1290–9.
128. Oura T, Yamashita K, Suzuki T, et al. Long-term hepatic allograft acceptance based on CD40 blockade by ASKP1240 in nonhuman primates. Am J Transplant 2012;12:1740–54.
129. Watanabe M, Yamashita K, Suzuki T, et al. ASKP1240, a fully human anti-CD40 monoclonal antibody, prolongs pancreatic islet allograft survival in nonhuman primates. Am J Transplant 2013;13:1976–88.
130. Song L, Ma A, Dun H, et al. Effects of ASKP1240 combined with tacrolimus or mycophenolate mofetil on renal allograft survival in Cynomolgus monkeys. Transplantation 2014;98:267–76.
131. Vincenti F, Yang H, Klintmalm G, et al. Clinical Outcomes in a Phase 1b, Randomized, Double-Blind, Parallel Group, Placebo-Controlled, Single-Dose Study of ASKP1240 in De Novo Kidney Transplantation. American Transplant Congress May 18–22, 2013 in Seattle, Washington. 2013.
132. Harland R, Klintmalm G, Yang H, et al. ASKP1240 in De Novo kidney transplant recipients. American Transplant Congress May 2–6, 2015 in Philadelphia, Pennsylvania. 2015.

133. Anil Kumar MS, Papp K, Tainaka R, et al. Randomized, controlled study of ble-selumab (ASKP1240) pharmacokinetics and safety in patients with moderate-to-severe plaque psoriasis. Biopharm Drug Dispos 2018;39:245–55.

134. O'Neill NA, Zhang T, Braileanu G, et al. Comparative evaluation of alphaCD40 (2C10R4) and alphaCD154 (5C8H1 and IDEC-131) in a nonhuman primate cardiac allotransplant model. Transplantation 2017;101:2038–47.

135. Aoyagi T, Yamashita K, Suzuki T, et al. A human anti-CD40 monoclonal antibody, 4D11, for kidney transplantation in cynomolgus monkeys: induction and mainte-nance therapy. Am J Transplant 2009;9:1732–41.

136. Cordoba F, Wieczorek G, Audet M, et al. A novel, blocking, Fc-silent anti-CD40 monoclonal antibody prolongs nonhuman primate renal allograft survival in the absence of B cell depletion. Am J Transplant 2015;15:2825–36.

137. Kitchens WH, Haridas D, Wagener ME. Integrin antagonists prevent costimula-tory blockade-resistant transplant rejection by CD8(+) memory T cells. Am J Transplant 2012;12:69–80.

138. Ford ML. T cell cosignaling molecules in transplantation. Immunity 2016;44: 1020–33.

139. Kitchens WH, Larsen CP, Ford ML. Integrin antagonists for transplant immuno-suppression: panacea or peril? Immunotherapy 2011;3:305–7.

140. Van Seventer GA, Shimizu Y, Horgan KJ, et al. The LFA-1 ligand ICAM-1 pro-vides an important costimulatory signal for T cell receptor-mediated activation of resting T cells. J Immunol 1990;144:4579–86.

141. Bachmann MF, McKall-Faienza K, Schmits R, et al. Distinct roles for LFA-1 and CD28 during activation of naive T cells: adhesion versus costimulation. Immunity 1997;7:549–57.

142. Isobe M, Suzuki J, Yamazaki S, et al. Acceptance of primary skin graft after treatment with anti-intercellular adhesion molecule-1 and anti-leukocyte func-tion-associated antigen-1 monoclonal antibodies in mice. Transplantation 1996;62:411–3.

143. Grazia TJ, Gill RG, Gelhaus HC Jr, et al. Perturbation of leukocyte function-associated antigen-1/intercellular adhesion molecule-1 results in differential out-comes in cardiac vs islet allograft survival. J Heart Lung Transplant 2005;24: 1410–4.

144. Arai K, Sunamura M, Wada Y, et al. Preventing effect of anti-ICAM-1 and anti-LFA-1 monoclonal antibodies on murine islet allograft rejection. Int J Pancreatol 1999;26:23–31.

145. Badell IR, Russell MC, Thompson PW, et al. LFA-1-specific therapy prolongs allograft survival in rhesus macaques. J Clin Invest 2010;120:4520–31.

146. Kitchens WH, Haridas D, Wagener ME, et al. Combined costimulatory and leukocyte functional antigen-1 blockade prevents transplant rejection mediated by heterologous immune memory alloresponses. Transplantation 2012;93: 997–1005.

147. Anderson DJ, Lo DJ, Leopardi F, et al. Anti-leukocyte function-associated anti-gen 1 therapy in a nonhuman primate renal transplant model of costimulation blockade-resistant rejection. Am J Transplant 2016;16:1456–64.

148. Samy KP, Anderson DJ, Lo DJ, et al. Selective targeting of high-affinity LFA-1 does not augment costimulation blockade in a nonhuman primate renal trans-plantation model. Am J Transplant 2017;17:1193–203.

149. Posselt AM, Bellin MD, Tavakol M, et al. Islet transplantation in type 1 diabetics using an immunosuppressive protocol based on the anti-LFA-1 antibody efalizu-mab. Am J Transplant 2010;10:1870–80.

150. Vincenti F, Mendez R, Pescovitz M, et al. A phase I/II randomized open-label multicenter trial of efalizumab, a humanized anti-CD11a, anti-LFA-1 in renal transplantation. Am J Transplant 2007;7:1770–7.

151. Schwab N, Ulzheimer JC, Fox RJ, et al. Fatal PML associated with efalizumab therapy: insights into integrin alphaLbeta2 in JC virus control. Neurology 2012;78:458–67 [discussion: 465].

152. Mages HW, Hutloff A, Heuck C, et al. Molecular cloning and characterization of murine ICOS and identification of B7h as ICOS ligand. Eur J Immunol 2000;30: 1040–7.

153. McAdam AJ, Chang TT, Lumelsky AE, et al. Mouse inducible costimulatory molecule (ICOS) expression is enhanced by CD28 costimulation and regulates differentiation of CD4+ T cells. J Immunol 2000;165:5035–40.

154. Yoshinaga SK, Whoriskey JS, Khare SD, et al. T-cell co-stimulation through B7RP-1 and ICOS. Nature 1999;402:827–32.

155. Haynes NM, Allen CD, Lesley R, et al. Role of CXCR5 and CCR7 in follicular Th cell positioning and appearance of a programmed cell death gene-1high germinal center-associated subpopulation. J Immunol 2007;179:5099–108.

156. Fazilleau N, McHeyzer-Williams LJ, Rosen H, et al. The function of follicular helper T cells is regulated by the strength of T cell antigen receptor binding. Nat Immunol 2009;10:375–84.

157. Sacquin A, Gador M, Fazilleau N. The strength of BCR signaling shapes terminal development of follicular helper T cells in mice. Eur J Immunol 2017;47: 1295–304.

158. Nanji SA, Hancock WW, Anderson CC, et al. Multiple combination therapies involving blockade of ICOS/B7RP-1 costimulation facilitate long-term islet allograft survival. Am J Transplant 2004;4:526–36.

159. Ozkaynak E, Gao W, Shemmeri N, et al. Importance of ICOS-B7RP-1 costimulation in acute and chronic allograft rejection. Nat Immunol 2001;2:591–6.

160. Nanji SA, Hancock WW, Anderson CC, et al. Combination therapy with anti-ICOS and cyclosporine enhances cardiac but not islet allograft survival. Transplant Proc 2003;35:2477–8.

161. Lo DJ, Anderson DJ, Song M, et al. A pilot trial targeting the ICOS-ICOS-L pathway in nonhuman primate kidney transplantation. Am J Transplant 2015; 15:984–92.

162. Sullivan BA, Tsuji W, Kivitz A, et al. Inducible T-cell co-stimulator ligand (ICOSL) blockade leads to selective inhibition of anti-KLH IgG responses in subjects with systemic lupus erythematosus. Lupus Sci Med 2016;3:e000146.

163. Gramaglia I, Weinberg AD, Lemon M, et al. Ox-40 ligand: a potent costimulatory molecule for sustaining primary CD4 T cell responses. J Immunol 1998;161: 6510–7.

164. Godfrey WR, Fagnoni FF, Harara MA, et al. Identification of a human OX-40 ligand, a costimulator of CD4+ T cells with homology to tumor necrosis factor. J Exp Med 1994;180:757–62.

165. Imura A, Hori T, Imada K, et al. The human OX40/gp34 system directly mediates adhesion of activated T cells to vascular endothelial cells. J Exp Med 1996;183: 2185–95.

166. Pippig SD, Pena-Rossi C, Long J, et al. Robust B cell immunity but impaired T cell proliferation in the absence of CD134 (OX40). J Immunol 1999;163: 6520–9.

167. Rogers PR, Song J, Gramaglia I, et al. OX40 promotes Bcl-xL and Bcl-2 expression and is essential for long-term survival of CD4 T cells. Immunity 2001;15: 445–55.
168. Zhang X, Xiao X, Lan P, et al. OX40 costimulation inhibits Foxp3 expression and Treg induction via BATF3-dependent and independent mechanisms. Cell Rep 2018;24:607–18.
169. Xiao X, Kroemer A, Gao W, et al. OX40/OX40L costimulation affects induction of Foxp3+ regulatory T cells in part by expanding memory T cells in vivo. J Immunol 2008;181:3193–201.
170. Vu MD, Xiao X, Gao W, et al. OX40 costimulation turns off Foxp3+ tregs. Blood 2007;110:2501–10.
171. Demirci G, Amanullah F, Kewalaramani R, et al. Critical role of OX40 in CD28 and CD154-independent rejection. J Immunol 2004;172:1691–8.
172. Kinnear G, Wood KJ, Marshall D, et al. Anti-OX40 prevents effector T-cell accumulation and CD8+ T-cell mediated skin allograft rejection. Transplantation 2010;90:1265–71.
173. Tsukada N, Akiba H, Kobata T, et al. Blockade of CD134 (OX40)-CD134L interaction ameliorates lethal acute graft-versus-host disease in a murine model of allogeneic bone marrow transplantation. Blood 2000;95:2434–9.
174. Kinnear G, Wood KJ, Fallah-Arani F, et al. A diametric role for OX40 in the response of effector/memory CD4+ T cells and regulatory T cells to alloantigen. J Immunol 2013;191:1465–75.

Genetic Polymorphism in Cytokines and Costimulatory Molecules in Stem Cell and Solid Organ Transplantation

Peter T. Jindra, PhD, D(ABHI)*, Matthew F. Cusick, PhD, D(ABHI)

KEYWORDS

- Single nucleotide polymorphisms • Transplantation • Co-stimulation • Cytokines
- Immune response • Rejection • Validation

KEY POINTS

- Single nucleotide polymorphisms in cytokines and costimulatory molecules have been shown to effect transplant outcomes.
- Interpretation of single nucleotide polymorphism findings has been difficult due to small population sizes and various approaches in their study design.
- There are a variety of bioinfomatic tools and functional assays available to provide meaningful SNP discovery.
- Most genome-wide association studies fail to validate candidate gene single nucleotide polymorphism associations with allo-human cell transplant outcomes.
- The genetic effects observed outside of the HLA region are more appropriate to understanding biological pathways rather than predicting clinical outcome.

INTRODUCTION

Transplantation triggers the immune system to mount a response to the allograft. In solid organ transplantation, the activated immune system through direct, semidirect, or indirect stimulation makes management with immunosuppression obligatory. However in hematopoietic stem cell transplantation (HSCT), the engrafted immune system must be allowed to function optimally to protect the recipient while not damaging the recipient. In an unrelated transplant, there are between 4 and 10 million gene variants

Disclosure Statement: The authors have nothing to disclose.
Department of Surgery, BCM Immune Evaluation Laboratory, One Baylor Plaza, MS: BCM504, Houston, TX 77030, USA
* Corresponding author.
E-mail address: Peter.Jindra@bcm.edu

between the donor and the recipient.[1] A fine balance must therefore be achieved to control the activation of the immune system.

T-cell activation involves an initial antigen recognition step in which a major histocompatibility complex (MHC) molecule presents a peptide antigen to a T-cell receptor. In addition, T-cell activation requires a second signal referred to as costimulation. The second signal is termed a positive costimulatory signal when 1, or more, T-cell surface receptors bind to certain ligands[2–5] and cause activation of T cells. These T-cell surface receptors and costimulatory molecules play a key role in determining the outcome of immune responses.[6–8] T cells may also receive negative costimulatory signals and T cells receiving this negative signal may fail to expand, be anergized, die by apoptosis, or be induced to become regulatory T cells.[9,10] An immune response additionally requires stimulation by cytokines for immune cells to perform various functions (referred to as signal 3).

On a human population level, the immune response varies among individuals, in that some individuals are strong responders whereas others respond poorly to non-self (weak responders). These phenotypic differences have a genetic component that drives the diversity in immune function. Although modern immunosuppression has decreased the incidence of acute rejection, chronic rejection and graft loss remain problematic.[11] Polymorphisms within HLA genes have been extensively studied in the context of transplantation[12] and clearly demonstrate the need to match donors and recipients. There has been a focus on expanding polymorphism studies to additional checkpoints in the immune response by including immune regulatory costimulatory molecules and cytokines.

There is a renewed interest in the interplay between positive and negative costimulatory signals as a key determinant of T-cell–mediated immune response in both solid organ transplantation and HSCT. Polymorphisms in the positive costimulatory molecule genes of B7 supergene family, including CD28/B7, inducible costimulator (ICOS or CD278), and the genes of the tumor necrosis factor (TNF) receptor (TNFR) family, including the OX40-OX40 L pathway genes, have been assessed for their clinical significance and mechanism of action in transplantation. Negative costimulatory molecules, in contrast, decrease T-cell proliferation and cytokine production, promote T-cell anergy or apoptosis, and induce the activity of regulatory T cells.[13] Targeting negative costimulatory molecules has been significantly associated with the attenuation of T-cell–mediated acute graft versus host disease (aGVHD).[14,15]

GENE VARIANTS IN COMMON POSITIVE COSTIMULATORY MOLECULES ASSOCIATED WITH TRANSPLANTATION OUTCOMES
CD28

The CD28 receptor is expressed on human CD4$^+$ T cells (80%) and CD8$^+$ T cells (50%) and its expression decreases with age.[16] It is required for the full activation of T cells. It functions to amply the T-cell receptor signal as well as activate unique signal transduction pathways leading to changes in T-cell gene expression programming. It is part of an increasingly complex combination of receptor–ligand interactions where a single receptor can bind multiple ligands (eg, B7-1 [CD80] and B7-2 [CD86]), each of which can bind multiple receptors such as ICOS and cytotoxic T-lymphocyte–associated protein 4 (CTLA-4). An analysis of the CD28 gene did not reveal any nonsynoymous or synonymous substitutions in the 4 exons that make up the coding region, suggesting low mutation rate and lack of coding single nucleotide polymorphisms (SNPs).[17] One of the first studies to determine the impact of CD28 gene polymorphism found no association of the polymorphism with liver transplant outcomes.[18] CD28

SNP rs3116496 T/C, located in the third intron, has been assessed in multiple studies and found to be associated with severe grade GVHD and acute rejection in kidney, but not liver, transplant recipients.[19,20] Additional small population studies of specific ethnic groups also found no association with between CD28 and rejection.[21] Interestingly, the haplotype TTGCACGC (a haplotype is a collection of mutually linked SNPs transmitted together), which comprises 8 SNPs from genes CD28, CTLA-4, ICOS and programmed cell death 1 (PD-1), respectively, all of which are located on chromosome 2, was found to be significantly higher in occurrence in cases of acute rejection.[21] Most transplantation studies lack the sample size for an immune haplotype analysis such as this. The study shows that, when specific SNPs are found to not be significant, they may need to be tested in the context of a complete genetic profile.

Inducible Costimulator

CD28, CTLA-4, and ICOS are located near each other on chromosome 2. ICOS is a costimulatory molecule that can bind to receptors other than CD80/CD86 on B cells and stimulate T cells during the late phase of T-cell activation. ICOS binds to its ligand B7H2. It serves also as a ligand for CD28 and CTLA-4.[22] ICOS stimulation can activate B-cell development and antibody production; however, blockade of the ICOS signaling pathway prolongs kidney graft survival in murine models.[22,23] When CD4$^+$ T cells were stimulated with plate-bound anti-CD3 and CD80, individuals having the CC genotype in SNP rs10932037 + 1624 C/T were found to have significantly more ICOS messenger RNA transcripts, compared with individuals with the CT genotype: no TT individuals were enrolled in this study.[24] This difference, which was observed at 1 and 3 hours, diminished after 6 hours, highlighting the transient nature of the response. SNP rs10932029 + 173 T/C affected the amount of messenger RNA of the competing CTLA-4 as well. In this case, the TT genotype individuals had increased full-length CTLA-4 messenger RNA transcripts at greater than 6 hours compared with those having the CT genotype.[24] In HSCT, this combination translated into worse overall survival.[25] In a cohort of 678 Finnish subjects receiving kidney transplants between 1999 and 2003, SNP rs10932037 + 1624 C/C was associated with a higher graft survival rate compared with TC or TT genotypes over a 7-year period. However, when corrected for multiple comparisons, no significant associations could be observed between rs10932037 and graft rejection.

Tumor Necrosis Factor Ligand Superfamily Member 4

The TNF ligand superfamily member 4 (TNFSF4, OX40 L)–TNF receptor superfamily member 4 (TNFRSF4, OX40) pathway represents one of the key positive costimulatory signals required for cell activation. TNFRSF4 is present on both activated CD4$^+$ and CD8$^+$ T cells, and its cognate ligand, TNFSF4, is expressed on dendritic cells, B cells, and activated endothelial cells.[26] Signaling through the TNFSF4–TNFRSF4 pathway facilitates T helper (Th) type 2 differentiation, enhances effector CD8$^+$ T-cell memory commitment, and promotes cytokine production.[27,28]

Gene polymorphisms in *TNFSF4* have been associated with HSCT and solid organ transplantation. These studies postulate that TNFSF4 is a major player in the T cell–antigen presenting cell interaction, leading to the activation of immune cells and production of proinflammatory cytokines and chemokines and, thereby, to active disease. Our dataset of 2570 donor–recipient pairs collected from 2 independent cohorts represents one of the largest SNP studies focused on TNFSF4 that provides information on each of clonal expansion of antigen-specific T cells, expansion of regulatory T cells, and generation of T-cell memory.[26,29] The CC genotype of TNFSF4 SNP rs10912564 was found to be associated with a higher likelihood of overall survival with less treatment-related mortality in our discovery cohort transplant patients between 1990 and 2002. This association lost significance when a more recent cohort from 2003 to 2007 having older patients, as well as when the DISCOVeRY-BMT (Determining the Influence of Susceptibility Conveying Variants Related to One Year mortality after Unrelated Donor Allogeneic Blood or Marrow Transplant) cohort 2000 to 2011[30] was considered. The obscuring of the effect of our SNP association by the ever-evolving field of clinical bone marrow transplantation sheds light on the challenge faced by genetic association studies in this field and virtually for all other fields for which therapies and standards of practice change over time.

A flow chart visualizing the essential key points involved in our SNP discovery is shown in **Fig. 1**. It is critical to determine the functional capacity of an SNP. SNPs are known to interact in gene promoter regions. However, noncoding intronic sequences also may contain functional SNPs that can enhance the transcription of genes, leading to disease associations.[31,32] Regulatory elements located in the first intron have been identified as sites of transcriptional regulation.[33] For example, assisted by the bioinformatics tool, F-SNP, a c-Myb binding site was identified as a possible functionally relevant site in the intron of *TNFSF4* gene with the major allele C nucleotide predicted to be a critical base required for c-Myb binding.[34,35] Additional web-based databases—RegulomeDB and HaploReg—allow users to retrieve information on DNA features and regulatory elements specific to the SNP of interest.[36,37]

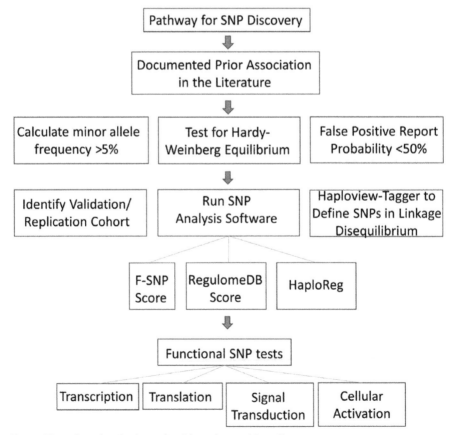

Fig. 1. Flow chart for single nucleotide polymorphism discovery.

Using a DNA protein interaction enzyme-linked immunosorbent assay, c-Myb was found to bind a 30 oligomer sequence of TNFSF4 containing the rs10912564 C allele. There was less binding when the C was substituted with a T. Computation algorithms in combination with functional assays form the basis of confirming functional relevance of a site. Even if associations between SNPs and complex diseases change owing to a variety of factors, information gained from functional studies at single polymorphic sites helps to expand the greater knowledge base of the human genome.

CD86

CD86 is constitutively expressed on antigen presenting cell and acts as a ligand in T-cell activation.[38] Karabon and colleagues[38] were the first to investigate the role of CD86 gene polymorphisms in HSCT outcomes in 295 patients receiving either related or unrelated HSCT. They selected 3 SNPs—rs1129055, rs9831894, and rs2715267—which were not in linkage association. HSCT outcomes could be analyzed individually or as a haplotype. Of note, SNP rs1129055 G/A at position +1057 is a genetic variant within exon 8 leading to an alanine to threonine substitution in the cytoplasmic tail, which is postulated to have potential phosphorylation activity, although this has not been confirmed. An intriguing feature about this work was the concept of gene-to-gene SNP interactions, specifically, gene-to-gene interaction between a receptor and a ligand. It was found that having a CD86 SNP rs1129055 GG genotype in donors and a CTLA-4 SNP CT60 GG genotype in recipients increased the risk of aGVHD by 2.73 times. The risk was upwards of 3-fold if the recipient had a CT60A+ allele. Increased activation of CD86 combined with increased soluble CTLA-4, which interferes with negative costimulation, favors T-cell activation. A synergy of functional SNPs can lead to robust alloimmune recognition. Gene-to-gene interaction can result from both SNPs being in either the recipient or the donor as a haplotype, or from a combination where 1 gene polymorphism is on the recipient and the other on the donor. Most studies would require greater sample sizes to generate enough power when making these multiple comparisons. In various studies of solid organ transplantation, alanine at the rs1129055 position has been shown to protect against acute rejection.[39,40] Specifically in liver transplantation, the rs1129055 A allele led to a decreased risk of acute rejection in 205 liver transplant recipients.[39] Among kidney transplant recipients, 168 were sequenced for SNP rs1129055,[40] and a significant association was found in a subpopulation of anti-HLA–positive recipients, where the AA genotype was expressed in 31.3% of the nonacute rejection cases and in 0% of the cases with acute rejection.[39] Of note, both reports were based on small sample populations and did not have validation cohorts or mechanism of action studies. A metaanalysis additionally confirmed a protective role in recipients of either the AA or the A allele for SNP rs1129055.[19]

GENE VARIANTS IN COMMON NEGATIVE COSTIMULATORY MOLECULES ASSOCIATED WITH TRANSPLANTATION OUTCOMES
Cytotoxic T-Lymphocyte–Associated Protein-4

CTLA, which is highly homologous to CD28, competes for binding to CD80/CD86 with higher affinity than CD28, thereby generating an inhibitory signal in T-cell activation.[41] SNPs in costimulatory molecules can also affect the way immunosuppression functions. Two of the SNPs in the CTLA4 gene, CT60A>G (rs3087243) in the 3'UTR and 49A>G (rs231775) in the first exon, have been associated with autoimmune diseases through modification to the production of the soluble form of CTLA4 or through a decrease in the amount of cell surface CTLA4, respectively.[42] Both polymorphisms have also been associated with differences in aGVHD incidence and also with overall survival after allogeneic stem cell transplantation.[43-45] Perez-Garcia and colleagues[43] were the first to report that a donor's *CTLA-4* SNP genotype CT60AA lead to the recipient developing aGVHD more frequently despite less relapse and higher overall survival compared with donors with a G allele (AG/GG). There was a dose-dependent increase in the level of soluble CTLA-4 transcript lacking exon 3 in individuals expressing the CT60 A allele. This soluble form competes with the full-length CTLA-4 isoform, which may disrupt the binding of full-length CTLA-4 to B7 ligands, thus inhibiting negative costimulation signals. More recent follow-up studies by Hossain failed to observe this association. Perez-Garcia and colleagues[46] used in vitro T-cell stimulation and CTLA-4 expression assays to generate a deeper understanding of CTLA SNP function. Full-length CTLA-4 is the predominant form produced, reaching maximal expression 72 hours after stimulation, whereas soluble CTLA-4, which reaches maximal expression 24 hours after stimulation, with the AA genotype having the highest level. The presence of the T allele at -1722T and -318T resulted in a synergistic increase in CTLA-4 transcription in gene promoter assays. Although the relevant transcription factors remain to be identified, nuclear factor of activated T cells may be involved, because it has been shown to be involved in downstream CTLA-4 signaling.[46]

Programmed Death-1/Programmed Death Ligand-1

The negative costimulatory PD-1–PD-L1 pathway plays a central role in suppressing the proliferation of autoreactive T cells and subsequent halting of the progression of autoimmune diabetes in NOD mice, suggesting a critical role for this pathway in inducing tolerance.[47-50] Various investigations have found that administration of anti–PD-L1 antibody[13,51,52] or blockade of PD-1 itself[52] resulted in an increased incidence of aGVHD by promoting the proliferation of alloreactive $CD4^+$ and $CD8^+$ T cells in mouse models. These studies provide strong evidence for the importance of the PD-1/PD-L1 system in aGVHD.

Within the transplant literature, gene polymorphisms have been shown also in the negative costimulatory molecule PD-1. Santos and colleagues[53] reported that homozygosity of PD-1.1 SNP (rs36084323 GG) in the promoter and the PD-1.3 SNP (rs11568821AA) in intron 4 were associated with an increased risk of grades II to IV GVHD, with a stronger association when combined as a haplotype (rs36084323 G + rs11568821 A). This association seems to be focused in the Caucasian population given that it is extremely rare in Asian and African populations. In a small Iranian population of 72 recipients, only SNP PD-1.9 (rs2227982 C/T) located in exon 5 showed a possible association.[21] Neither study provided mechanistic data to support SNP association with the disease.

GENE VARIANTS IN COMMON CYTOKINES ASSOCIATED WITH TRANSPLANTATION OUTCOMES
Transforming Growth Factor-β1

The multifunctional cytokine, transforming growth factor β1 (TGF-β1), has been implicated in models of transplantation because of the many roles it plays in wound healing, leading to scarring and fibrosis.[54] *TGFB1*, with 7 exons and 6 introns, is mapped to chromosome 19q13.1–13.3, and the expression of *TGFB1* to produce TGF-β1 is related to SNPs of the gene. *TGFB1* contains 2 SNPs within exon 1, +869 C/T at codon 10 (coding(c).29C>T, rs1800470) and +915 G/C at codon 25 (c.74G>C, rs1800471) that contribute to variation in TGF-β1 production both in vitro and in serum.[55] In cardiac transplantation, the TGF-β1 polymorphism, +915 C/G, was validated in 2 studies showing that donor GG genotype leads to a higher expression of

TGF-β1, leading to coronary vasculopathy (CV). C allele carriers, associated with low/intermediate production of this cytokine, are less susceptible to CV development, whereas the presence of the GG genotype (high TGF-β1 production) is a significant risk factor for CV development (hazard ratio, 3.01; P = .042).[56] The mean time of CV development was found to be 1240.5 days in GG homozygotes in comparison with 2266.5 days in C allele carriers. The second study examined 147 patients and 134 transplant donors with the focus on SNPs at positions +915 and +869 of the TGF-β1 gene.[57] The results of the previous work were confirmed with regard to GG homozygous donors (but not recipients) with TGF-β1 polymorphism at position +915 G/C. This effect seems to be related to chronic disease. Other investigations studying +915 SNP at acute timepoints, that is, 12 months, did not see an association[58,59]; however, +869 SNP was strongly associated.

Overall, a metaanalysis of 8 studies was performed by Liu and colleagues[60] on 1038 renal transplant recipients. Neither polymorphism +915 nor +869 alone was found to be significant as a stand-alone SNP. However, as a haplotype, T/T G/G and T/C G/G genotypes, respectively, were associated with higher production of TGF-β1, and increased susceptibility to coronary artery disease after kidney transplantation as reported by Nikolova and colleagues.[61] In contrast, a study of 105 pediatric kidney recipients between 1983 and 1999 found no correlation between intrarenal TGF-β1 expression and the +915 and +869 genotypes. TGF-β1 was observed in control healthy kidneys.[62] They observed a predicted an increase in TGF-β1 only for +869 T/C and attributed it to the basal state of cytokine production and to a gene–environment interaction related to chronic allograft dysfunction, leading to loss of significance.[62] In the area of HSCT, a study that included 245 patient/donor pairs analyzed TGF-β1 SNPs at positions +29 and +74 in myeloablative sibling HSCT. The +29 CC recipients had a significant increase in nonrelapse mortality owing to GVHD and sinusoidal obstruction syndrome, whereas recipients with donors carrying the +29 TT genotype had increased relapse rate and decreased overall survival.[63]

Tumor Necrosis Factor-α

TNF-α is a proinflammatory cytokine produced mainly by monocytes/macrophages at sites of inflammation.[64] Once released, TNF-α causes endothelial cell activation and a variety of cellular changes, including heightened MHC and adhesion molecule expression, which facilitates recruitment and activation of leukocytes to an allograft. The TNF-α gene is located in the HLA class III region. A gene variant of TNF-alpha, −308 A/G, with alteration in the promoter region has been characterized. The presence of the A allele is associated with increased transcriptional activity and TNF-α production. Its concentration is increased in solid organ allografts undergoing acute rejection. Some studies have found an association between the −308A allele and graft rejection, although others have not.[65–67] This inconclusiveness may be attributed to sample selection over different periods of time, the standard of clinical care for induction, and posttransplant immunosuppression changes over time. The study did not include hyperimmunized or retransplanted patients. The study by Sanchez-Fructuoso and colleagues[68] analyzed the outcome in 439 kidney transplant patients from 2005 to 2012, 27% of whom had developed acute rejection. The study focused on first transplants with no preformed antibodies and patients were randomly separated into a discovery and validation cohort. In the discovery cohort, the −308 A allele was significantly associated with acute kidney graft rejection (GA/AA 35% vs GG 16%; P = .003) and confirmed in their validation cohort. The effect was strengthened in −308 A allele carriers not treated with thymoglobulin for induction. When considering immunosuppression strategies, patients with the high producer −308 A genotype may benefit from thymoglobulin induction to inhibit proinflammatory TNF-α release by macrophages that may drive a series of events leading to graft rejection.

Interferon-γ

Interferon (IFN)-γ +874 A/T is associated with an increased risk of cytomegalovirus infection among Hispanic renal transplant recipients.[69] Through functional enzyme-linked immunosorbent assay testing, the TT genotype recipients were found to have had high levels of IFN-γ, compared with the AA genotype recipients.[69] This SNP has not been associated with kidney rejection, yet the high expression TT genotype was associated with the development of the bronchiolitis obliterans syndrome in lung transplant recipients.[70]

Interleukin-1β

Within kidney transplant studies, no association was found between IL-1β −511 C/T and acute rejection.[71] Other studies looking at an additional SNP variant, +3954, also did not find a significant association.[72]

Interleukin-4

IL-4 is an essential polyfunctional cytokine that stimulates a variety of cell types including T cells, B cells, and mast cells. In B cells, IL-4 drives proliferation and class switching.[73] IL-4 has GATA3 and signal transducer and activator of transcription 5 binding sites in its second intron that are essential for priming T cells to become IL-4 producers.[73] IL-4 polymorphisms have been associated with the clinical course after heart transplantation. In a study published in 2002 by Bijlsma and colleagues,[74] the authors failed to find any relationships between the presence of the IL-4 -590 SNP in donors and occurrence of graft rejection.

Interleukin-6

IL-6 is a cytokine produced by activated cells of the vascular endothelium, monocytes, macrophages, T lymphocytes, natural killer cells, and mast cells.[75] Its special role in the development of ischemic heart disease stems from the fact that it participates in the acute phase response and is secreted by mast cells constituting atherosclerotic plaques (local effect). IL-6 −174 G/C SNP was suggested to be an important risk factor for CV. The average time until the first confirmation of CV was 2.8 years for CC homozygotes, 3.9 years for CG heterozygotes, and 5.3 years for GG homozygotes.[76] Kaplan-Meier analysis confirmed earlier CV development in CC homozygotes. In the fifth year, 100% had confirmed CV, whereas this rate for the GG group was approximately 60%. In lung transplantation, high-expression polymorphism −174 (GG or GC) significantly increased the risk and faster development of bronchiolitis obliterans syndrome compared with the low expression −174 (CC) polymorphism.[77]

Interleukin-10

IL-10 pleiotropic antiinflammatory cytokine are involved in inhibiting the production of proinflammatory cytokines by monocytes and macrophages via the downregulation of MHC class I and costimulatory molecule secretion. IL-10 can favor a Th2 immune response to decrease inflammatory mechanisms and cytokine release.[78] Lin and colleagues[79] have discussed the role of IL-10 and IL-10 receptor SNPs in GVHD in a cohort of 953 HLA-identical sibling donor–recipient pairs. They found that IL-10 592 A*, in combination with a G allele in the donor IL-10Rβ c238 G, was associated with a significantly lower risk of severe aGVHD. This finding highlights an interesting dynamic where the combination of donor and recipient genotypes in the cytokine and its receptor can have an influence on transplant outcome. The IL-10 592 A* effect may be greater given its complete linkage disequilibrium with the presence of a 5-SNP IL-10 promoter haplotype T-C-A-T-A (−3575T, −2763C, −1082A, −819T, and −592A). Any SNP within this promoter haplotype has the potential to be the causal variant of IL-10 gene regulation. A systematic review of these sites for function was not performed. Although the exact molecular mechanism remains to be elucidated, the true causal variant may involve these sites in the promoter region. Additional studies using multivariate analysis of IL-10 polymorphisms at positions −1082 G/A, −819 C/T, and −592 C/A in a small cohort of 74 allogeneic sibling HSCT donors and 93 recipients revealed that the GCC haplotype had a lower risk of aGVHD (P = .05).[80] However, this same association was not observed in other studies.[81] Furthermore, inconclusive results of IL-10 SNPs have been reviewed in HSCT and kidney transplantation.[82] The IL-10 SNPs at positions −1082 G/A, −819 C/T, and −592 C/A were also examined in heart transplant recipients.[83] The authors divided the study group (65 individuals) into the following haplotype subgroups: GCC, which is associated with high IL-10 production (high producer), and ATA, which is associated with low IL-10 production (low producer). Based on International Society of Heart and Lung Transplant rejection criteria, which include endomyocardial biopsy and histopathology findings to stage severity (0, 1 A/B, 2, 3 A/B, 4),[84] patient groups with stages 2 and 3 A/B with moderate and severe rejection, respectively, had a significantly lower percentage of high IL-10 producer GCC haplotype group than patients with mild rejection stage 1A respectively (28.6% vs 22.6% vs 80%; $P<.01$). The authors concluded that the genotype associated with high IL-10 production seems to be a significant protective factor against heart transplant rejection.[85] In lung transplantation, although no association was found between IL-10 −592 A/C and acute rejection, the −592 CC genotype in combination with −819 CC had a significantly decreased risk of infection.[70]

Interleukin-17

Th-17 cells are a subset of Th cells and are labeled as such based on their ability to produce and secrete IL-17, a proinflammatory cytokine.[86] Genetic variation in IL-17 promoter region has been functionally associated with aGVHD in unrelated bone marrow transplant, and the focus has been on SNP rs2275913 G/A at position −197 in the promoter region of the *IL-17* gene. This location has a binding motif for nuclear factor of activated T cells, which represents a possible mechanism for IL-17 cytokine gene expression regulation. *In vitro* studies stimulating peripheral blood mononuclear cells with anti-CD3/CD28 show a dose-dependent increase of IL-17 production in 197A allele individuals. The 197A allele had higher promoter activity and more affinity to the transcription factor nuclear factor of activated T cells when examining nuclear extracts compared with 197G.[87] Individuals with the 197A allele produce significantly more IL-17 than individuals with the 197G allele. This SNP highlights the important factors when considering SNP selection, including strong evidence of clinical involvement.

Interleukin-23

The IL-23 receptor (IL-23R) is a type I cytokine receptor formed as a heterodimer with IL-12 receptor beta1 and an IL-12 receptor beta2–related molecule.[86] The *IL23R* gene is mapped to chromosome 1p31. IL-23R functions to differentiate the Th cell response. It associates constitutively with Janus kinase 2 (JAK2) and binds signal transducer and activator of transcription 3 in a ligand-dependent manner. IL-23 is a potent proinflammatory cytokine involved in chronic autoimmune responses and induces a Th1 response in T cells, thereby releasing IFN-γ, activating proliferation, and generating Th17 cells. The IL-23 uncommon coding variant 1142G>A rs11209026 is a nonsynonymous SNP and has been shown to determine susceptibility in inflammatory bowel disease.[88] It confers strong protection against Crohn's disease.[89,90] In a study by Elmaagacli and colleagues[91] examining 221 matched sibling donor and 186 matched unrelated donor patients, donors expressing the G polymorphism were found to have a decreased risk of aGVHD in both cohorts, the polymorphism conferring a strong protection against the occurrence of severe aGVHD.

ETHNIC/RACIAL EFFECT ON COSTIMULATORY AND CYTOKINE SINGLE NUCLEOTIDE POLYMORPHISMS

Most genetic polymorphism studies have used study samples from European ancestry in an attempt to minimize the amount of variability. This method narrows the potential analysis of SNPs. Girnita and colleagues[92] performed a multicenter study that included Caucasian, African American, and Hispanic populations. Note that the minor allele frequency of SNPs has the potential to fluctuate when different ethnic groups are genotyped. In their analysis, they found that African Americans have a genetic background that is proinflammatory with a lower regulatory responsiveness. African Americans exhibited a greater prevalence of genotypes associated with low expression of IFN-γ (SNP +874 T/A; 24% vs 45.7%, P<.001) and IL-10 (SNP ATA/ ATA; 33% vs 57.1%; $P = .052$). African Americans also exhibited an increased prevalence of the GG genotype associated with the production of higher levels of IL-6, compared with the genotype having the C allele at position -174 G/C (82.9% vs 38.1%; P<.001). The IL-6 (-174 G/C) allele frequency was found to vary greatly among racial groups. Additional population studies have shown that the -174 G/C IL-6 allele was more heterozygous than homozygous in Caucasians. The minor C allele was found to be lowest in frequency in African Americans followed by Hispanics, and highest in Caucasians, which display the most diversity.[93] In the studies of Japanese population this SNP was nonpolymorphic expressing only the G allele.[93]

GENOME-WIDE ASSOCIATION STUDIES IN TRANSPLANTATION COHORTS

Although costimulatory molecules and cytokines play a pivotal role in the activation of the immune system, they do not seems to be routinely identified in genome-wide association studies (GWAS) studies of transplantation. By and large, only in single candidate gene study approaches have these immune regulatory molecules been found to be significant. When the first large-scale GWAS, with 139 SNPs including several chemokines and cytokines, was performed using 2094 complete renal transplant pairs with a validation cohort of 5866, outside of HLA region, no strong donor or recipient genetic SNPs were found to be associated with long- or short-term allograft survival.[94] Many published studies have concentrated on immune-related genes under the assumption that the risk to the allograft is generated by genetic variation in the immune response. A potential reason for this lack of SNP influence in immune response genes could be due to the fact that all transplant recipients are on immunosuppressive regiments. These patients have depressed immune systems, which levels the playing field between the strong and the weak immune responders.[95] Interestingly, the most promising genetic factors found in the study were related to extracellular matrix and cell growth and motility, the latter processes being essential basic cellular functions and thus conserved. Costimulation and cytokine production being dependent on MHC–T-cell receptor interactions, which is different in every individual, too much noise is created in the system for any single SNP association to remain significant. Overall, the genetic effects outside of the HLA region are more appropriate to understand biological pathways rather than predicting clinical outcome.

The use of GWAS has provided a powerful platform to simultaneously analyze millions of SNPs in a transplant cohort with the goal of identifying causal genetic variants of allograft rejection or graft failure and of predicting outcome. Currently, there are insufficient numbers of transplant recipients to study these genetic signals. Overall, many studies investigating the correlation between specific SNPs and transplant outcomes have been inconclusive when follow-up studies were attempted to validate the initial finding.[96] Given the complex nature of the disease, gene–gene and gene–environment interactions make association approaches minimalistic. A multitude of repetitive factors could explain the inconsistent results including the study population, batch effects, experimental conditions, insufficient power owing to small sample size, publication bias, correction for multiple comparisons, and validation cohort. GWAS allows simultaneously study of all the potential candidate gene variants in 1 cohort.

To confirm multiple candidate SNPs in cytokines and costimulatory molecules previously documented to be associated with chronic GVHD, 3 large cohorts of GWAS with European ancestry were generated.[97] One such cohort is the Fred Hutchinson Cancer Research Center cohort, which includes 3918 donor–recipient pairs from 1990 to 2011. The other 2 cohorts are DISCOVeRY-BMT cohorts from the Center of International Blood and Marrow Transplant Research. Of these, cohort I includes 1656 recipients who received a first HLA-A, HLA-B, and HLA-C, DRB1, DQB1-matched unrelated human cell transplant for the treatment of acute lymphoblastic leukemia, acute myeloid leukemia, or myelodysplastic syndrome between 2000 and 2008. The cohort includes 1601 donor samples. Cohort II included 527 recipients who were selected by the same criteria as cohort I, but had human cell transplant between 2009 and 2011, plus 351 patients who received their HLA-A, -B, -C, -DRB1 match, but not DQB1 match. This cohort included 514 donor samples. SNPs in cytokines and costimulatory molecules IL-1R, IL-2 IL-6, IL-10, CTLA-4, and TNF-α were not replicated. The authors note that a more defined criteria for chronic GVHD developed by the National Institutes of Health Consensus Development Project would help to ensure that recipients are accurately classified thereby ensuring that replicate studies use the same criteria for diagnosis. They recommend also expanding the number of SNPs evaluated to include ones capable of altering the immune response with the caveat that GWAS incur a statistical penalty for multiple comparisons. They highlight 5 considerations when generating an association study:

1. Number of SNPs in the study,
2. Minimum minor allele frequency,
3. Anticipated effect size,
4. Available numbers of donor–recipient pairs, and
5. Need to replicate and new discoveries in an independent cohort.

FUTURE DIRECTIONS IN GENETIC POLYMORPHISM STUDIES

The solution may involve gathering a multitude of samples from around the world with detailed history to have sufficient power to observe effects of gene polymorphisms or haplotypes and the ability to control for multiple variables. iGeneTrain is an international consortium set up for sharing and for metaanalyzing genetic and phenotypic data from transplant cohorts worldwide.[98] Data are collected from multiple institutions and characterized to increase statistical power for identifying causal genetic regions outside of HLA. True biomarker discovery may require a systems biology approach using various high-throughput omics techniques within a transplant study population (**Fig. 2**).[99] A single polymorphism in costimulatory molecules or cytokines may function as part of a whole human system response to the complex nature of an allograft.

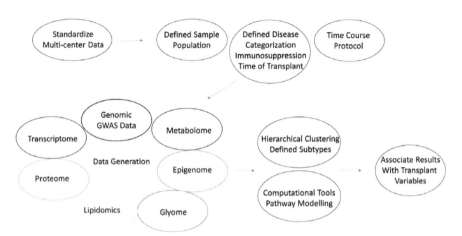

Fig. 2. Systems biology approach to immune regulatory gene effects in transplantation.

ACKNOWLEDGMENTS

The authors would like to thank Jane E. Libbey, MS, for copyediting and proofreading of the article.

REFERENCES

1. iGeneTRAiN. Igenetrain- an overview. 2015; 1. Available at: http://igenetrain.org/igenetrain-an-overview/. Accessed August 1, 2018.
2. Sayegh MH. Looking into the crystal ball: kidney transplantation in 2025. Nat Clin Pract Nephrol 2009;5(3):117.
3. Linsley PS, Ledbetter JA. The role of the CD28 receptor during T cell responses to antigen. Annu Rev Immunol 1993;11:191–212.
4. Bluestone JA. New perspectives of CD28-B7-mediated T cell costimulation. Immunity 1995;2:555–9.
5. Rothstein DM, Sayegh MH. T-cell costimulatory pathways in allograft rejection and tolerance. Immunol Rev 2003;196:85–108.
6. Ambruzova Z, Mrazek F, Raida L, et al. Association of IL-6 gene polymorphism with the outcome of allogeneic haematopoietic stem cell transplantation in Czech patients. Int J Immunogenet 2008;35(4–5):401–3.
7. Azarian M, Busson M, Lepage V, et al. Donor CTLA-4 +49 A/G*GG genotype is associated with chronic GVHD after HLA-identical haematopoietic stem-cell transplants. Blood 2007;110(13):4623–4.
8. Tseng LH, Storer B, Petersdorf E, et al. IL10 and IL10 receptor gene variation and outcomes after unrelated and related hematopoietic cell transplantation. Transplantation 2009;87(5):704–10.
9. Khoury SJ, Sayegh MH. The roles of the new negative T cell costimulatory pathways in regulating autoimmunity. Immunity 2004;20(5):529–38.
10. Sandner SE, Clarkson MR, Salama AD, et al. Mechanisms of tolerance induced by donor-specific transfusion and ICOS-B7h blockade in a model of CD4+ T-cell-mediated allograft rejection. Am J Transplant 2005;5(1):31–9.
11. Tantravahi J, Womer KL, Kaplan B. Why hasn't eliminating acute rejection improved graft survival? Annu Rev Med 2007;58:369–85.

12. Leeaphorn N, Pena JRA, Thamcharoen N, et al. HLA-DQ mismatching and kidney transplant outcomes. Clin J Am Soc Nephrol 2018;13(5):763–71.
13. Boenisch O, Sayegh MH, Najafian N. Negative T-cell costimulatory pathways: their role in regulating alloimmune responses. Curr Opin Organ Transplant 2008;13(4):373–8.
14. Via CS, Rus V, Nguyen P, et al. Differential effect of CTLA4Ig on murine graft-versus-host disease (GVHD) development: CTLA4Ig prevents both acute and chronic GVHD development but reverses only chronic GVHD. J Immunol 1996; 157(9):4258–67.
15. Schuchmann M, Meyer RG, Distler E, et al. The programmed death (PD)-1/PD-ligand 1 pathway regulates graft-versus-host-reactive CD8 T cells after liver transplantation. Am J Transplant 2008;8(11):2434–44.
16. Esensten JH, Helou YA, Chopra G, et al. CD28 costimulation: from mechanism to therapy. Immunity 2016;44(5):973–88.
17. Matsushita M, Tsuchiya N, Oka T, et al. New polymorphisms of human CD80 and CD86: lack of association with rheumatoid arthritis and systemic lupus erythematosus. Genes Immun 2000;1(7):428–34.
18. Marder BA, Schroppel B, Lin M, et al. The impact of costimulatory molecule gene polymorphisms on clinical outcomes in liver transplantation. Am J Transplant 2003;3(4):424–31.
19. Han FF, Fan H, Wang ZH, et al. Association between co-stimulatory molecule gene polymorphism and acute rejection of allograft. Transpl Immunol 2014; 31(2):81–6.
20. Iravani-Saadi M, Karimi MH, Yaghobi R, et al. Polymorphism of costimulatory molecules (CTLA4, ICOS, PD.1 and CD28) and allogeneic hematopoietic stem cell transplantation in Iranian patients. Immunol Invest 2014;43(4):391–404.
21. Niknam A, Karimi MH, Geramizadeh B, et al. Polymorphisms of the Costimulatory Genes CTLA-4, CD28, PD-1, and ICOS and outcome of kidney transplants in Iranian patients. Exp Clin Transplant 2017;15(3):295–305.
22. Harada H, Salama AD, Sho M, et al. The role of the ICOS-B7h T cell costimulatory pathway in transplantation immunity. J Clin Invest 2003;112(2):234–43.
23. Ozkaynak E, Gao W, Shemmeri N, et al. Importance of ICOS-B7RP-1 costimulation in acute and chronic allograft rejection. Nat Immunol 2001;2(7):591–6.
24. Kaartinen T, Lappalainen J, Haimila K, et al. Genetic variation in ICOS regulates mRNA levels of ICOS and splicing isoforms of CTLA4. Mol Immunol 2007;44(7): 1644–51.
25. Wu J, Tang JL, Wu SJ, et al. Functional polymorphism of CTLA-4 and ICOS genes in allogeneic hematopoietic stem cell transplantation. Clin Chim Acta 2009; 403(1–2):229–33.
26. Hori T. Roles of OX40 in the pathogenesis and the control of diseases. Int J Hematol 2006;83(1):17–22.
27. Mousavi SF, Soroosh P, Takahashi T, et al. OX40 costimulatory signals potentiate the memory commitment of effector CD8+ T cells. J Immunol 2008;181(9): 5990–6001.
28. Ishii N, Ndhlovu LC, Murata K, et al. OX40 (CD134) and OX40 ligand interaction plays an adjuvant role during in vivo Th2 responses. Eur J Immunol 2003;33(9): 2372–81.
29. Hippen KL, Harker-Murray P, Porter SB, et al. Umbilical cord blood regulatory T-cell expansion and functional effects of tumor necrosis factor receptor family members OX40 and 4-1BB expressed on artificial antigen-presenting cells. Blood 2008;112(7):2847–57.

30. Karaesmen E, Rizvi AA, Preus LM, et al. Replication and validation of genetic polymorphisms associated with survival after allogeneic blood or marrow transplant. Blood 2017;130(13):1585–96.

31. Ozaki K, Ohnishi Y, Iida A, et al. Functional SNPs in the lymphotoxin-alpha gene that are associated with susceptibility to myocardial infarction. Nat Genet 2002; 32(4):650–4.

32. Bassuny WM, Ihara K, Sasaki Y, et al. A functional polymorphism in the promoter/ enhancer region of the FOXP3/Scurfin gene associated with type 1 diabetes. Immunogenetics 2003;55(3):149–56.

33. Reddy CD, Reddy EP. Differential binding of nuclear factors to the intron 1 sequences containing the transcriptional pause site correlates with c-myb expression. Proc Natl Acad Sci U S A 1989;86(19):7326–30.

34. Lee PH, Shatkay H. F-SNP: computationally predicted functional SNPs for disease association studies. Nucleic Acids Res 2008;36(Database issue):D820–4.

35. Ogata K, Morikawa S, Nakamura H, et al. Solution structure of a specific DNA complex of the Myb DNA-binding domain with cooperative recognition helices. Cell 1994;79(4):639–48.

36. Boyle AP, Hong EL, Hariharan M, et al. Annotation of functional variation in personal genomes using RegulomeDB. Genome Res 2012;22(9):1790–7.

37. Ward LD, Kellis M. HaploReg v4: systematic mining of putative causal variants, cell types, regulators and target genes for human complex traits and disease. Nucleic Acids Res 2016;44(D1):D877–81.

38. Karabon L, Markiewicz M, Chrobot K, et al. The influence of genetic variations in the CD86 gene on the outcome after allogeneic hematopoietic stem cell transplantation. J Immunol Res 2018;2018:3826989.

39. Marin LA, Moya-Quiles MR, Miras M, et al. Evaluation of CD86 gene polymorphism at +1057 position in liver transplant recipients. Transpl Immunol 2005; 15(1):69–74.

40. Krichen H, Sfar I, Bardi R, et al. CD86 +1057G>A polymorphism and susceptibility to acute kidney allograft rejection. Iran J Kidney Dis 2011;5(3):187–93.

41. Schildberg FA, Klein SR, Freeman GJ, et al. Coinhibitory pathways in the B7-CD28 ligand-receptor family. Immunity 2016;44(5):955–72.

42. Ueda H, Howson JM, Esposito L, et al. Association of the T-cell regulatory gene CTLA4 with susceptibility to autoimmune disease. Nature 2003;423(6939): 506–11.

43. Perez-Garcia A, De la Camara R, Roman-Gomez J, et al. CTLA-4 polymorphisms and clinical outcome after allogeneic stem cell transplantation from HLA-identical sibling donors. Blood 2007;110(1):461–7.

44. Piccioli P, Balbi G, Serra M, et al. CTLA-4 +49A>G polymorphism of recipients of HLA-matched sibling allogeneic stem cell transplantation is associated with survival and relapse incidence. Ann Hematol 2010;89(6):613–8.

45. Metaxas Y, Bertz H, Spyridonidis A, et al. CT60 single-nucleotide polymorphism as a surrogate marker for donor lymphocyte infusion outcome after allogeneic cell transplantation for acute leukemia. Bone Marrow Transplant 2012;47(3):411–5.

46. Perez-Garcia A, Osca G, Bosch-Vizcaya A, et al. Kinetics of the CTLA-4 isoforms expression after T-lymphocyte activation and role of the promoter polymorphisms on CTLA-4 gene transcription. Hum Immunol 2013;74(9):1219–24.

47. Kobayashi M, Takaori-Kondo A, Fukunaga K, et al. Lentiviral gp34/OX40L gene transfer into dendritic cells facilitates alloreactive CD4+ T-cell response in vitro. Int J Hematol 2004;79(4):377–83.

48. Linton PJ, Bautista B, Biederman E, et al. Costimulation via OX40L expressed by B cells is sufficient to determine the extent of primary CD4 cell expansion and Th2 cytokine secretion in vivo. J Exp Med 2003;197(7):875–83.

49. Kato H, Kojima H, Ishii N, et al. Essential role of OX40L on B cells in persistent alloantibody production following repeated alloimmunizations. J Clin Immunol 2004;24(3):237–48.

50. Copper GF, Herskovits E. A Bayesian method for the induction of probabilistic networks from data. Machine Learn 1992;9:309–47.

51. Yang J, Popoola J, Khandwala S, et al. Critical role of donor tissue expression of programmed death ligand-1 in regulating cardiac allograft rejection and vasculopathy. Circulation 2008;117(5):660–9.

52. Blazar BR, Carreno BM, Panoskaltsis-Mortari A, et al. Blockade of programmed death-1 engagement accelerates graft-versus-host disease lethality by an IFN-gamma-dependent mechanism. J Immunol 2003;171(3):1272–7.

53. Santos N, Rodriguez-Romanos R, de la Camara R, et al. PD-1 genotype of the donor is associated with acute graft-versus-host disease after HLA-identical sibling donor stem cell transplantation. Ann Hematol 2018;97(11):2217–24.

54. Meng XM, Nikolic-Paterson DJ, Lan HY. TGF-beta: the master regulator of fibrosis. Nat Rev Nephrol 2016;12(6):325–38.

55. Dunning AM, Ellis PD, McBride S, et al. A transforming growth factorbeta1 signal peptide variant increases secretion in vitro and is associated with increased incidence of invasive breast cancer. Cancer Res 2003;63(10):2610–5.

56. Densem CG, Hutchinson IV, Cooper A, et al. Polymorphism of the transforming growth factor-beta 1 gene correlates with the development of coronary vasculopathy following cardiac transplantation. J Heart Lung Transplant 2000;19(6):551–6.

57. Densem CG, Mutlak AS, Pravica V, et al. A novel polymorphism of the gene encoding furin, a TGF-beta1 activator, and the influence on cardiac allograft vasculopathy formation. Transpl Immunol 2004;13(3):185–90.

58. Holweg CT, Baan CC, Niesters HG, et al. TGF-beta1 gene polymorphisms in patients with end-stage heart failure. J Heart Lung Transplant 2001;20(9):979–84.

59. Bijlsma FJ, van der Horst AA, Tilanus MG, et al. No association between transforming growth factor beta gene polymorphism and acute allograft rejection after cardiac transplantation. Transpl Immunol 2002;10(1):43–7.

60. Liu K, Liu X, Gu S, et al. Association between TGFB1 genetic polymorphisms and chronic allograft dysfunction: a systematic review and meta-analysis. Oncotarget 2017;8(37):62463–9.

61. Nikolova PN, Ivanova MI, Mihailova SM, et al. Cytokine gene polymorphism in kidney transplantation–impact of TGF-beta 1, TNF-alpha and IL-6 on graft outcome. Transpl Immunol 2008;18(4):344–8.

62. Melk A, Henne T, Kollmar T, et al. Cytokine single nucleotide polymorphisms and intrarenal gene expression in chronic allograft nephropathy in children. Kidney Int 2003;64(1):314–20.

63. Berro M, Palau Nagore MV, Rivas MM, et al. Transforming growth factor-beta1 functional polymorphisms in myeloablative sibling hematopoietic stem cell transplantation. Bone Marrow Transplant 2017;52(5):739–44.

64. Kalliolias GD, Ivashkiv LB. TNF biology, pathogenic mechanisms and emerging therapeutic strategies. Nat Rev Rheumatol 2016;12(1):49–62.

65. Sankaran D, Asderakis A, Ashraf S, et al. Cytokine gene polymorphisms predict acute graft rejection following renal transplantation. Kidney Int 1999;56(1):281–8.

66. Alakulppi NS, Kyllonen LE, Jantti VT, et al. Cytokine gene polymorphisms and risks of acute rejection and delayed graft function after kidney transplantation. Transplantation 2004;78(10):1422–8.

67. Breulmann B, Bantis C, Siekierka M, et al. Influence of cytokine genes polymorphisms on long-term outcome in renal transplantation. Clin Transplant 2007; 21(5):615–21.

68. Sanchez-Fructuoso AI, Perez-Flores I, Valero R, et al. The polymorphism -308G/A of tumor necrosis factor-alpha gene modulates the effect of immunosuppressive treatment in first kidney transplant subjects who suffer an acute rejection. J Immunol Res 2016;2016:2197595.

69. Vu D, Shah T, Ansari J, et al. Interferon-gamma gene polymorphism +874 A/T is associated with an increased risk of cytomegalovirus infection among Hispanic renal transplant recipients. Transpl Infect Dis 2014;16(5):724–32.

70. Mu HJ, Xie P, Chen JY, et al. Association of TNF-alpha, TGF-beta1, IL-10, IL-6, and IFN-gamma gene polymorphism with acute rejection and infection in lung transplant recipients. Clin Transplant 2014;28(9):1016–24.

71. Ding S, Xie J, Wan Q. Association between cytokines and their receptor antagonist gene polymorphisms and clinical risk factors and acute rejection following renal transplantation. Med Sci Monit 2016;22:4736–41.

72. Bhat MA, Parry MA, Nissar S, et al. Association of IL1 beta gene polymorphism and allograft functions in renal transplant recipients :a case control study from Kashmir Valley. BMC Nephrol 2017;18(1):111.

73. Paul WE. History of interleukin-4. Cytokine 2015;75(1):3–7.

74. Bijlsma FJ, vanKuik J, Tilanus MG, et al. Donor interleukin-4 promoter gene polymorphism influences allograft rejection after heart transplantation. J Heart Lung Transplant 2002;21(3):340–6.

75. Tanaka T, Narazaki M, Kishimoto T. IL-6 in inflammation, immunity, and disease. Cold Spring Harb Perspect Biol 2014;6(10):a016295.

76. Densem CG, Ray M, Hutchinson IV, et al. Interleukin-6 polymorphism: a genetic risk factor for cardiac transplant related coronary vasculopathy? J Heart Lung Transplant 2005;24(5):559–65.

77. Lu KC, Jaramillo A, Lecha RL, et al. Interleukin-6 and interferon-gamma gene polymorphisms in the development of bronchiolitis obliterans syndrome after lung transplantation. Transplantation 2002;74(9):1297–302.

78. Trifunovic J, Miller L, Debeljak Z, et al. Pathologic patterns of interleukin 10 expression–a review. Biochem Med (Zagreb) 2015;25(1):36–48.

79. Lin MT, Storer B, Martin PJ, et al. Relation of an interleukin-10 promoter polymorphism to graft-versus-host disease and survival after hematopoietic-cell transplantation. N Engl J Med 2003;349(23):2201–10.

80. Karabon L, Wysoczanska B, Bogunia-Kubik K, et al. IL-6 and IL-10 promoter gene polymorphisms of patients and donors of allogeneic sibling hematopoietic stem cell transplants associate with the risk of acute graft-versus-host disease. Hum Immunol 2005;66(6):700–10.

81. Azarpira N, Ramzi M, Aghdaie MH, et al. Interleukin-10 gene polymorphism in bone marrow transplant recipients. Exp Clin Transplant 2008;6(1):74–9.

82. Morgun A, Shulzhenko N, Gerbase-DeLima M. IL-10 gene polymorphisms in transplantation. Austin (Tx): Madame Curie Bioscience Database Landes Bioscience; 2000.

83. McDaniel OD, Roten PD, Yamout SZ, et al. Cytokine gene polymorphism might affect the outcome of clinical rejection in cardiac transplantation. J Appl Res 2004;4(1):68–80.

84. Billingham ME, Cary NR, Hammond ME, et al. A working formulation for the standardization of nomenclature in the diagnosis of heart and lung rejection: Heart Rejection Study Group. The International Society for Heart Transplantation. J Heart Transplant 1990;9(6):587–93.

85. McDaniel DO, Barber WH, Nguyan C, et al. Combined analysis of cytokine genotype polymorphism and the level of expression with allograft function in African-American renal transplant patients. Transpl Immunol 2003;11(1):107–19.

86. Gaffen SL, Jain R, Garg AV, et al. The IL-23-IL-17 immune axis: from mechanisms to therapeutic testing. Nat Rev Immunol 2014;14(9):585–600.

87. Espinoza JL, Takami A, Nakata K, et al. A genetic variant in the IL-17 promoter is functionally associated with acute graft-versus-host disease after unrelated bone marrow transplantation. PLoS One 2011;6(10):e26229.

88. Duerr RH, Taylor KD, Brant SR, et al. A genome-wide association study identifies IL23R as an inflammatory bowel disease gene. Science 2006;314(5804):1461–3.

89. Rioux JD, Xavier RJ, Taylor KD, et al. Genome-wide association study identifies new susceptibility loci for Crohn disease and implicates autophagy in disease pathogenesis. Nat Genet 2007;39(5):596–604.

90. Feagan BG, Sandborn WJ, Gasink C, et al. Ustekinumab as induction and maintenance therapy for Crohn's disease. N Engl J Med 2016;375(20):1946–60.

91. Elmaagacli AH, Koldehoff M, Landt O, et al. Relation of an interleukin-23 receptor gene polymorphism to graft-versus-host disease after hematopoietic-cell transplantation. Bone Marrow Transplant 2008;41(9):821–6.

92. Girnita DM, Webber SA, Ferrell R, et al. Disparate distribution of 16 candidate single nucleotide polymorphisms among racial and ethnic groups of pediatric heart transplant patients. Transplantation 2006;82(12):1774–80.

93. Ivanova M, Ruiqing J, Kawai S, et al. IL-6 SNP diversity among four ethnic groups as revealed by bead-based liquid array profiling. Int J Immunogenet 2011;38(1):17–20.

94. Hernandez-Fuentes MP, Franklin C, Rebollo-Mesa I, et al. Long- and short-term outcomes in renal allografts with deceased donors: a large recipient and donor genome-wide association study. Am J Transplant 2018;18(6):1370–9.

95. Kerman RH, Floyd M, Van Buren CT, et al. Improved allograft survival of strong immune responder-high risk recipients with adjuvant antithymocyte globulin therapy. Transplantation 1980;30(6):450–4.

96. Colhoun HM, McKeigue PM, Davey Smith G. Problems of reporting genetic associations with complex outcomes. Lancet 2003;361(9360):865–72.

97. Martin PJ, Fan W, Storer BE, et al. Replication of associations between genetic polymorphisms and chronic graft-versus-host disease. Blood 2016;128(20):2450–6.

98. International Genetics & Translational Research in Transplantation Network (iGeneTRAiN). Design and implementation of the international genetics and translational research in transplantation network. Transplantation 2015;99(11):2401–12.

99. Bontha SV, Maluf DG, Mueller TF, et al. Systems biology in kidney transplantation: the application of multi-omics to a complex model. Am J Transplant 2017;17(1):11–21.

MicroRNAs and Transplantation

Zahraa Khan, MD[a,b], Manikkam Suthanthiran, MD[a,b],
Thangamani Muthukumar, MD[a,b],*

KEYWORDS

• miRNA • Biomarkers • Rejection • Kidney transplantation

KEY POINTS

• MicroRNAs (miRNAs) are small, noncoding, single-stranded RNAs that regulate protein coding genes.
• Common methods for detecting and quantifying specific individual miRNAs include real-time quantitative polymerase chain reaction, Northern blot, and in situ hybridization. Common methods for global profiling of miRNAs include microarrays, TaqMan low density arrays, nCounter miRNA expression assay, and RNA sequencing.
• Cellular and extracellular miRNAs are emerging as robust biomarkers of allograft status.

INTRODUCTION

Small RNAs are less than 200 nucleotides in length and usually do not translate into a protein. A major function of small RNAs is gene silencing. There are 3 families of small RNAs that regulate gene expression in animals: microRNAs (miRNAs), small interfering RNAs (siRNAs), and piwi-interacting RNAs (piRNAs). miRNAs are single-stranded RNAs, ~20 to 22 nucleotides in length, and play a pivotal role in the regulation of protein-coding genes. siRNAs are ~21 nucleotides long and mediate posttranscriptional suppression of transcripts and transposons and contribute to antiviral defense. piRNAs are 24 to 30 nucleotides long, and their main function is to silence

Disclosure Statement: Supported in part by awards from the National Institutes of Health (NIH MERIT Award, R37-AI051652 to M. Suthanthiran, K08-DK087824 and R03-DK105270 to T. Muthukumar, and UL1TR000457 Clinical and Translational Science Center Award to Weill Cornell Medical College), and by an award from the American Society of Transplantation (AST-Faculty Development Grant to T. Muthukumar).
[a] Division of Nephrology and Hypertension, Department of Medicine, New York-Presbyterian–Weill Cornell Medicine, 525 East 68th Street, Box 3, New York, NY 10065, USA; [b] Division of Nephrology and Hypertension, Department of Transplantation Medicine, New York-Presbyterian–Weill Cornell Medicine, 525 East 68th Street, Box 3, New York, NY 10065, USA
* Corresponding author.
E-mail address: mut9002@med.cornell.edu

Clin Lab Med 39 (2019) 125–143
https://doi.org/10.1016/j.cll.2018.10.003
0272-2712/19/© 2018 Elsevier Inc. All rights reserved.

transposable elements in germline cells.[1] The current miRBase sequence database (released March 2018; http://www.mirbase.org/), a searchable online repository of published miRNA sequences and associated annotations maintained by researchers at the University of Manchester, reported 2654 mature miRNAs in the human genome. miRNAs influence the development and function of immune cells, modulate innate and adaptive immune responses, and are emerging as robust biomarkers in transplantation as well as targets for therapeutic intervention. Herein, the authors briefly review the biogenesis and function of the miRNAs and provide an overview of the tools to quantify miRNAs in tissues and body fluids. They then summarize data regarding miRNA expression patterns in kidney transplant recipients.

NOMENCLATURE

Human miRNAs are designated by the suffix "hsa." Mature miRNA is designated as "miR," whereas the gene is designated as "mir."[2] The numbering of genes is sequential (eg, mir-22 was the next miRNA published after mir-21). Mature sequences that are identical but originate from distinct precursor sequences and genomic loci are designated with numbered suffixes (eg, hsa-miR-121-1 and hsa-miR-121-2). Closely related mature sequences that are near-identical except for one or 2 nucleotides are designated by letter suffixes (eg, has-miR-121a and has-miR-121b). When cloning studies identify 2 miRNAs that originate from the same predicted precursor, the mature sequence that is less abundant is designated with a star symbol (eg, hsa-miR-21*). When there are insufficient data to determine which mature sequence is the predominant one, the miRNAs are designated based on their 3' arm origin (eg, hsa-miR-142-3p) or 5' arm origin (hsa-miR-142-5p).[2,3] The first miRNA discovered in humans, let-7, does not follow the naming convention for historical reasons.[2]

BIOGENESIS

Based on their genomic location, miRNA genes can be intergenic or intronic. Intergenic miRNAs are found in genomic regions that are distinct from known transcription units. These miRNAs can be monocistronic with their own promoters or polycistronic, where more than one miRNA is transcribed as a cluster with a shared promoter. Intronic miRNAs are found in the introns of annotated genes, both protein-coding and noncoding. They use the same promoter as their host genes. Rarely, genes encoding miRNAs are located in the exon. miRNAs are transcribed in the nucleus by RNA polymerase II. Initially, the transcription results in an ~80-nucleotide-long nascent transcript called pri-miR, which is 5' capped and 3' polyadenylated.[4] pri-miR is processed in the nucleus by an RNAse III-like enzyme, *Drosha*, in concert with DGCR8 (DiGeorge Syndrome Critical Region 8), to an ~65-nucleotide-long nascent transcript termed pre-miR. *Exportin 5*, a nuclear export factor, exports the pre-miR into the cytoplasm,[5] where it is cleaved by another RNAse III-like enzyme, *Dicer*, to form short (~22 nt) ds-RNA duplexes. One of the strands of the duplex is incorporated into the RNA-induced silencing complex (RISC) and guided to the target messenger RNAs (mRNAs). The other strand of the duplex is degraded. Pairing between the mature single-stranded miRNA and its target mRNA takes place in association with the Argonaute family of proteins in the RISC.[6]

In addition to the canonical biogenesis described above, there are several noncanonical pathways of miRNA biogenesis: (i) a 7-methylguanosine(m^7G)-capped pre-miR can be generated directly through transcription, bypassing Drosha processing, and exported to cytoplasm; (ii) a small RNA precursor (*mitron*) can be generated through mRNA splicing and debranching, also bypassing the Drosha-mediated processing step, folded into pre-miR and exported to the cytoplasm; (iii) some small nucleolar RNAs can be cleaved to produce pre-miR; (iv) terminal uridylyltransferase–dependent group II pri-miR produces pre-miR with a shorter 3′ overhang that undergoes monouridylation in the cytoplasm for Dicer processing; and (v) a Dicer-independent pathway in which a short pre-miR is produced by Drosha and is exported directly and loaded to Argonaute protein without Dicer processing.[1]

FUNCTION

The core of the RISC is composed of an Argonaute protein (Ago4 in mammals) and GW182 protein (TNRC6A-C in mammals). The seed sequence of an miRNA, a stretch of 6 nucleotides spanning nucleotide 2 to 7, determines the mRNA target recognition. Base-pairing between the miRNA seed sequence and complementary sequence in the 3′ untranslated region or coding region of the target mRNA is responsible for mRNA degradation or inhibition of translation.[7] miRNA bound to target mRNA directs cleavage at the site resulting in mRNA degradation. miRNA bound to target mRNA at multiple sites causes translational repression.[8] A single miRNA can target multiple protein-coding mRNAs, and many miRNAs can work synergistically or competitively to target a single mRNA. Thus, miRNAs regulate diverse physiologic processes, such as cell development, differentiation, proliferation, and apoptosis, as well as pathologic processes, such as oncogenesis and immune rejection.[9]

In addition to the intracellular regulatory function, the presence of nuclease-resistant extracellular miRNAs has been identified in all biological fluids. Although spiked-in synthetic miRNAs are susceptible to quick degradation in the body fluids, extracellular miRNAs resist such degradation. The extracellular miRNAs are protected from RNase degradation by packaging them into membrane vesicles, including apoptotic bodies, microvesicles, and exosomes, by complexing with argonaute protein-positive ribonucleoprotein particles, or, rarely, with high-density lipoproteins. It is not clear whether these secreted miRNAs simply represent cellular byproducts or participate in cell-to-cell communication.[10]

QUANTIFICATION

Several inherent characteristics of mature miRNAs make their detection with high sensitivity and specificity technically demanding.[11,12] For example, mature miRNAs lack 5′ cap and 3′ poly(A) tail, features that would facilitate their selective purification. The small size of mature miRNAs makes conventional polymerase chain reaction (PCR) assays difficult because of the inability of primers to bind to such small templates. Moreover, miRNAs are heterogeneous in their GC content, which results in a relatively large interval of melting temperatures of nucleic acid duplexes for the population of miRNAs. The target sequence in the mature miRNA is also present in the pri-miR and pre-miR. Finally, miRNAs within the same family may differ by a single nucleotide. There are 3 common methods for the detection and quantification of specific individual miRNAs in tissues, cells, or fluids including circulating body fluids: (i) real-time quantitative PCR, (ii) Northern blot, and (iii) in situ hybridization. There are 4 common methods for global profiling of miRNAs: (i) microarrays, (ii) TaqMan low density arrays (TLDA), (iii) nCounter miRNA expression assay, and (iv) RNA sequencing.

Real-Time Quantitative Polymerase Chain Reaction

The stem-loop primer design is the main ingredient that overcomes the challenge of amplifying ∼22 nucleotide miRNAs by PCR (eg, Megaplex miRNA assay,

ThermoFisher Scientific). The stem-loop primer consists of a constant portion that forms a stem-loop and extends the ~22 nucleotide miRNA to more than ~60 nucleotides to allow for subsequent traditional PCR assay.[13] The stem-loop primer also consists of a variable 6-nucleotide extension that is the reverse complement of the last 6 nucleotides on the 3' end of miRNA of interest. The stacked bases in the stem-loop design, compared with a linear design, provide thermal stability and spatial constraint, thereby minimizing errors in primer binding. During amplification, the miRNA is reverse transcribed using the stem-loop primer. Next, an miRNA-specific forward primer, a universal reverse primer that is specific for the stem-loop portion, and a labeled probe are used to initiate a typical real-time PCR assay. In addition to the stem-loop primer design, a poly(T) adaptor PCR can also be used for quantifying miRNAs. In this method, total RNAs, including miRNAs, are extended by a poly(A) tailing reaction using poly(A) polymerase.[14] The miRNA with a poly(A) tail is converted into complementary DNA (cDNA) and then PCR-amplified using an miRNA-specific forward primer and a universal poly(T) adaptor reverse primer (eg, miScript II; Qiagen).

Detection of the PCR product is achieved by fluorescent probes–based TaqMan method or DNA binding cyanine dye–based SYBR Green method. In the TaqMan method, an oligonucleotide probe is constructed containing a reporter fluorescent dye on the 5' end and a quencher dye on the 3' end. In an intact probe, the proximity of the quencher dye greatly reduces the fluorescence emitted by the reporter dye by fluorescence resonance energy transfer through space. In the presence of target sequence, the probe anneals downstream from one of the primer sites and is cleaved by the 5' nuclease activity of Taq DNA polymerase as this primer is extended. The cleavage of the probe separates the reporter dye from the quencher dye, increasing the reporter dye signal, and removes the probe from the target strand, allowing primer extension to continue to the end of the template strand. In the SYBR Green method, the dye immediately binds to all double-stranded DNA present in the sample and to each new copy of double-stranded DNA during PCR amplification. The increase in fluorescence intensity is proportionate to the amount of PCR product produced. TaqMan probes have higher sensitivity and specificity for the target miRNA but must be designed for each miRNA of interest.

Quantification of the amplified PCR product is achieved by relative quantification (comparative C_T method) or by absolute quantification (standard curve method).[15] The quantitative endpoint for real-time PCR is the threshold cycle (C_T), defined as the PCR cycle at which the fluorescent signal of the reporter dye crosses an arbitrarily placed threshold. The numerical value of the C_T is inversely related to the amount of amplicon in the reaction. In the comparative C_T method, the data are presented as fold change (FC) in expression, where $FC = 2^{-\Delta\Delta \ CT}$. To compare a gene of interest in a given sample, $FC = 2^{-\Delta\Delta \ CT} = [(C_T$ gene of interest $- C_T$ internal control) sample A $- (C_T$ gene of interest $- C_T$ internal control) sample B]. The comparative C_T method makes several assumptions, including that the efficiency of the PCR is close to 1 and the PCR efficiency of the target gene is similar to the internal control gene.[15] When performing statistical analysis, statistical tests should not be run on the raw C_T data, and standard deviation should always be calculated after $2^{-\Delta\Delta \ CT}$, $2^{-\Delta \ CT}$, or 2^{-CT}.

In the standard curve method, the absolute quantity is determined using an external calibration curve, and the data are presented relatively compared with a defined unit of interest (eg, copies per microgram of total RNA). The authors have developed a standard curve method, using a PCR-generated 73-bp mouse Bak amplicon as the standard, for the absolute quantification of mRNAs and miRNAs (**Fig. 1**).[16–18] To use a single Bak standard curve to quantify all genes of interest,

Stock Solution

Serial Dilutions

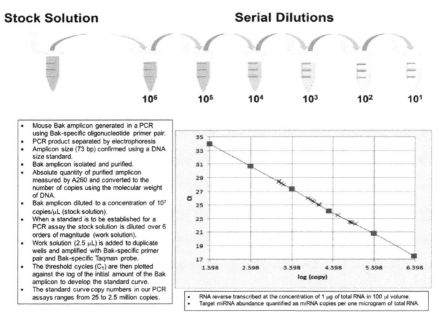

10^6 10^5 10^4 10^3 10^2 10^1

- Mouse Bak amplicon generated in a PCR using Bak-specific oligonucleotide primer pair.
- PCR product separated by electrophoresis
- Amplicon size (73 bp) confirmed using a DNA size standard.
- Bak amplicon isolated and purified.
- Absolute quantity of purified amplicon measured by A260 and converted to the number of copies using the molecular weight of DNA.
- Bak amplicon diluted to a concentration of 10^7 copies/μL (stock solution).
- When a standard is to be established for a PCR assay the stock solution is diluted over 6 orders of magnitude (work solution).
- Work solution (2.5 μL) is added to duplicate wells and amplified with Bak-specific primer pair and Bak-specific Taqman probe.
- The threshold cycles (C_T) are then plotted against the log of the initial amount of the Bak amplicon to develop the standard curve.
- The standard curve copy numbers in our PCR assays ranges from 25 to 2.5 million copies.

- RNA reverse transcribed at the concentration of 1 μg of total RNA in 100 μl volume.
- Target miRNA abundance quantified as miRNA copies per one microgram of total RNA.

Fig. 1. Development of a Bak amplicon-based standard curve for absolute quantification of mRNAs and miRNAs by real-time quantitative PCR assay. A universal standard curve for absolute quantification of mRNAs and miRNAs by quantitative PCR assay was developed in the authors' laboratory by synthesizing and quantifying a customized Bak amplicon template.

the authors ensured that the amplification efficiency of target genes is greater than 90% so that there is minimal bias due to different amplification efficiencies of target genes and the Bak amplicon.

In droplet digital PCR method (Bio-Rad Laboratories), the sample for PCR is partitioned into thousands of nanoliter-size samples encapsulated into oil droplets before amplification.[19] At the end of the PCR reaction, PCR-positive and PCR-negative droplets are counted. Each droplet either contains or does not contain the nucleic acid of interest. Poisson distribution is assumed to estimate the number of molecules in the reaction. Droplet digital PCR provides absolute quantification based on the principles of sample partitioning and Poisson statistics, thus overcoming the normalization and calibrator issues. It is relatively insensitive to potential PCR inhibitors and directly provides the copies of target per microliter of reaction. Droplet digital PCR is an end-point analysis, and the absolute quantification relies on the presence or absence of fluorescence in each droplet, rather than the fluorescence levels during the reaction. These factors offer the advantage of direct and independent quantification of DNA without standard curves.[19] The current droplet digital PCR system (QX100 and QX200) is compatible with TaqMan probes but not with SYBR Green dye.

Northern Blot

RNA is denatured and separated by urea polyacrylamide gel electrophoresis, transferred to nylon membrane, fixed, and hybridized with labeled DNA or RNA probes. Target miRNAs with sequences complementary to the probe are detected. Locked-nucleic acid probes are widely used because these are stable and specific and have no radioactive contamination (eg, miRCURY LNA miRNA detection probes;

Qiagen). These nucleotides are nucleotides in which the furanose ring of the ribose sugar is chemically locked in a $3'$-*endo* (North) conformation, with an extra methylene bridge connecting the $2'$ oxygen and $4'$ carbon, thus increasing its hybridization properties.[20]

In Situ Hybridization

In situ hybridization technology allows for detection of specific nucleic acid sequences in tissue samples at the cellular level. Because of their increased thermal stability, locked-nucleic acids are used to generate short nucleotide probes with high melting temperature required for in situ hybridization. miRNA in situ hybridization is technically challenging, and various modifications for fixation and permeabilization, hybridization, washing, and sequence amplification and detection are available.[21]

Microarrays

Modified oligonucleotide probes antisense to miRNAs are anchored on microscopic glass slides. miRNAs in a given sample are biotinylated and are captured on the microarray by the oligonucleotide probes in hybridization. Streptavidin-Phycoerythrin is then used for detecting the biotinylated miRNA (eg, GeneChip miRNA array; Thermo-Fisher Scientific). The hybridized microarray slide is scanned to measure the relative gene expression of each miRNA captured on the slide. Several technical variants of miRNA arrays have been independently developed. These variants differ in oligonucleotide probe design, probe immobilization chemistry, sample labeling, and microarray chip signal-detection methods.[22]

TaqMan Low-Density Arrays

TLDA (ThermoFisher Scientific), which are based on TaqMan stem-loop PCR, are available in 3 forms: 96-well pates, 384-well microfluidic cards, and OpenArray plates. The wells in all 3 formats are preloaded with miRNA primers and TaqMan fluorogenic probes. After the cDNA sample and TaqMan Master Mix are loaded on to the wells, the plate/card is placed in a thermal cycler for PCR. miRNA expression level is reported using the comparative C_T ($\Delta\Delta C_T$) method. TaqMan OpenArray contains 754 human miRNA sequences and enables generation of miRNA profile of up to 48 samples in a single working day.

nCounter microRNA Expression Assay

The NanoString technology is based on direct molecular barcoding and digital detection of target molecules using a pair of color-coded probes and requires minimal sample intervention. The "direct" refers to the process of counting individual tagged nucleic acids without any need for amplification, and the "digital" refers to the capacity to use absolute and specific quantification, independent of relative measures like intensity or amplification cycles. The miRNAs are ligated with unique oligonucleotide tags. The probe pair consists of a Reporter Probe, which carries a signal on its $5'$ end, and a Capture Probe, which carries biotin on its $3'$ end. During hybridization, probe pairs are used in large excess, such that each miRNA with oligonucleotide tag finds a probe pair. The hybridization mixture containing miRNA/probe complexes is allowed to bind to magnetic beads complementary to sequences on the Capture Probe. After washing, the Capture Probes and miRNA/probe complexes are eluted off the beads and are hybridized to magnetic beads complementary to sequences on the Reporter Probe. The purified target/probe complexes are eluted off the beads and immobilized on the cartridge for data collection. The digital images are processed, and the barcode counts are tabulated.

RNA Sequencing

Next-generation sequencing methods offer several advantages over microarray or PCR assays, including discovery of novel small RNAs, detection of single nucleotide polymorphisms, distinguishing of different isoforms, a better signal-to-noise ratio than microarrays, and a higher throughput than PCR or Northern blotting. Sequencing also allows comprehensive quantification of gene expression over a dynamic range (no upper or lower limit) compared with other techniques.[23] The steps involved in sequencing include small RNA isolation, cDNA library preparation, and sequencing.

In a typical library preparation protocol, adapters are ligated to the RNAs followed by reverse transcription and PCR amplification.[24] Serious biases may be introduced during the adapter ligation steps due to RNA sequence/structure effects resulting in the preferential ligation of certain small RNAs with a given adapter sequence.[25] An approach to neutralize this effect and improve the fidelity of sequencing results is randomization of adapter sequences close to the ligation junction. Instead of modifying the adapters, bias suppression has been attempted also through optimizing reaction conditions. In one such approach, polyethylene glycol, a macromolecular crowding agent known to increase ligation efficiency and reduce bias, is used. Another concern is the formation of adapter dimers. Currently available library preparation kits use either strategies to eliminate excess 3′ adapter before 5′ adapter ligation, including purification steps, or complementary oligonucleotides that inactivate the 3′ adapter. Some protocols use polyadenylation instead of ligation for 3′ adapter addition. Multiple A residues are added to the 3′ end using poly(A) polymerase. Then, a 5′ adapter is ligated either directly to the RNA or to the nascent cDNA after reverse transcription. Certain newer protocols eliminate ligation bias by avoiding adapter ligation altogether through adding 3′ adapter by polyadenylation and 5′ adapter by reverse transcriptase template-switching.

A robust protocol for small RNA sequencing using barcoded 3′ adapters (multiple unique sequences at the 5′ end of the 3′ adapter oligonucleotides), that allows for pooling of multiple RNA samples, was initially reported a decade ago.[24,26,27] TruSeq (Illumina) small RNA library preparation, which allows for pooling of multiple RNA samples, is a commonly used protocol used for small RNA sequencing. After isolation of total RNA from the sample, synthetic oligonucleotide adapters of known sequence are ligated to the 3′ and 5′ ends of the small RNA pool using T4 RNA ligases. The adapters introduce primer-binding sites for reverse transcription and PCR amplification. The amplification is performed with 2 primers that anneal to the adapter ends. This step selectively enriches RNA fragments with adapter molecules on both ends. Subsequently, the cDNA construct is purified, and the library is normalized before sequencing. Using unique index adapter sequences, samples can be multiplexed, with up to 48 libraries combined in a single lane. The index is added at the amplification step following reverse transcription. Libraries are pooled immediately before gel purification or after gel purification. Other small RNA library preparation protocols that are compatible with Illumina sequencing platform include BIOO Scientific NEXTflex small RNA sequencing kit (PerkinElmer), NEBNext small RNA library prep set (New England BioLabs), SMARTer smRNA-seq kit (TaKaRa), and CATS small RNA seq kit (Diagenode).[25] In the Illumina sequencing platform, the library is loaded into a flow cell with a lawn of surface-bound oligonucleotides complementary to the adapters. The 3′ and 5′ adapters of each cDNA library fragment bind to complementary oligonucleotides forming a "bridge" that allows priming and PCR amplification of the cDNA fragment sandwiched between the 2 adapters.[28] Millions of copies of unique sequence clusters are produced that serve as single-stranded templates for sequencing. Based on the sequence of the template, fluorescently labeled 2'-deoxy-nucleoside 5'-triphosphates are added to the growing chain. The addition of a single nucleotide leads to emission of a characteristic fluorescent signal. The wavelength and intensity of emission identify the base. The length of the read depends on the number of sequencing cycles. The reads are sorted based on the index sequence and aligned to a reference transcript to produce a transcription map with the level of expression of each gene.

MicroRNA EXPRESSION PATTERNS IN KIDNEY TRANSPLANT RECIPIENTS

Kidney transplantation has evolved from a risky experimental procedure to a treatment of choice for patients with end-stage kidney disease. However, allograft destructive immune response may occur at any time during the life span of the kidney transplant despite the use of potent immunosuppressive drugs. The mechanistic pathways of rejection, both acute and chronic, are being resolved. The Banff classification of allo-graft pathology captures well the multiple pathways of immune rejection in the kidney allograft.[29]

The authors have proposed a time-line model to illustrate immune rejection of kidney allograft as a continuum, with initial events identified by molecular perturbations before the late histologic changes.[30] In this conceptualization, molecular biomarkers serve not only a diagnostic role but also as an anticipatory, treatment response-predictive and prognostic role. The hypothesis that early intervention is efficacious is an important rationale for the development of molecular monitoring strategies. miRNAs play a pivotal role in the development, maturation, and function of the cells of the innate and adaptive immune system. Because miRNAs are stable and present in high abundance, they have emerged as attractive biomarkers to assess kidney allograft status.

Table 1 is a summary of published studies on miRNA expression patterns observed in human kidney transplant recipients. Recent reviews have addressed the role of miR-NAs in other solid organ transplants and in hematopoietic cell transplantation.[31–33] The authors' first study of global profiling of mature human miRNAs in kidney allograft re-cipients with or without acute rejection (AR) in the allografts used TLDA. Among the 365 mature human miRNAs analyzed in the training set (4 normal biopsies and 3 AR biopsies), 174 ± 7 miRNAs (48%) were expressed in the biopsy samples.[17] Unsuper-vised hierarchical clustering of miRNA expression patterns correctly classified the normal allograft biopsies and the AR biopsies (Fig. 2). In a validation set of 26 kidney allograft biopsies (9 AR and 17 normal allograft biopsies), the authors validated a sub-set of differentially expressed miRNAs using targeted PCR assays. Their analysis involving receiver operating characteristic curve showed that AR can be predicted accurately using intragraft levels of miR-142-5p or miR-155 (area under the curve 0.99 and 0.98, respectively; $P<.0001$). The authors found a positive association be-tween intragraft levels of CD3 (T-cell coreceptor) mRNA or CD20 (B-cell molecule) mRNA and intragraft levels of miR-142-5p, miR-155, or miR-223, miRNAs that were overexpressed in AR. They also found a positive association between intragraft levels of NKCC2 (tubular cotransporter) mRNA and intragraft levels of miR-10b, miR-30a-3p, or let-7c, miRNAs that were underexpressed in AR (Fig. 3). To address whether the altered expression of miRNAs in AR biopsies is due to relative proportions of immune cells and kidney parenchymal cells or due to altered regulation of miRNAs within the cells themselves, the authors quantified the abundance of differentially expressed miRNAs in normal human peripheral blood mononuclear cells (PBMC) and in normal human renal tubular epithelial cells (HREC). They also investigated whether stimulation

Table 1
Published studies on microRNA expression in human kidney transplants

PMID (Journal)	First Author, Year	Specimen	Profiling Technique	Targeted or Global Profiling	Platform	Company	Patients/Diagnosis	Major Findings
18346642 (*Transpl Immunol*)	Sui, 2008	Biopsy tissue	Microarray	Global	LNA-based miChip	University of Heidelberg, Germany	3 AR &	AR: 8 miRNAs up & 12 miRNAs down
			PCR	Targeted			3 Native kidney control (RNA pooled in each group)	PCR for 2 miRNAs AR: up- miR-320 Down- miR-324-3p
19289845 (*Proc Natl Acad Sci USA*)	Anglicheau et al,[17] 2009	Biopsy tissue (RNAlater)	PCR (TLDA)	Global	Taqman miRNA	Applied Biosystems/ ThermoFisher	3 AR & 4 normal	ACR: 10 miRNAs up & 43 miRNAs down
			PCR	Targeted	Taqman miRNA		9 AR & 17 normal	PCR done for 6 miRNAs AR: up- miR-142-5p, miR-155, & miR-223 Down- miR-10b, miR-30a-3p, & let-7c
21794090 (*Am J Transplant*)	Scian, 2011	Biopsy tissue (RNAlater)	Microarray	Global	Sentrix Universal BeadChip array	Illumina	13 IFTA & 5 normal	Differential expression: 56 miRNAs
			PCR	Targeted	Taqman miRNA	Applied Biosystems/ ThermoFisher	32 IFTA & 13 normal	IFTA: up- miR-32 & miR-142-3p Down- miR-107, miR-204, & miR-211
		Urine	PCR	Targeted	Taqman miRNA	Applied Biosystems/ ThermoFisher	7 IFTA & 7 normal	IFTA: up- miR-142-3p. Down- miR-204 & miR-211

(continued on next page)

Table 1
(continued)

PMID (Journal)	First Author, Year	Specimen	Profiling Technique	Targeted or Global Profiling	Platform	Company	Patients/Diagnosis	Major Findings
21812927 (*Am J Transplant*)	Lorenzen, 2011	Urine	PCR	Targeted	Taqman miRNA	Applied Biosystems/ThermoFisher	68 ACR & 20 stable	ACR: Up- miR-10a Down- miR-10b & miR-210
23131772 (*Transplantation*)	Ben-Dov et al,[18] 2012	Biopsy tissue (RNAlater)	RNA Seq	Global	Sequencing by synthesis Taqman miRNA	Illumina / Applied Biosystems/ThermoFisher	3 IFTA & 4 normal / 10 IFTA & 8 normal	IFTA: 9 miRNAs up & 0 miRNAs down / IFTA up: miR-21, miR-21*, & miR-142-3p
23469132 (*PLoS One*)	Glowacki, 2013	Serum	PCR	Targeted	Taqman miRNA	Applied Biosystems/ThermoFisher	42 IFTA	Severe IFTA: up- miR-21
23511211 (*Transplantation*)	Wilflingseder, 2013	Biopsy tissue (FFPE)	Microarray	Global	GeneChip	Affymetrix/ThermoFisher	10 stable, 14 DGF, 30 ACR, 11 ABMR	DGF vs stable: 7 miRNAs up & 0 down / ACR vs stable: 4 miRNAs up & 18 down / ABMR vs stable: 6 miRNAs up & 0 down
24025639 (*Kidney Int*)	Maluf, 2014	Urine cells	Microarray	Global	GeneChip	Affymetrix/ThermoFisher	IFTA 10 & 12 normal	Differential expression: 22 miRNAs
			PCR	Targeted	Taqman miRNA	Applied Biosystems/ThermoFisher	IFTA 7 & normal 10	IFTA: up- miR-142-3p, down- miR-125b, miR-203, miR-204, & miR-211
			PCR	Targeted	Taqman miRNA	Applied Biosystems/ThermoFisher	Longitudinal: 41 good graft function & 25 poor graft function	Differential expression: miR-99a, miR-140-3p, miR-142-3p, miR-200*, & miR-200b

24731148 (Am J Transplant)	Li, 2014	Plasma	PCR	Targeted	Taqman miRNA	Applied Biosystems/ThermoFisher	31 BK viremia & 15 normal	BK viremia: up- bkv-miR-B1-5p & bkv-miR-B1-3p
25659925 (Exp Cell Res)	Liu, 2015	Biopsy tissue	RNA-Seq	Global	Pyrosequencing	454 Life Sciences/Roche	15 AR & 15 normal	Differential expression: 75 miRNAs
				Targeted	Taqman miRNA	Applied Biosystems/ThermoFisher		PCR done for miR-10b AR: down- miR-10b
26002284 (Transp Immunol)	Soltaninejad, 2015	Biopsy tissue (RNAlater)	PCR	Targeted	Taqman miRNA	Applied Biosystems/ThermoFisher	17 TCMR & 18 no rejection	TCMR: up- miR-142-5p, miR-142-3p, miR-155, & miR-223
		PBMC	PCR	Targeted	Taqman miRNA			TCMR: up- miR-142-3p & miR-223
26154388 (Transplantation)	Vitalone, 2015	Biopsy tissue	PCR	Targeted	Taqman miRNA	ThermoFisher	29 AR & 68 no AR	AR: up- miR-25, & miR-142-3p, & miR-342-3p. Down- miR-10b, miR-181a, miR-192, miR-204, miR-215, & miR-615-3p
26734715 (PLoS One)	MgGuinness, 2016	Biopsy tissue (pretransplant, RNAlater)	PCR	Targeted	Taqman miRNA	Applied Biosystems/ThermoFisher	27 DGF 67 no DGF	DGF: down- miR-125b & miR-217
26444957 (Transplantation)	Matz, 2016	Whole blood (PAXgene tube)	Microarray	Global	miRXplore microarray	Miltenyi Biotec	4 TMVR & 4 stable	Differential expression: 23 miRNAs
			PCR	Targeted	Taqman miRNA	Life Technologies/ThermoFisher	PCR: 24 TMVR & 137 all other diagnoses	TMVR: down- miR-15a, miR-15b, miR-16, miR-103a, miR-106a, & miR-107

(continued on next page)

Table 1
(continued)

PMID (Journal)	First Author, Year	Specimen	Profiling Technique	Targeted or Global Profiling	Platform	Company	Patients/Diagnosis	Major Findings
27663089 (*Transpl Immunol*)	Matz, 2016	Plasma	PCR	Targeted	Taqman miRNA	Life Technologies/ThermoFisher	39 TCMR & 40 stable	TCMR: down- miR-15b, miR-103a, & miR-106a
27521993 (*Clin Biochem*)	Vahed, 2017	Urine cells	PCR	Targeted	Stem loop primers/iCycler iQ system	Bio-Rad	23 IFTA, 24 stable, & 15 non-Tx healthy	IFTA (vs non-Tx healthy): up- miR-21 & miR-142-3p Down- miR-200b
27323802 (*Biomarkers*)	Iwasaki, 2017	PBMC	Microarray	Global	miRCURY LNA microarray	Exiqon/Qiagen	11 Normal, 11 DSA + normal, 6 DSA + w/ graft dysfunction (RNA pooled in each group)	Differential expression: 9 miRNAs
				Targeted	Taqman miRNA	Applied Biosystems/ThermoFisher		Normal: up- miR-142-5p
				Targeted	Taqman miRNA	Applied Biosystems/ThermoFisher	22 Normal, 10 subclinical cABMR, 13 DSA + w/ no graft dysfunction w/ other histology, 9 clinical cABMR	Clinical cABMR: up- miR-486-5p
28380212 (*Braz J Med Biol Res*)	Domenico, 2017	PBMC Urine cells	PCR	Targeted Targeted	Taqman miRNA Taqman miRNA	Applied Biosystems/ThermoFisher	23 AR, 18 ATN, 8 stable	ATN: up- miR-142-3p ATN: up- miR-142-3p

PMID (Journal)	Author, Year	Sample	Method		Platform	Vendor	Samples	Findings
28455659 (Int Urol Nephrol)	Vahed, 2017	Plasma	PCR	Targeted	miRCURY LNA	Exiqon/Qiagen	26 IFTA & 27 stable	IFTA: up- miR-21, miR-142-3p, & miR-155
28880456 (Br J Clin Pharmacol)	Milan, 2017	Urine cells	PCR	Targeted	miRCURY LNA Roche LightCycler 480	Exiqon/Qiagen Roche	8 AR & 72 no AR	AR: up- miR-142-3p & miR-155-5p Down- miR-210-3p
29267352 (PLoS One)	Kim, 2017	Urine exosomes	PCR	Targeted	Taqman miRNA	Applied Biosystems/ ThermoFisher	13 BK virus nephropathy & 67 other histology	BK virus nephropathy: up- bkv-miR-B1-5p
29518695 (J Clin Virol)	Virtanen, 2018	Plasma	PCR	Targeted	Taqman miRNA	Applied Biosystems/ ThermoFisher	9 BK viremia (serial samples) & 2 normal	BK viremia: up- bkv-miR-B1-5p & bkv-miR-B1-3p

Abbreviations: ABMR, antibody mediated rejection; ACR, acute cellular rejection; cABMR, chronic antibody-mediated rejection; DGF, delayed graft function; DSA, donor-specific antibodies; FFPE, formalin-fixed paraffin embedded; IFTA, interstitial fibrosis and tubular atrophy; PMID, PubMed identifier; TCMR, T-cell–mediated rejection; TMVR, T-cell–mediated vascular rejection; Tx, transplant.

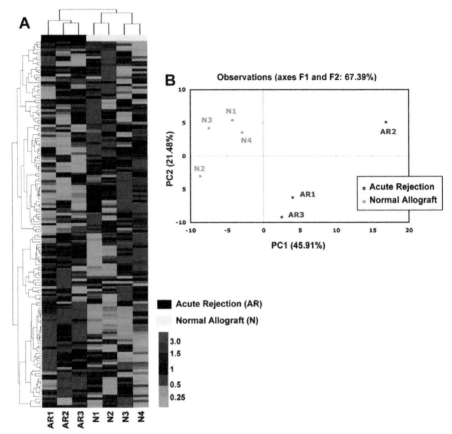

Fig. 2. Clustering analysis of miRNA expression differentiates AR biopsies from normal allograft biopsies of human kidney allografts. Unsupervised hierarchical clustering (*A*) and principal component analysis (*B*) of miRNA expression in 7 human kidney allograft biopsies (3 AR and 4 normal) were examined using TLDA. Two major clusters accurately divided the AR biopsies from normal allograft biopsies. Principal component analysis confirmed the separation of AR samples from normal allograft biopsies. (*From* Anglicheau D, Sharma VK, Ding R, et al. MicroRNA expression profiles predictive of human renal allograft status. Proc Natl Acad Sci U S A 2009;106(13):5331; with permission.)

of PBMCs or HRECs altered the level of expression of miRNAs. They found that the miRNAs overexpressed in AR biopsies (miR-142-5p, miR-155, and miR-223) were all expressed at a higher level in normal human PBMCs compared with miRNAs underexpressed in AR biopsies (miR-30a-3p, miR-10b, or let-7c). Stimulation of PBMCs with the mitogen phytohemagglutinin (PHA) resulted in an increase in the abundance of miR-155 and a decrease in miR-223, let-7c, or miR-142-5p. Quantification of miRNAs in primary cultures of HRECs showed that miR-30a-3p, miR-10b, or let-7c is expressed at a higher level in HRECs compared with PBMCs, and that stimulation of HRECs with cell-free supernatants of PHA-activated PBMCs results in a decrease in the abundance of miR-30a-3p. The authors' in vitro studies suggest the possibility that the altered expression of miRNAs in AR biopsies may be due to the altered regulation of miRNAs within the infiltrating immune cells and the resident kidney parenchymal cells themselves.[17]

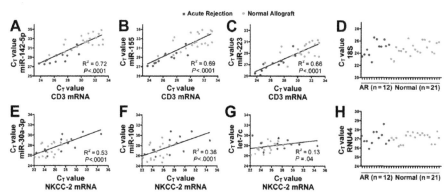

Fig. 3. Positive association between miRNAs and mRNAs in human kidney allograft biopsies. The relationship between the intragraft levels of miRNA and mRNA is shown. A strong positive association between the levels of CD3 mRNA and the levels of miRNAs overexpressed in AR biopsies was found: (*A*) miR-142-5p; (*B*) miR-155; or (*C*) miR-223. A positive association between kidney tubule-specific NKCC-2 mRNA and miRNAs underexpressed in AR biopsies was also observed: (*E*) miR-30a-3p; (*F*) miR-10b; or (*G*) let-7c. The mean (± standard deviation) C_T values of the endogenous control for mRNAs (18S rRNA) (*D*) and for miRNAs (RNU44 small nucleolar RNA) (*H*) were similar between the groups. (*From* Anglicheau D, Sharma VK, Ding R, et al. MicroRNA expression profiles predictive of human renal allograft status. Proc Natl Acad Sci U S A 2009;106(13):5332; with permission.)

In the first study of human kidney allograft biopsy miRNA sequencing,[18] the authors characterized the miRNA expression profiles of 3 biopsies with fibrosis and 4 normal allograft biopsies using barcoded deep-sequencing of a cDNA library prepared from multiplexed RNA by the method developed by Hafner and colleagues.[26,27] Among the differentially expressed miRNAs, 2 sequence families (miR-21 and miR-142-3p) showed expression exceeding 0.1% of total miRNA, suggesting that they may be causally involved in the fibrotic process.[18] Inspection of kidney miRNA profiles in relation to profiles obtained from kidney cell lines, PBMCs, and cultured fibroblasts suggested that occurrence of miR-142-3p in fibrosis samples is due to leukocyte infiltration, whereas miR-21 is likely upregulated in kidney parenchymal cells (**Fig. 4**). The authors used an independent cohort of 18 kidney-transplant recipients (10 fibrosis and 8 normal) to validate, by targeted PCR assay, a subset of differentially expressed miRNAs identified by global profiling.

IDENTIFYING microRNA TARGETS

There are 2 ways in which targets of miRNAs are identified: computational methods and experimental methods. Computational methods rely on the identification of phylogenetically conserved matches to the miRNA seed sequence.[34] Different miRNA-target prediction algorithms predict targets with different techniques and criteria, such as base pairing, target accessibility, and evolutionary conservation of target site.[35] Once targets are predicted, the next step is to infer the miRNA functions. Computational methods to reveal functions of miRNAs involve annotating the functions of miRNA through functional enrichment analysis using their target mRNA; identifying the coexpressed miRNA/mRNA groups, either at the sequence level or by integrating sequence and expression profiles of miRNAs and mRNAs; and inferring functional miRNA-mRNA regulatory modules, which are regulatory networks of miRNAs and their target mRNAs in specific biological processes.[35] Experimental methods

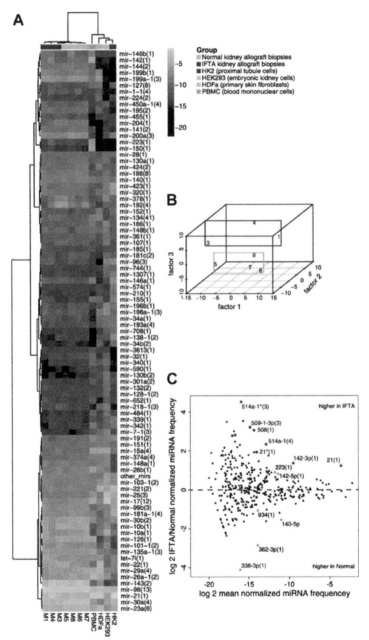

Fig. 4. MiRNA profiles generated by small RNA sequencing distinguish human kidney allograft biopsies with fibrosis from normal allograft biopsies. FDR, False Discovery Rate; MA plot, MA plot should be called as such. M stands for log-intensity ratios (M-values) and A stands for log-intensity averages (A-values). It is traditionally called as MA plot and not by any other name. This figure depicts the miRNA profiles generated by small RNA sequencing. (*A*) Hierarchical clustering and heat map representation of kidney allograft biopsies with fibrosis (IFTA, interstitial fibrosis and tubular atrophy) and normal allograft biopsies, human PBMC, HDFa (primary skin fibroblast), HEK293 cells (human embryonic

```
Forward: Score: 140.000000  Q:2 to 9  R:10 to 32 Align Len (7) (100.00%) (100.00%)

  miR-21:      3' cagttgtagtcagacTATTCGAt 5'
                                |||||||
  SMAD7:       5' tgtttagactt taacATAAGCTa 3'

  Energy:  -8.980000 kCal/Mol

Scores for this hit:
>sf-hsa-miR-21(1)    slc5941 chr18  140.00    -8.98    2 9  10 32    7   100.00%   100.00%
```

Fig. 5. miRNA target identification. SMAD7 was identified as an miR-21 target by querying a published Argonaute PAR-CLIP. Dataset: aligned and scored by the miRanda algorithm (microrna.org). Colored "t" represents a position found to be cross-linked according to PAR-CLIP T to C transition signature. (*From* Ben-Dov IZ, Muthukumar T, Morozov P, et al. MicroRNA sequence profiles of human kidney allografts with or without tubulointerstitial fibrosis. Transplantation 2012;94(11):1086–94; with permission.)

are based on immunoprecipitation of the miRNA effector complex, followed by sequencing-based identification of its interacting RNAs. Cross-linking immunoprecipitation (CLIP) methods involve UV irradiation of tissues, organisms, or cells, for covalently cross-linking miRNA targets to the Argonaute proteins. The cross-linked RNAs are reduced in size, amplified by PCR, and then sequenced for the identification of Argonaute tags that contain miRNA binding sites on target mRNAs. One such method for human cell lines, photoactivatable ribonucleoside-enhanced cross-linking and immunoprecipitation (PAR-CLIP), is based on the incorporation of photoreactive ribonucleoside analogues into nascent RNA transcripts by living cells. Irradiation of the cells induces cross-linking of photoreactive nucleoside-labeled cellular RNAs to interacting RNA-binding proteins. Immunoprecipitation of RNA-binding proteins of interest is followed by isolation of the cross-linked and coimmunoprecipitated RNA, which is sequenced.[36]

In the authors' miRNA sequencing of kidney allograft biopsies with fibrosis, they focused on miR-21 and searched for possible targets among transcripts that were coimmunoprecipitated with Argonaute 1 to 4 (*EIF2C1-4*) proteins. The authors queried a published dataset of mRNA clusters from pooled PAR-CLIP experiments on FLAG/HA-tagged Argonaute proteins in human embryonic kidney HEK293 cells for miR-21 binding sites. They found enrichment for 7-mer (ATAAGCT) and 8-mer (GATAAGCT) seed-complementary sequences of miR-21 and identified SMAD7 as an miR-21 target[18] (**Fig. 5**). SMAD7 has been shown to inhibit the fibrotic effect of transforming growth factor-β (TGF-β), a potent fibrogenic cytokine involved in repair following tissue injury, by blocking SMAD2 activation. This finding provides further credence to a TGF-β-centric hypothesis in the pathogenesis of chronic nephropathy/rejection (manifested histologically as interstitial fibrosis and tubular atrophy) of the kidney allograft.[37,38] In this hypothesis, which integrates immune and nonimmune events in the pathogenesis of allograft fibrosis, TGF-β represents a critical and self-perpetuating event for the progressive damage to the kidney allograft and attendant decline in graft function.[37,38]

---

kidney cells), and HK2 cells (kidney proximal tubule cells) according to merged miRNA profiles. (*B*) Multidimensional scaling showing separation of IFTA biopsies from normal biopsies. (*C*) MA plot showing the differentially expressed miRNA sequence families. Colored data points represent $P<.05$ (red points signify in addition false discovery rate adjusted $P<0.1$). (*From* Ben-Dov IZ, Muthukumar T, Morozov P, et al. MicroRNA sequence profiles of human kidney allografts with or without tubulointerstitial fibrosis. Transplantation 2012;94(11):1089; with permission.)

SUMMARY

miRNAs have emerged as robust molecular markers for assessing human kidney allograft status. In addition, miRNA expression patterns have provided mechanistic insights for kidney allograft dysfunction and are attractive targets for intervention. However, several challenges remain before they can be applied for managing kidney transplant recipients. Similar to the multicenter Clinical Trials in Organ Transplantation 04 that validated urinary cell mRNA profiles for diagnosing AR of kidney allograft,[39] large, well-designed, multicenter trials are needed to assess the usefulness of miRNAs in clinical organ transplantation. The authors are optimistic of the progress thus far and anticipate clinical trials for testing miRNA-based management strategies in kidney transplant recipients.

REFERENCES

1. Ha M, Kim VN. Regulation of microRNA biogenesis. Nat Rev Mol Cell Biol 2014; 15(8):509–24.
2. Ambros V, Bartel B, Bartel DP, et al. A uniform system for microRNA annotation. RNA 2003;9(3):277–9.
3. Desvignes T, Batzel P, Berezikov E, et al. miRNA nomenclature: a view incorporating genetic origins, biosynthetic pathways, and sequence variants. Trends Genet 2015;31(11):613–26.
4. Cai X, Hagedorn CH, Cullen BR. Human microRNAs are processed from capped, polyadenylated transcripts that can also function as mRNAs. RNA 2004;10(12): 1957–66.
5. Yi R, Qin Y, Macara IG, et al. Exportin-5 mediates the nuclear export of pre-microRNAs and short hairpin RNAs. Genes Dev 2003;17(24):3011–6.
6. Wahid F, Shehzad A, Khan T, et al. MicroRNAs: synthesis, mechanism, function, and recent clinical trials. Biochim Biophys Acta 2010;1803(11):1231–43.
7. Vidigal JA, Ventura A. The biological functions of miRNAs: lessons from in vivo studies. Trends Cell Biol 2015;25(3):137–47.
8. He L, Hannon GJ. MicroRNAs: small RNAs with a big role in gene regulation. Nat Rev Genet 2004;5(7):522–31.
9. Anglicheau D, Muthukumar T, Suthanthiran M. MicroRNAs: small RNAs with big effects. Transplantation 2010;90(2):105–12.
10. Turchinovich A, Tonevitsky AG, Burwinkel B. Extracellular miRNA: a collision of two paradigms. Trends Biochem Sci 2016;41(10):883–92.
11. Benes V, Castoldi M. Expression profiling of microRNA using real-time quantitative PCR, how to use it and what is available. Methods 2010;50(4):244–9.
12. de Planell-Saguer M, Rodicio MC. Analytical aspects of microRNA in diagnostics: a review. Anal Chim Acta 2011;699(2):134–52.
13. Chen C, Ridzon DA, Broomer AJ, et al. Real-time quantification of microRNAs by stem-loop RT-PCR. Nucleic Acids Res 2005;33(20):e179.
14. Shi R, Chiang VL. Facile means for quantifying microRNA expression by real-time PCR. Biotechniques 2005;39(4):519–25.
15. Schmittgen TD, Livak KJ. Analyzing real-time PCR data by the comparative C(T) method. Nat Protoc 2008;3(6):1101–8.
16. Muthukumar T, Dadhania D, Ding R, et al. Messenger RNA for FOXP3 in the urine of renal-allograft recipients. N Engl J Med 2005;353(22):2342–51.
17. Anglicheau D, Sharma VK, Ding R, et al. MicroRNA expression profiles predictive of human renal allograft status. Proc Natl Acad Sci U S A 2009;106(13):5330–5.

18. Ben-Dov IZ, Muthukumar T, Morozov P, et al. MicroRNA sequence profiles of human kidney allografts with or without tubulointerstitial fibrosis. Transplantation 2012;94(11):1086–94.
19. Hindson CM, Chevillet JR, Briggs HA, et al. Absolute quantification by droplet digital PCR versus analog real-time PCR. Nat Methods 2013;10(10):1003–5.
20. Obernosterer G, Martinez J, Alenius M. Locked nucleic acid-based in situ detection of microRNAs in mouse tissue sections. Nat Protoc 2007;2(6):1508–14.
21. Nielsen BS. MicroRNA in situ hybridization. Methods Mol Biol 2012;822:67–84.
22. Liu CG, Calin GA, Volinia S, et al. MicroRNA expression profiling using microarrays. Nat Protoc 2008;3(4):563–78.
23. Wang Z, Gerstein M, Snyder M. RNA-Seq: a revolutionary tool for transcriptomics. Nat Rev Genet 2009;10(1):57–63.
24. Hafner M, Landgraf P, Ludwig J, et al. Identification of microRNAs and other small regulatory RNAs using cDNA library sequencing. Methods 2008;44(1):3–12.
25. Dard-Dascot C, Naquin D, d'Aubenton-Carafa Y, et al. Systematic comparison of small RNA library preparation protocols for next-generation sequencing. BMC Genomics 2018;19(1):118.
26. Hafner M, Renwick N, Brown M, et al. RNA-ligase-dependent biases in miRNA representation in deep-sequenced small RNA cDNA libraries. RNA 2011;17(9):1697–712.
27. Hafner M, Renwick N, Farazi TA, et al. Barcoded cDNA library preparation for small RNA profiling by next-generation sequencing. Methods 2012;58(2):164–70.
28. Illumina. In-depth NGS introduction. Available at: https://www.illumina.com/science/technology/next-generation-sequencing.html. Accessed August 10, 2018.
29. Haas M, Loupy A, Lefaucheur C, et al. The Banff 2017 Kidney Meeting Report: revised diagnostic criteria for chronic active T cell-mediated rejection, antibody-mediated rejection, and prospects for integrative endpoints for next-generation clinical trials. Am J Transplant 2018;18(2):293–307.
30. Anglicheau D, Suthanthiran M. Noninvasive prediction of organ graft rejection and outcome using gene expression patterns. Transplantation 2008;86(2):192–9.
31. Hamdorf M, Kawakita S, Everly M. The potential of MicroRNAs as novel biomarkers for transplant rejection. J Immunol Res 2017;2017:4072364.
32. Tomuleasa C, Fuji S, Cucuianu A, et al. MicroRNAs as biomarkers for graft-versus-host disease following allogeneic stem cell transplantation. Ann Hematol 2015;94(7):1081–92.
33. Mas VR, Dumur CI, Scian MJ, et al. MicroRNAs as biomarkers in solid organ transplantation. Am J Transplant 2013;13(1):11–9.
34. Seitz H. Issues in current microRNA target identification methods. RNA Biol 2017;14(7):831–4.
35. Liu B, Li J, Cairns MJ. Identifying miRNAs, targets and functions. Brief Bioinform 2014;15(1):1–19.
36. Hafner M, Landthaler M, Burger L, et al. PAR-CliP–a method to identify transcriptome-wide the binding sites of RNA binding proteins. J Vis Exp 2010;(41) [pii:2034].
37. Sharma VK, Bologa RM, Xu GP, et al. Intragraft TGF-beta 1 mRNA: a correlate of interstitial fibrosis and chronic allograft nephropathy. Kidney Int 1996;49(5):1297–303.
38. Muthukumar T, Lee JR, Dadhania DM, et al. Allograft rejection and tubulointerstitial fibrosis in human kidney allografts: interrogation by urinary cell mRNA profiling. Transplant Rev (Orlando) 2014;28(3):145–54.
39. Suthanthiran M, Schwartz JE, Ding R, et al. Urinary-cell mRNA profile and acute cellular rejection in kidney allografts. N Engl J Med 2013;369(1):20–31.

Biomarkers in Fetomaternal Tolerance

Sudipta Tripathi, PhD[a], Indira Guleria, PhD, D(ABHI)[b],*

KEYWORDS

- Biomarkers • Allograft • Fetomaternal tolerance • Tregs • Bregs • MDSCs • miRNA

KEY POINTS

- Acceptance of the fetus expressing allogeneic paternal antigens by the mother is a physiologic model of transplantation tolerance.
- The fetus is not rejected, suggesting that certain tolerance mechanisms are in place to achieve successful pregnancy.
- A majority of the studies to understand the mechanism of allograft acceptance during pregnancy have focused on immune mediators presented locally at the uteroplacental interface.
- Research on identifying biomarkers for fetomaternal tolerance in the peripheral blood is only beginning and regulatory T cells, regulatory B cells, and myeloid-derived suppressor cells have emerged as potential candidates.
- An ideal biomarker would be a noninvasive protein signature in the blood that correlates with pregnancy outcomes.

INTRODUCTION

The fetus represents a foreign entity to the maternal immune system, yet this "natural" allograft is not normally rejected, thereby indicating the existence of active tolerance mechanisms that prevent rejection. Different mechanisms have been proposed to account for tolerance at the fetomaternal interface (FMI). Molecules involved in apoptosis of maternal leukocytes and negative signals delivered to activated T cells by regulatory costimulatory pathways, which can also act as natural inhibitors for effector T-cell expansion, have been shown critical for maintaining tolerance at the FMI in murine models of allogeneic pregnancy. A balance between anti-inflammatory cytokines, such as transforming growth factor (TGF)-β; interleukin (IL)-10; and proinflammatory

Disclosure Statement: The authors have nothing to disclose.

[a] Transplantation Research Center, Harvard Medical School, LMRC #316, 221 Longwood Avenue, Boston, MA 02115, USA; [b] HLA Tissue Typing Laboratory, Renal Transplant Program, Division of Renal Medicine, Transplantation Research Center, Harvard Medical School, Brigham and Women's Hospital, 75 Francis Street, PBB 161G, Boston, MA 02115, USA
* Corresponding author.
E-mail address: iguleria@bics.bwh.harvard.edu

cytokines, such as IL-17, and suppression of immune response by regulatory immune cells, such as regulatory T cells (Tregs) and myeloid-derived suppressor cells (MDSCs), seems to play an important role in maintaining successful pregnancy in both mice and humans. This review summarizes the data on regulatory cells, cytokines, and costimulatory molecules and discusses the status of new candidates, such as exosomes and microRNAs (miRNAs), as potential biomarkers to predict successful or unfavorable pregnancy outcomes.

FETOMATERNAL CROSS-TALK

Fetomaternal cross-talk at the tissue level occurs in the placenta. The placenta is composed of both fetal cells and maternal cells. Extravillous trophoblasts (EVTs), the cells of fetal origin, interact with the decidual cells of maternal origin and modulate the tolerance at the FMI. The EVTs uniquely express HLA-G, a nonclassical major histocompatibility complex class I molecule.[1] HLA-G plays an important role in embryo implantation and establishment of tolerance at the FMI by promoting a tolerogenic decidual natural killer cell (dNK) population during interaction between the EVTs and dNK cells.[2] HLA-G is also known to modulate the immune response of decidual macrophages, T cells, and B cells during pregnancy.[2] Decidual cells express Fas ligand, which contributes toward the maintenance of tolerance by inducing apoptosis of infiltrating leukocytes that express Fas receptor.[3]

DYSFUNCTION AT THE FETOMATERNAL INTERFACE RESULTS IN FETAL LOSS

Decidualization of the human endometrium is essential for the establishment of successful pregnancy. Decidualization controls the invasion of trophoblasts and generates the FMI.[4] Tolerance to the fetus is maintained at the FMI by the interactions between the cells of fetal and maternal origin. Dysfunction at the FMI results in impaired fetal development or loss. This has been attributed to poor trophoblast invasion and/or dysregulated placental function. Cellular stress within the placenta increases the release of several factors into the maternal circulation. Many of these factors can be detected in the peripheral circulation and may serve as surrogate markers of loss of tolerance at the FMI. Dysregulated cellular interactions at the FMI release soluble factors. Factors released in the early stage may differ from those released in the late stages of pregnancy. This should be taken into consideration while evaluating possible surrogate candidates for biomarkers of tolerance of the fetus. Expression levels of both HLA-G and Fas ligand can be predictive of successful immunoregulation at the FMI. Circulating levels of either of these molecules, however, in the periphery may not predicate the interactions at the FMI.

IMPLANTATION WINDOW, DECIDUALIZATION, AND INFLUX OF SPECIFIC IMMUNE CELLS

Endometrial receptivity primarily driven by hormones during implantation window can be detected by specific expression patterns of integrins, mucins, osteopontin, and heparin-binding epidermal growth factor–like growth factor.[5] There is also a customized transcriptomic signature of 238 endometrial receptivity–related genes available that can be used as a diagnostic tool.[6] This unique transcriptomic signature can be valuable in treatment of recurrent implantation failure.

Implantation followed by decidualization provides nutritional support and controlled invasion of trophoblast.[7] These 2 events lead to an influx of specific cell types like monocytes and macrophages and an abundance of natural killer (NK) cells.[8] These immune cells, specifically uterine macrophages and uterine NK cells, play a key role in the successful implantation and decidualization of the embryo.[9] For example, both uterine macrophages and uterine NK cells together with uterine dendritic cells (DCs) are known to be important in establishment and maintenance of the state of tolerance toward the fetus.

NATURAL KILLER CELLS

Accumulation of a unique subset of NK cells in the decidua is associated with early stages of pregnancy in both humans and mice. These dNK cells are devoid of cytotoxic properties and secrete large amounts of cytokines, chemokines, and angiogenic factors, which play an important role in establishing successful placentation and vascular remodeling, thus underscoring that these factors play a pivotal role in successful pregnancy.[10-12] The dNK cells are known to interact with several other decidual cell populations and create a microenvironment of immune regulation conducive to maintenance of tolerance at the FMI. Absence or depletion of dNK cells is associated with fetal loss both in mice and humans. The authors have shown that a change in the phenotype of the dNK cells of mice results in dysregulation of tolerance to the fetus in mice.[13] Furthermore, it has been reported by Fu and colleagues[14] that dNK cells promote immune tolerance and successful pregnancy by dampening inflammatory type 17 helper T cells (T_H17) via interferon (IFN)-γ secreted by the CD56[bright]CD27[+] NK subset. This NK cell–mediated regulatory response is lost in patients who experience recurrent spontaneous abortions and exhibit a prominent T_H17 response and extensive local inflammation. This local inflammatory response further affects the regulatory function of NK cells, leading to the eventual loss of maternal-fetal tolerance. Furthermore, dNK cells can regulate tolerance at the FMI also by interacting with DCs and Tregs.[15-17] Recently, a novel CD49a[+]Eomes[+] subset of NK cells that secreted growth-promoting factors, including pleiotrophin and osteoglycin, was identified in both humans and mice. It was shown that interaction between HLA-G and dNK cell receptor Ig-like transcript 2 helps promote the ability of CD49a[+]Eomes[+] NK cells to secrete growth-promoting factors. Adoptive transfer of induced CD49a[+]Eomes[+] NK cells was shown to reverse impaired fetal growth and rebuild an appropriate local microenvironment.[18]

Although it is evident from literature that dNK cells are one of the most important regulators of tolerance at the FMI, the change in the influx of dNK at the FMI is not reflected in the periphery and is not a reliable biomarker of tolerance.

MACROPHAGES

Decidual macrophages are the dominant professional antigen-presenting cells in the decidua, comprising 20% to 30% of the local leukocyte population. Owing to their remarkable phenotypic plasticity, decidual macrophages can participate in diverse activities during pregnancy.[19] At baseline, decidual macrophages are characterized by an immunosuppressive phenotype and polarization toward the M2 phenotype that supports fetomaternal tolerance.[20] Their function, however, is not restricted to immune tolerance and extends to those, such as recognition and clearance of infection, clearance of apoptotic debris, and tissue remodeling. Decidual macrophages largely function as tissue-resident macrophages that are crucial for maintaining homeostasis and reproductive success.[21,22] Two distinct subsets of CD14[+] decidual macrophages have been identified in first-trimester decidual tissue, namely CD11c[hi] and CD11c[lo], among which the CD11c[hi] subset is likely to be the major antigen-presenting cells in the decidua.[23] A more recent study has identified 3 decidual macrophage subsets. These subsets are CCR2-CD11c[lo] (CD11c[low], approximately 80%), CCR2-CD11c[hi]

(CD11c^{high}, approximately 5%), and CCR2$^+$CD11c^{hi} (CD11c^{high}, 10%–15%), which maintain an inflammatory balance at the leading edge of trophoblast invasion during the first trimester of human pregnancy to facilitate the clearance of pathogen infection as well as maintain the homeostasis of the FMI.[24] Various molecular mechanisms by which decidual macrophages maintain tolerance have been described. Decidual macrophages are able to suppress T-cell IFN-γ production via B7-H1:PD-1 interactions.[25] Interactions with HLA-G[26] and decidua-derived vascular endothelial growth factor from endometrial stromal cells are other mechanisms by which decidual macrophages contribute to the maintenance of tolerance at the FMI.[27] Similar to dNK cells, however, the effects of decidual macrophages are confined to the local FMI milieu and not reflected in the periphery, thereby preventing any noninvasive method to detect the regulation of tolerance at the FMI by these cells.

MYELOID-DERIVED SUPPRESSOR CELLS

MDSCs have been described and characterized in human decidua. These cells express a CD33$^+$ HLA-DR$^-$ phenotype; secrete inducible nitric oxide synthase, arginase, and indoleamine dioxygenase; and are capable of suppressing T-cell proliferation.[28] Decidual and peripheral MDSC populations are also associated with tolerance to the fetus. In patients with fetal loss, a decrease in functionally suppressive MDSC cell population was observed in both endometrium and peripheral blood.[29] Also it has been shown that granulocytic MDSCs (G-MDSCs), a CD15$^+$ subset of MDSCs with granulocytic-like characteristics,[30,31] maintain fetomaternal tolerance by inducing Foxp3 expression in Tregs in humans.[32] Similar observations in mice demonstrate that G-MDSCs expand rapidly in the uteri of mice during normal healthy pregnancy, and their frequency is reduced in models of spontaneous fetal loss.[32] Other studies also show the role of MDSCs in maintenance of tolerance at the FMI in mice. For instance, MDSCs expand in the decidua of pregnant mice, and depletion of MDSCs results in fetal loss.[33,34] MDSCs have pleiotropic effects and have been shown to affect T-cell proliferation,[35–37] regulate NK-cell cytotoxicity,[38–40] induce Treg cells in vivo,[41–43] and induce T-cell and/or Treg-cell apoptosis.[41] Some of the mechanisms by which MDSCs mediate immunosuppression are shown in **Fig. 1**. The existing data from literature suggest that it is possible to detect a change in the peripheral MDSC compartment that reflects the regulation/dysregulation of tolerance at the FMI. A more detailed phenotypic and functional characterization of the peripheral MDSC compartment, however, is necessary to define the subpopulations that most accurately reflect the changes at the FMI. It is also important to understand the accuracy of the correlation between maintenance of tolerance at the FMI and the changes in the periphery during different stages of pregnancy when a single marker is used as a predictor. This is due to the fact that cellular interactions in early and late stages of pregnancy differ greatly.

DENDRITIC CELLS

Uterine DCs are reported to have a potential trophic role in the peri-implantation period. Uterine DCs play a crucial role in embryo implantation and decidualization as shown in mice and are essential specifically during the implantation window.[44] In mice, 2 different subsets of uterine DCs are described. Both appear to be immature. In humans the uterine DCs appear to be mature and are predominantly of the myeloid DC type-2 subset.[45] A detailed discussion of the role of uterine DCs in establishing and maintaining tolerance at the FMI is described by Tagliani and Erlebacher.[46] Uterine DCs are a comparatively smaller cell population at the FMI and the population size

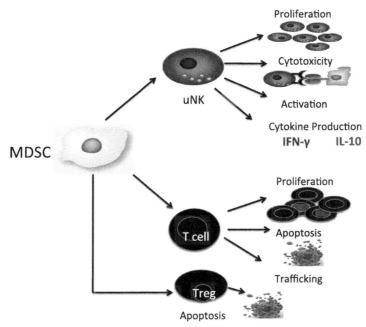

Fig. 1. Model for proposed MDSC-induced regulation of tolerance at FMI. MDSCs have the ability to affect the function of uterine NK (uNK) cells and T cells. MDSCs can regulate uNK cells by suppressing their proliferation, activation, cytotoxicity, and/or cytokine release. MDSCs can suppress the proliferation, apoptosis and/or trafficking of T cells. Any or all of these suppressive effects of MDSCs could be playing a role in maintaining tolerance at the FMI.

may or may not change substantially to predict dysregulation of tolerance. This cell population is not an ideal choice for a biomarker.

REGULATORY T CELLS

Although tolerance to fetus is attributed mostly to the molecular mechanisms occurring at the local FMI, peripheral Tregs also play a significant role in the maintenance of tolerance at the FMI. An extensive review of Tregs in pregnancy is discussed elsewhere.[47] It has been shown previously in humans that Tregs increase in the periphery during pregnancy and a deficit in number of Tregs leads to fetal loss both in mice and humans.[48,49] Adoptive transfer of Tregs has also been shown to prevent fetal loss both in mice and humans.[50,51] Maintenance of tolerance of the fetus by Tregs occurs mostly through the production of TGF-β and IL-10. It has also been shown that production of TGF-β and IL-10 is associated with high heme-oxygenase 1 (HO-1) and low IL-17 production at the FMI, leading to tolerance of the fetus.[50] Persistence of paternal antigens is involved in generation and expansion of Tregs.[52] Samstein and colleagues[53] have reported that peripheral Tregs expand in response to paternal antigens and eventually accumulate in the placenta. Furthermore, it has been reported that trophoblast cells also are involved in the generation and expansion of Tregs at the FMI.[22] Based on these studies, a simplistic diagram showing Treg-mediated immunosuppression is shown in **Fig. 2**. Although expansion of peripheral Tregs is associated with pregnancy, a direct reflection of dysregulation of tolerance at the FMI may not be predicted accurately from the change in the peripheral Treg

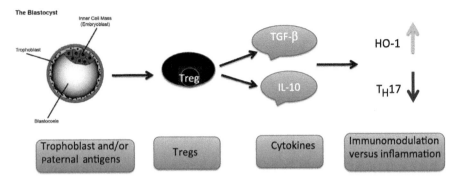

Fig. 2. Proposed model for Treg-mediated immunoregulation at the FMI. In response to paternal antigens and/trophoblasts, Tregs are induced locally as well as in the periphery. Tregs, via secretion of anti-inflammatory cytokines, TGF-β and IL-10, create an environment conducive to well-being of the fetus by modulating the secretion of anti-inflammatory molecule (HO-1) ([*upward green arrow*] up-regulation) and proinflammatory (T$_H$17) cells ([*upside-down red arrow*] down-regulation).

population. Tregs play a major role in the maintenance of fetomaternal tolerance but are not an ideal choice as a standalone biomarker.

REGULATORY B CELLS

Regulatory B cells (Bregs), as one of the major cellular sources of IL-10, play an important role in the maintenance of tolerance at the FMI. In mice, IL-10–secreting regulatory B10 cells increase during normal healthy pregnancy. These cells are capable of preventing fetal loss in murine models of spontaneous abortion.[54] IL-10–producing B cells have also been reported to increase in human pregnancy. These cells have been shown capable of suppressing CD4[+] T cells.[55] Furthermore, it has been shown that marginal zone B cells are induced and expanded only in normal healthy pregnancy.[56] The peripheral B-cell compartment undergoes quantitative changes late in normal pregnancy and postpartum and Bregs are present in significantly higher numbers in postpartum than in nonpregnant women.[57] Bregs contribute to the maintenance of tolerance at the FMI by secreting IL-10 as well as by interacting with Tregs and DCs. An endocrine-modulated feedback loop highlighting the Breg-Treg–tolerogenic DC interface for the induction of maternal immune tolerance has also been proposed.[58] Bregs in the periphery may reflect accurately the regulation of tolerance in late pregnancy and postpartum but not in the early stages.[57] This suggests that there is a distinct possibility that early stage biomarkers of tolerance dysregulation may be different from that of late-stage biomarkers. This also suggests that monitoring of a combination of Bregs, Tregs, and MDSC expansion during pregnancy together with other parameters may act as potential markers to predict fetal loss.

COSIGNALING MOLECULES

Cosignaling molecules (CTLA-4, PD-1/PDL-1, and T-cell immunoglobulin and mucin domain-containing 3 (TIM-3)) and other molecules like galectin, cytokines, miRNA, hormones (human chorionic gonadotropin), and complement have been found involved in maintaining tolerance at the FMI and assisting decidual vascular remodeling. It has been hypothesized that dysregulation of these molecules could lead to pregnancy complications and pregnancy loss.[59] The pregnancy hormone, human chorionic gonadotropin, determines fetal fate by regulating maternal innate and adaptive immune responses, thereby allowing the acceptance of the foreign fetal antigens.[60] Similarly, the PD1/PDL1 signaling pathway also regulates tolerance at FMI by maintaining equilibrium between the frequency of Tregs and T_H17 cells.[61] A more detailed discussion on the role of PD1/PDL1 pathway in pregnancy is discussed Tripathi and Guleria,[62] and Guleria and colleageus.[63] ICOS, another costimulatory molecule, promotes tolerance at the FMI by regulating CD8 effector T-cell responses.[64] (TIM-3) proteins have also been shown by the authors' group to be critical in maintaining fetomaternal tolerance by innate immune cells.[13,65]

Detailed analysis of expression levels of cosignaling molecules on various populations and subpopulations of cells during different stages of pregnancy may also reflect the status of tolerance regulation at the FMI. An assessment of tolerance, therefore, may involve conducting multiparametric analyses of cosignaling molecule expression and identifying the markers that reflect the changes at the FMI most accurately in the periphery. Furthermore, peripheral cytokine production profile can also be combined together to generate a multiparametric biomarker panel that predicts and reflects accurately the regulation/dysregulation of tolerance at the FMI. In line with this concept for a need to study a battery of biomarkers, a recent study suggests a positive role for Tregs, CTLA-4, and TGF-β and a negative role for IL-6, TNF-α, and T_H17 in fetomaternal tolerance.[66] These observations were made when comparing data obtained from peripheral blood samples from women with recurrent abortion versus healthy pregnant controls.

OTHER POTENTIAL CANDIDATES OF BIOMARKER (EXOSOMES AND microRNAs AS BIOMARKERS)

Circulating exosomes contain proteins and RNAs that are representative of the cell of origin, including surface and cytoplasmic protein, messenger RNA, and miRNA.[67] Exosomes have recently gained rapid recognition as biomarkers for various diseases, accurately predicting disease progression as well as monitoring therapies. During pregnancy, the placenta releases exosomes into the maternal circulation from as early as 6 weeks of gestation. Exosomes/extracellular vesicles of placental origin can be detected in a variety of body fluids, including urine and blood, and have been identified in the maternal circulation.[68] Moreover, the number of exosomes across gestation is higher in complications of pregnancies, such as preeclampsia and gestational diabetes mellitus, compared with normal pregnancies. Release of exosomes is regulated by factors that include both oxygen tension and glucose concentration and correlates with placental mass and perfusion. The concentration of placenta-derived exosomes in maternal plasma increases progressively during gestation. Exosomes isolated from maternal plasma are bioactive in vitro and are incorporated into target cells by endocytosis. Although the functional significance of placental exosomes in pregnancy remains to be fully elucidated, available data support a role in normal placental development and maternal immune tolerance. Changes in the release of placenta-derived and non–placenta-derived exosomes, their concentration in maternal plasma, composition, and bioactivity have been reported to be associated with pregnancy complications.[69] Specific placenta-derived exosomal material has been proposed to contribute to maintenance of tolerance at the FMI.[70] Monitoring exosomes, both in the amniotic fluid and the maternal peripheral circulation, may indicate the regulation of the immune tolerance at the FMI much more accurately than surrogate markers that partially reflect the changes.

Noninvasive biomarkers in maternal blood, such as circulating miRNAs, are promising molecules and have been shown to predict pregnancy disorders. miRNAs are noncoding short RNAs that regulate mRNA expression by repressing the translation or cleaving the transcript. miRNAs are released to the extracellular systemic circulation via exosomes. Specific placental miRNAs have been detected in maternal plasma in different ways depending on whether the pregnancy is normal or pathologic or if there is no pregnancy.[71] The miRNAs associated with human placenta were significantly elevated in sera from pregnant women, and their levels were shown to correlate with the stage of pregnancy.[72]

In addition to exosomes and miRNAs, measurement of ratio of maternal circulating angiogenesis biomarker soluble FMS-like tyrosine kinase-1 (sFlt-1) (an antiangiogenic factor)/placental growth factor (PIGF) (an angiogenic factor) can reflect the antiangiogenic balance that characterizes pregnancy disorder, such as incipient or overt preeclampsia. A meta-analysis suggested that sFlt-1/PIGF ratio is 80% sensitive in predicting preeclampsia in both high-risk and low-risk patients,[73] suggesting that the ratio can be a valuable biomarker.

Collectively the data point to the fact that circulating levels of certain exosomes, miRNAs, and antiangiogenic factors in the blood could predict fetal acceptance or rejection.

NONINVASIVE METHODS TO DETECT A BIOMARKER

Multiparameter immunophenotyping together with systems biology is currently used to identify and define immune signatures for various diseases. This may also be a possible approach to detect any surrogate change in the peripheral immune compartment that reflects the dysregulation of tolerance at the FMI.

An ideal biomarker should be a single parameter that can be detected noninvasively and can predict the outcome/endpoint of the disease or treatment with utmost accuracy. In fetomaternal tolerance, however, where multiple local interactions contribute to the maintenance of tolerance and are redundant, it is difficult to identify a single parameter in the peripheral circulation that absolutely reflects the changes at the FMI. In addition, the mechanisms of tolerance vary between different stages of pregnancy. Hence, efforts toward finding a robust biomarker(s) for fetal acceptance and rejection is challenging because biomarkers for tolerance during early pregnancy versus late pregnancy are likely different. Therefore, a multiparametric biomarker panel that can be detected in the peripheral circulation in early pregnancy and/or late pregnancy may be a better approach to finding a noninvasive method to predict the regulation/dysregulation of tolerance at the FMI.

SUMMARY

Review of the available data suggests that there is an enormous need to formulate new studies to further research in the area of noninvasive biomarkers for fetomaternal tolerance. Despite significant data on biomarkers in the local milieu (placenta and uterus), few studies have explored biomarkers in the periphery (blood and serum). Prospective studies, including serum and blood profiling, need to be undertaken to identify biomarkers of tolerance and rejection during pregnancy so that patients with pregnancy disorders, such as miscarriage and recurrent spontaneous abortion, can be managed better.

Once a panel of tolerogenic markers is identified and validated in a fetomaternal model, this panel could be tested in other models of solid organ transplant because published data suggest that the molecule and pathways in these 2 models overlap; hence, data from fetomaternal tolerance/pregnancy have the potential to be extrapolated to other transplant models.

REFERENCES

1. Kovats S, Main EK, Librach C, et al. A class I antigen, HLA-G, expressed in human trophoblasts. Science 1990;248:220–3.
2. Ferreira LMR, Meissner TB, Tilburgs T, et al. HLA-G: at the interface of maternal-fetal tolerance. Trends Immunol 2017;38:272–86.
3. Hunt JS, Vassmer D, Ferguson TA, et al. Fas ligand is positioned in mouse uterus and placenta to prevent trafficking of activated leukocytes between the mother and the conceptus. J Immunol 1997;158:4122–8.
4. Okada H, Tsuzuki T, Murata H. Decidualization of the human endometrium. Reprod Med Biol 2018;17:220–7.
5. Aghajanova L, Hamilton AE, Giudice LC. Uterine receptivity to human embryonic implantation: histology, biomarkers, and transcriptomics. Semin Cell Dev Biol 2008;19:204–11.
6. Koot YE, van Hooff SR, Boomsma CM, et al. An endometrial gene expression signature accurately predicts recurrent implantation failure after IVF. Sci Rep 2016;6:19411.
7. Wang H, Dey SK. Roadmap to embryo implantation: clues from mouse models. Nat Rev Genet 2006;7:185–99.
8. Lobo SC, Huang ST, Germeyer A, et al. The immune environment in human endometrium during the window of implantation. Am J Reprod Immunol 2004;52:244–51.
9. Hofmann AP, Gerber SA, Croy BA. Uterine natural killer cells pace early development of mouse decidua basalis. Mol Hum Reprod 2014;20:66–76.
10. Le Bouteiller P. Human decidual NK cells: unique and tightly regulated effector functions in healthy and pathogen-infected pregnancies. Front Immunol 2013;4:404.
11. Chaouat G. Inflammation, NK cells and implantation: friend and foe (the good, the bad and the ugly?): replacing placental viviparity in an evolutionary perspective. J Reprod Immunol 2013;97:2–13.
12. Jabrane-Ferrat N, Siewiera J. The up side of decidual natural killer cells: new developments in immunology of pregnancy. Immunology 2014;141:490–7.
13. Tripathi S, Chabtini L, Dakle PJ, et al. Effect of TIM-3 blockade on the immunophenotype and cytokine profile of murine uterine NK cells. PLoS One 2015;10:e0123439.
14. Fu B, Li X, Sun R, et al. Natural killer cells promote immune tolerance by regulating inflammatory TH17 cells at the human fetomaternal interface. Proc Natl Acad Sci U S A 2013;110:E231–40.
15. Leno-Duran E, Munoz-Fernandez R, Olivares EG, et al. Liaison between natural killer cells and dendritic cells in human gestation. Cell Mol Immunol 2014;11:449–55.
16. Sharma S. Natural killer cells and regulatory T cells in early pregnancy loss. Int J Dev Biol 2014;58:219–29.
17. Lash GE, Robson SC, Bulmer JN. Review: functional role of uterine natural killer (uNK) cells in human early pregnancy decidua. Placenta 2010;31(Suppl):S87–92.
18. Fu B, Zhou Y, Ni X, et al. Natural killer cells promote fetal development through the secretion of growth-promoting factors. Immunity 2017;47:1100–11013 e6.

19. Ning F, Liu H, Lash GE. The role of decidual macrophages during normal and pathological pregnancy. Am J Reprod Immunol 2016;75:298–309.

20. Nagamatsu T, Schust DJ. The contribution of macrophages to normal and pathological pregnancies. Am J Reprod Immunol 2010;63:460–71.

21. Brown MB, von Chamier M, Allam AB, et al. M1/M2 macrophage polarity in normal and complicated pregnancy. Front Immunol 2014;5:606.

22. Svensson-Arvelund J, Mehta RB, Lindau R, et al. The human fetal placenta promotes tolerance against the semiallogeneic fetus by inducing regulatory T cells and homeostatic M2 macrophages. J Immunol 2015;194:1534–44.

23. Houser BL, Tilburgs T, Hill J, et al. Two unique human decidual macrophage populations. J Immunol 2011;186:2633–42.

24. Jiang X, Du MR, Li M, et al. Three macrophage subsets are identified in the uterus during early human pregnancy. Cell Mol Immunol 2018;15:1027–37.

25. Sayama S, Nagamatsu T, Schust DJ, et al. Human decidual macrophages suppress IFN-gamma production by T cells through costimulatory B7-H1:PD-1 signaling in early pregnancy. J Reprod Immunol 2013;100:109–17.

26. Shakhawat A, Shaikly V, Elzatma E, et al. Interaction between HLA-G and monocyte/macrophages in human pregnancy. J Reprod Immunol 2010;85:40–6.

27. Wheeler KC, Jena MK, Pradhan BS, et al. VEGF may contribute to macrophage recruitment and M2 polarization in the decidua. PLoS One 2018;13:e0191040.

28. Bartmann C, Junker M, Segerer SE, et al. CD33(+)/HLA-DR(neg) and CD33(+)/HLA-DR(+/-) cells: rare populations in the human decidua with characteristics of MDSC. Am J Reprod Immunol 2016;75:539–56.

29. Nair RR, Sinha P, Khanna A, et al. Reduced myeloid-derived suppressor cells in the blood and endometrium is associated with early miscarriage. Am J Reprod Immunol 2015;73:479–86.

30. Kusmartsev S, Su Z, Heiser A, et al. Reversal of myeloid cell-mediated immunosuppression in patients with metastatic renal cell carcinoma. Clin Cancer Res 2008;14:8270–8.

31. Liu CY, Wang YM, Wang CL, et al. Population alterations of L-arginase- and inducible nitric oxide synthase-expressed CD11b+/CD14(-)/CD15+/CD33+ myeloid-derived suppressor cells and CD8+ T lymphocytes in patients with advanced-stage non-small cell lung cancer. J Cancer Res Clin Oncol 2010;136:35–45.

32. Kang X, Zhang X, Liu Z, et al. Granulocytic myeloid-derived suppressor cells maintain feto-maternal tolerance by inducing Foxp3 expression in CD4+CD25- T cells by activation of the TGF-beta/beta-catenin pathway. Mol Hum Reprod 2016;22:499–511.

33. Pan T, Liu Y, Zhong LM, et al. Myeloid-derived suppressor cells are essential for maintaining feto-maternal immunotolerance via STAT3 signaling in mice. J Leukoc Biol 2016;100:499–511.

34. Zhao H, Kalish F, Schulz S, et al. Unique roles of infiltrating myeloid cells in the murine uterus during early to midpregnancy. J Immunol 2015;194:3713–22.

35. Dardalhon V, Anderson AC, Karman J, et al. Tim-3/galectin-9 pathway: regulation of Th1 immunity through promotion of CD11b+Ly-6G+ myeloid cells. J Immunol 2010;185:1383–92.

36. Gabrilovich DI, Nagaraj S. Myeloid-derived suppressor cells as regulators of the immune system. Nat Rev Immunol 2009;9:162–74.

37. Bronte V, Serafini P, De Santo C, et al. IL-4-induced arginase 1 suppresses alloreactive T cells in tumor-bearing mice. J Immunol 2003;170:270–8.

38. Liu C, Yu S, Kappes J, et al. Expansion of spleen myeloid suppressor cells re-presses NK cell cytotoxicity in tumor-bearing host. Blood 2007;109:4336–42.

39. Hoechst B, Voigtlaender T, Ormandy L, et al. Myeloid derived suppressor cells inhibit natural killer cells in patients with hepatocellular carcinoma via the NKp30 receptor. Hepatology 2009;50:799–807.

40. Li H, Han Y, Guo Q, et al. Cancer-expanded myeloid-derived suppressor cells induce anergy of NK cells through membrane-bound TGF-beta 1. J Immunol 2009;182:240–9.

41. Huang B, Pan PY, Li Q, et al. Gr-1+CD115+ immature myeloid suppressor cells mediate the development of tumor-induced T regulatory cells and T-cell anergy in tumor-bearing host. Cancer Res 2006;66:1123–31.

42. Pan PY, Ma G, Weber KJ, et al. Immune stimulatory receptor CD40 is required for T-cell suppression and T regulatory cell activation mediated by myeloid-derived suppressor cells in cancer. Cancer Res 2010;70:99–108.

43. Serafini P, Mgebroff S, Noonan K, et al. Myeloid-derived suppressor cells pro-mote cross-tolerance in B-cell lymphoma by expanding regulatory T cells. Cancer Res 2008;68:5439–49.

44. Plaks V, Birnberg T, Berkutzki T, et al. Uterine DCs are crucial for decidua forma-tion during embryo implantation in mice. J Clin Invest 2008;118:3954–65.

45. Collins MK, Tay CS, Erlebacher A. Dendritic cell entrapment within the pregnant uterus inhibits immune surveillance of the maternal/fetal interface in mice. J Clin Invest 2009;119:2062–73.

46. Tagliani E, Erlebacher A. Dendritic cell function at the fetomaternal interface. Expert Rev Clin Immunol 2011;7:593–602.

47. Guerin LR, Prins JR, Robertson SA. Regulatory T-cells and immune tolerance in pregnancy: a new target for infertility treatment? Hum Reprod Update 2009;15:517–35.

48. La Rocca C, Carbone F, Longobardi S, et al. The immunology of pregnancy: reg-ulatory T cells control maternal immune tolerance toward the fetus. Immunol Lett 2014;162:41–8.

49. Shima T, Sasaki Y, Itoh M, et al. Regulatory T cells are necessary for implantation and maintenance of early pregnancy but not late pregnancy in allogeneic mice. J Reprod Immunol 2010;85:121–9.

50. Alijotas-Reig J, Llurba E, Gris JM. Potentiating maternal immune tolerance in pregnancy: a new challenging role for regulatory T cells. Placenta 2014;35:241–8.

51. Wang WJ, Liu FJ, Xin L, et al. Adoptive transfer of pregnancy-induced CD4+CD25+ regulatory T cells reverses the increase in abortion rate caused by interleukin 17 in the CBA/JxBALB/c mouse model. Hum Reprod 2014;29:946–52.

52. Zenclussen ML, Thuere C, Ahmad N, et al. The persistence of paternal antigens in the maternal body is involved in regulatory T-cell expansion and fetal-maternal tolerance in murine pregnancy. Am J Reprod Immunol 2010;63:200–8.

53. Samstein RM, Josefowicz SZ, Arvey A, et al. Extrathymic generation of regulatory T cells in placental mammals mitigates fetomaternal conflict. Cell 2012;150:29–38.

54. Jensen F, Muzzio D, Soldati R, et al. Regulatory B10 cells restore pregnancy toler-ance in a mouse model. Biol Reprod 2013;89:90.

55. Rolle L, Memarzadeh Tehran M, Morell-Garcia A, et al. Cutting edge: IL-10-producing regulatory B cells in early human pregnancy. Am J Reprod Immunol 2013;70:448–53.

56. Muzzio DO, Ziegler KB, Ehrhardt J, et al. Marginal zone B cells emerge as a critical component of pregnancy well-being. Reproduction 2016;151:29–37.

57. Lima J, Martins C, Leandro MJ, et al. Characterization of B cells in healthy pregnant women from late pregnancy to post-partum: a prospective observational study. BMC Pregnancy Childbirth 2016;16:139.

58. Guzman-Genuino RM, Diener KR. Regulatory B cells in pregnancy: lessons from autoimmunity, graft tolerance, and cancer. Front Immunol 2017;8:172.

59. Xu YY, Wang SC, Li DJ, et al. Co-signaling molecules in fetomaternal immunity. Trends Mol Med 2017;23:46–58.

60. Schumacher A. Human chorionic gonadotropin as a pivotal endocrine immune regulator initiating and preserving fetal tolerance. Int J Mol Sci 2017;18 [pii: E2166].

61. D'Addio F, Riella LV, Mfarrej BG, et al. The link between the PDL1 costimulatory pathway and Th17 in fetomaternal tolerance. J Immunol 2011;187:4530–41.

62. Tripathi S, Guleria I. Role of PD1/PDL1 pathway, and TH17 and treg cells in maternal tolerance to the fetus. Biomed J 2015;38:25–31.

63. Guleria I, Khosroshahi A, Ansari MJ, et al. A critical role for the programmed death ligand 1 in fetomaternal tolerance. J Exp Med 2005;202:231–7.

64. Riella L, Dada S, Chabtini L, et al. B7h (ICOS L) maintains tolerance at the fetomaternal interface. Am J Pathol 2013;182(6):2204–13.

65. Chabtini L, Mfarrej B, Mounayar M, et al. TIM-3 regulates innate immune cells to induce fetomaternal tolerance. J Immunol 2013;190:88–96.

66. Qian J, Zhang N, Lin J, et al. Distinct pattern of Th17/Treg cells in pregnant women with a history of unexplained recurrent spontaneous abortion. Biosci Trends 2018;12:157–67.

67. Salomon C, Rice GE. Role of exosomes in placental homeostasis and pregnancy disorders. Prog Mol Biol Transl Sci 2017;145:163–79.

68. Sarker S, Scholz-Romero K, Perez A, et al. Placenta-derived exosomes continuously increase in maternal circulation over the first trimester of pregnancy. J Transl Med 2014;12:204.

69. Mitchell MD, Peiris HN, Kobayashi M, et al. Placental exosomes in normal and complicated pregnancy. Am J Obstet Gynecol 2015;213:S173–81.

70. Pillay P, Moodley K, Moodley J, et al. Placenta-derived exosomes: potential biomarkers of preeclampsia. Int J Nanomedicine 2017;12:8009–23.

71. Tsochandaridis M, Nasca L, Toga C, et al. Circulating microRNAs as clinical biomarkers in the predictions of pregnancy complications. Biomed Res Int 2015; 2015:294954.

72. Gilad S, Meiri E, Yogev Y, et al. Serum microRNAs are promising novel biomarkers. PLoS One 2008;3:e3148.

73. Agrawal S, Cerdeira AS, Redman C, et al. Meta-analysis and systematic review to assess the role of soluble FMS-Like tyrosine kinase-1 and placenta growth factor ratio in prediction of preeclampsia: the SaPPPhirE study. Hypertension 2018;71: 306–16.

Novel Targets of Immunosuppression in Transplantation

Ho Sik Shin, MD, PhD[a], Ivica Grgic, MD[b], Anil Chandraker, MD[c],*

KEYWORDS

- T cell - B cell - Plasma cell - Complement - Immunosuppression - Transplantation
- Novel - Target

KEY POINTS

- It is increasingly recognized that calcineurin inhibitors (CNI), such as cyclosporine and tacrolimus, are not ideal immunosuppressive agents.
- Side effects, including increased rates of infection, hypertension, and malignancy, can be severe.
- Thus, in the past decade, there has been much focus on the development of novel therapeutic agents and strategies designed to replace or minimize CNI exposure in transplant patients.
- This article reviews potential novel targets in T cells, alloantibody-producing B cells, plasma cells, and complement in transplantation.

INTRODUCTION

Since the first successful kidney transplantation in 1954, the short-term success rate of transplantation has improved due to advances in immunosuppressive therapy and a more comprehensive understanding of the alloimmune response.[1] However, less progress has been made in the past 2 decades at reducing the long-term attrition rate of allografts, much of which is attributed to a chronic alloimmune response.[2]

Disclosure Statement: The authors have nothing to disclose.
I. Grgic was supported by the Deutsche Forschungsgemeinschaft and grants from the Philipps-University Marburg, University Medical Center Giessen and Marburg, and the Von Behring-Roentgen- Foundation.
a Renal Division, Department of Internal Medicine, Gospel Hospital, Kosin University College of Medicine, 262 Gamcheon-ro, Seo-gu, Busan 49267, Republic of Korea; b Department of Internal Medicine and Nephrology, University Hospital, Giessen and Marburg, Philipps-University Marburg, Baldinger Strasse 1, Marburg 35033, Germany; c Transplantation Research Center, Renal Division, Brigham and Women's Hospital, Harvard Medical School, 221 Longwood Avenue, Boston, MA 02215, USA
* Corresponding author.
E-mail address: achandraker@bwh.harvard.edu

The mechanisms for these processes are not fully understood, but are thought to represent the culmination of a complex interaction between inherent donor and recipient characteristics, the posttransplant course, subclinical humoral and cellular rejection, and long-term calcineurin inhibitor (CNI) exposure.[3]

It is increasingly recognized that the CNIs cyclosporine and tacrolimus, although the mainstay of most immunosuppressive protocols, are not ideal immunosuppressive agents. Side effects, including increased rates of infection, hypertension, malignancy, and nephrotoxicity, can be severe.[4] Thus, there is a need for the development of new immunosuppressive agents and strategies that can replace or minimize CNI exposure in transplant patients.

This article reviews potential novel targets in T cells, alloantibody-producing B cells, plasma cells, and complement in transplantation.

EMERGING DRUGS FOR PREVENTING T-CELL-MEDIATED REJECTION IN TRANSPLANTATION
Voclosporin (ISA247)

Voclosporin is a novel oral semisynthetic analogue of cyclosporine with a modification at the first amino acid residue of the molecule (**Fig. 1**).[5] In the phase 2b PROMISE study, a multicenter study of Volcosporin versus Tacrolimus, 334 de novo kidney transplant patients were randomized to receive 3 different doses of voclosporin (0.4, 0.6, or 0.8 mg/kg body weight, twice daily) or standard tacrolimus (0.5 mg/kg body weight, twice daily), in addition to an interleukin-2 (IL-2) receptor antagonist, mycophenolate mofetil (MMF), and a steroid. No difference was found in the incidence of biopsy-proven acute rejection (BPAR) between the voclosporin groups (10.7%, 9.1%, and 2.3% for low, medium, and high doses, respectively) and the tacrolimus

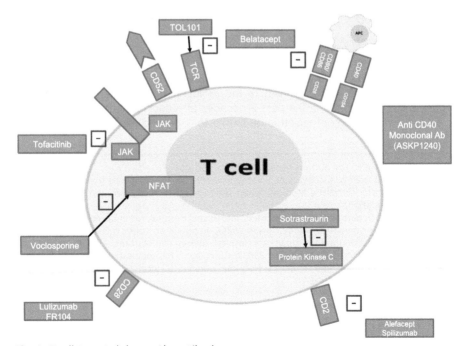

Fig. 1. T-cell-targeted drugs. Ab, antibody.

group (5.8%), within the first 6 months. Renal function 6 months after transplantation showed a slightly inferior estimated glomerular filtration rate (eGFR) for high-dose voclosporin when compared with standard tacrolimus ($P = .049$). The incidence of hypertension and other adverse events was not different, but low-dose voclosporin was associated with fewer incidence of new onset diabetes. This study, which was 6 months long, suggests that voclosporin is as potent as tacrolimus in preventing acute rejection, with similar renal allograft function in the low- and medium-exposure groups, and its use is potentially associated with a reduced incidence of new onset diabetes after transplantation.[6] The Special Access for the Use of Voclosporin for Kidney Transplant study (NCT01236287) is listed as an active renal transplantation trial wherein subjects previously participating in the PROMISE study may be eligible to continue to receive voclosporin. The last update posted in clinicaltrials.gov was on February 28, 2018.

Tofacitinib

Tofacitinib, also known as CP-690550, is a Janus kinase 3 (JAK3) inhibitor. JAKs are associated with several cytokine receptors. Upon cytokine-receptor binding, JAKs are activated, leading to phosphorylation of the receptor, which provides the docking sites for signal transducers and activators of transcription. By inhibiting JAK3, tofacitinib suppresses signaling of various cytokines, including IL-2, -4, -7, -9, -15, and -21.[7]

In a pilot study of de novo kidney transplant recipients, patients were randomized to receive either tacrolimus or tofacitinib (15 or 30 mg, twice daily) in addition to MMF. Although eGFR was found to be similar across all 3 groups, a higher incidence of BK virus nephropathy and cytomegalovirus (CMV) disease was observed in patients receiving high-dose tofacitinib, potentially a reflection of "over-immunosuppression."[8]

In renal transplant clinical trials in humans, tofacitinib has been found to be noninferior to cyclosporine with regard to rejection rates and graft survival. A phase 2b trial randomized low to moderate risk de novo kidney transplant patients to receive cyclosporine or tofacitinib at 2 different intensities. With tofacitinib, there was a lower rate of new onset diabetes after transplantation, but there was a trend toward more infections, including CMV and BK virus nephritis. The incidence of BPAR at 6 months was similar across the 3 groups. The measured GFRs at 12 months were higher for the tofacitinib groups compared with the cyclosporine group (65 vs 54 mL/min), with higher rates of serious infections and posttransplant lymphoproliferative disorder (PTLD) observed in the more intensive tofacitinib group.[9] Tofacitinib was equivalent to cyclosporine in preventing acute rejection and was associated with improved renal function and less chronic allograft histologic injury, but produced considerable side effects. A post hoc analysis demonstrated that patients with below-median exposure to tofacitinib had a comparable rejection risk, improved renal function, and similar risk of serious infections and PTLD compared with the patients in the cyclosporine group.[10] An extension study (72 months) showed that tofacitinib continued to be effective in preventing allograft rejection, with a better outcome for renal function (10–15 mL/min/1.73 m^2 higher eGFR with tofacitinib vs cyclosporine), but at similar rates of chronic allograft injury.[11]

Sotrastaurin (AEB071)

Sotrastaurin is an oral protein kinase C inhibitor selective for kinases that are important for early T-cell activation.[12] Initial studies using rodents and primates demonstrated the potential for this agent to prevent allograft rejection.[13,14] In a phase 2 randomized trial of low-risk kidney transplant recipients comparing sotrastaurin with cyclosporine, a higher failure rate was observed with the use of sotrastaurin.[15] In a phase 2 randomized trial of the efficacy of sotrastaurin plus tacrolimus after de novo kidney transplantation, mean heart rates were faster with higher sotrastaurin doses. Furthermore, discontinuations due to adverse events, including gastrointestinal adverse events, were more common. Fewer patients in the sotrastaurin groups experienced leukopenia than in the mycophenolic acid group (1.3–5.5 vs 16.5%). Sotrastaurin 200 and 300 mg had comparable efficacy to mycophenolic acid in preventing rejection, and there was no significant difference in renal function between the groups.[16]

Anti-CD40 Monoclonal Antibody

Both CD40 and CD154 are expressed on antigen-presenting and activated T cells and are potential targets for development of antibodies. However, the latter is also found on platelets, and the development of an anti-CD154 monoclonal antibody (mAb) was halted due to an unacceptably high rate of thrombotic events.[17] A fully humanized immunoglobulin G4 (IgG4) antibody to CD40 (ASKP1240) is currently undergoing clinical studies.[18] A phase 1b study in de novo kidney transplant patients showed that ASKP1240 was well tolerated at different doses ranging from 50 to 500 mg.[19] A phase 2 study is currently ongoing comparing the efficacy and safety of ASKP1240 combined with CNI-free, CNI-minimization, or standard-of-care CNI regimens. Early results showed comparable efficacy between ASKP1240 with CNI minimization and standard-of-care CNI, whereas ASKP1240 alone was associated with a higher risk of BPAR. Of note, there were no thromboembolic events observed with the use of ASKP1240.[20] Recruitment of patients for the Study to Assess the Efficacy and Safety of ASKP1240 in de Novo Kidney Transplant Recipients (NCT01780844) was completed on April 21, 2017, and results are awaited.

Lulizumab (FR104)

Selective targeting of CD28 might represent an effective immunomodulation strategy by preventing T-cell costimulation, while favoring co-inhibition because inhibitory signals transmitted through CTLA-4, PD-L1, and B7 would not be affected. Emerging evidence suggests that selective blockade of CD28 signals in the presence of preserved inhibitory CTLA-4 signaling may be beneficial in orchestrating and fine-tuning antigen-specific CD8β T-cell responses, thus potentially mitigating unwanted immune reactions in transplantation.[21]

A new generation of single-chain anti-CD28 molecules has been engineered to selectively target, but not activate, CD28. Examples include FR104, a pegylated humanized Fab fragment, and lulizumab, a pegylated anti-CD28 domain antibody that has shown promising results in preclinical models of transplantation.[22] In a nonhuman primate renal allograft study, FR104 reinforced immunosuppression in both CNI-low and CNI-free protocols, without the need of steroids. Accumulation of intragraft T-regulatory cells suggested the promotion of immunoregulatory mechanisms. Selective CD28 antagonists might become an alternative CNI-sparing strategy to B7 antagonists for kidney transplant recipients.[23]

Siplizumab

Siplizumab is a humanized mAb targeting the T lymphocyte CD2 antigen. It has been tested as an induction agent in one of the first human studies of renal allograft tolerance after combined bone marrow and kidney transplantation from HLA single-haplotype mismatched living related donors that had resulted in chimerism.[24] A study examining the safety profile, pharmacokinetics, and pharmacodynamics of siplizumab in renal allograft recipients showed an acceptable safety profile. Detectable siplizumab concentrations were maintained for days after the second dose at the 2 highest dose levels.[25]

TOL101

TOL101 is a highly selective murine IgM mAb directed against the $\alpha\beta$ T-cell receptor. Unlike other T-cell targets (eg, CD3), the $\alpha\beta$ T-cell receptor has no known intracellular signaling domains and may thus represent a target to neutralize T cells in a "silent," nonmitogenic fashion. A study investigating the pharmacokinetics and pharmacodynamics of TOL101 showed its pharmacologic profile was somewhat versatile, allowing for daily dosing without immunogenicity concerns.[26] In a first-in-human phase 2 trial investigating the safety and efficacy of TOL101 in induction to prevent renal transplant rejection, there were no cases of patient or graft loss. Few significant adverse events were reported, with one case of nosocomial pneumonia. There were 5 BPARs (13.9%); however, no donor-specific antibodies (DSAs) were detected. Overall, TOL101 was well tolerated.[27]

Potential Development Issues

With novel drugs, one can anticipate potential difficulties. These difficulties may be due to the direct effects of the drug in question, or a class effect that is inherent, in this case, immunosuppression. This class effect is likely to be unavoidable.

Several agents have fallen by the wayside because of the imbalance between efficacy and side effects. Efalizumab, an antilymphocyte function-associated antigen 1 molecule that inhibits lymphocyte migration, was withdrawn due to an increased risk of progressive multifocal leukoencephalopathy and PTLD in renal transplant recipients.[28] Another induction agent, alefacept, a CD2-lymphocyte function-associated antigen 3 costimulation inhibitor, was also withdrawn from further development. In a phase 2 study of alefacept versus placebo in renal transplant recipients receiving tacrolimus, MMF, and corticosteroids, no difference in efficacy was found when compared with placebo, but a higher rate of malignancy was observed in the alefacept arm.[29] Finally, the development of sotrastaurin for use in the transplant setting had been halted because of suboptimal efficacy.

The fact that only a few agents have been approved in the last decade highlights the difficulties associated with developing novel immunosuppressive therapies in transplantation. This stagnation is compounded further by the lack of sensitive biomarkers that can help predict, diagnose, and monitor rejection and measure the degree of immunosuppression.

EMERGING DRUGS/COMPOUNDS TO TARGET ALLOANTIBODY-PRODUCING B AND PLASMA CELLS IN TRANSPLANTATION
B-Cell-Targeted Drugs

B-cell depletion
B-cell depletion has been achieved through splenectomy or via the administration of the anti-CD52 antibody, alemtuzumab (CAMPATH-1H), anti-thymocyte globulin (both of which deplete T cells in addition to B cells), and the anti-CD20 antibody, rituximab (**Fig. 2**). Rituximab has been used as part of desensitization strategies in ABO and HLA-incompatible transplantation, and for the treatment of acute and chronic antibody-mediated rejection (ABMR). A randomized controlled trial (RITUX ERAH) of 38 patients with acute ABMR suggested no additional benefit when patients were treated with a regimen of plasmapheresis, intravenous immunoglobulin, and corticosteroids.[30]

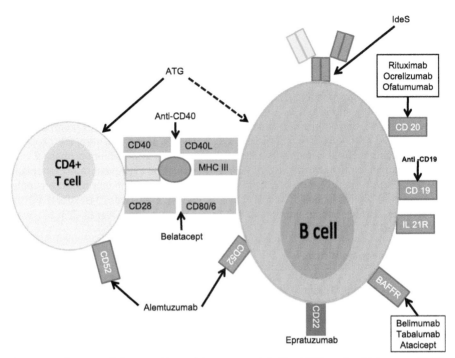

Fig. 2. B-cell-targeted drugs. ATG, antithymocyte globulin; MHC, major histocompatibility complex.

Additional B-cell-specific mAbs, including a humanized anti-CD20 antibody (ofatumumab) and those binding to other B-cell antigens,[31] as well as bispecific antibodies that target 2 molecules on the B cell, for example, CD19 and CD22, have also been developed to treat hematological malignancies,[32] but have yet to be applied to transplantation. Recently, the first case report of using ofatumumab in kidney transplantation (ABO incompatible) was reported. The results showed that the patient tolerated administration of the drug without signs of adverse effects and with good clinical efficacy. Thus, ofatumumab is a valid alternative B-cell-depleting agent.[33]

Modulation of B-cell activation
One attractive target for affecting B-cell activation is the cytokine B-cell activating factor (BAFF), because blocking mAbs targeting BAFF have already been developed for treating autoimmunity. In transplantation, BAFF-deficient mice had extended cardiac allograft survival,[34] and BAFF blockade (in combination with rapamycin at induction) resulted in long-term survival of major histocompatibility complex-disparate islet allografts.[35] The authors and others have identified circulating BAFF as a potential biomarker for humoral alloimmunity; high-circulating BAFF is associated with the development of DSAs[36] and ABMR.[37] BAFF neutralization has been tested as a desensitization strategy (see discussion on plasma cells later), but in terms of its use in targeting B cells, the results of a phase 2 pilot study using belimumab in non-sensitized patients in the first 6 months after kidney transplantation showed that belimumab might be a useful adjunct to standard-of-care immunosuppression in renal transplantation, with no major increased risk of infection, and potential beneficial effects on humoral alloimmunity (clinicaltrials.gov identifier: NCT01536379).[38]

B cells also express several inhibitory receptors, including CD22 and FcgRIIB, that, if cross-linked, recruit phosphatases that terminate activating signaling and may, therefore, also be useful in inhibiting humoral alloimmunity. Epratuzumab, a humanized anti-CD22 antibody, has been used in lupus and induces some depletion of naive and transitional B cells, producing a 35% reduction in total B-cell numbers. However, it can also inhibit B-cell activation and proliferation.[39]

The IgG-degrading enzyme of *Streptococcus pyogenes*, IdeS, is an endopeptidase that has specificity for human IgG and, when infused intravenously, results in rapid cleavage of IgG. It has been harnessed as a tool to degrade DSA in sensitized patients,[40] but may also have utility in preventing B-cell activation by cleaving the B-cell receptor.[41] The results of a recent study, [IdeS (Imlifidase)]: A Novel Agent That Cleaves Human IgG and Permits Successful Kidney Transplantation Across High-strength Donor-specific Antibody, showed that IdeS may provide a groundbreaking new method of desensitization for patients who otherwise might have no hope for receiving a lifesaving transplant.[42]

Plasma Cell-Targeted Drugs

Germinal center disruption

The most promising target for germinal center disruption is costimulatory blockade (eg, inhibiting CD40-CD40L or CD28-CD80/86 interactions) (**Fig. 3**). Long-term follow-up data from the BENEFIT and BENEFIT-Ext studies have demonstrated a significant reduction in the development of de novo DSA in belatacept (a CTLA4 fusion protein that inhibits the CD28-CD80/86 pathway)-treated patients.[43]

Follicular helper T (Tfh) cells provide critical support for germinal center B cells. De Graav and colleagues[44] quantified circulating Tfh cells in transplant recipients and found the highest numbers in patients with preformed DSAs. Ex vivo, peripheral Tfh

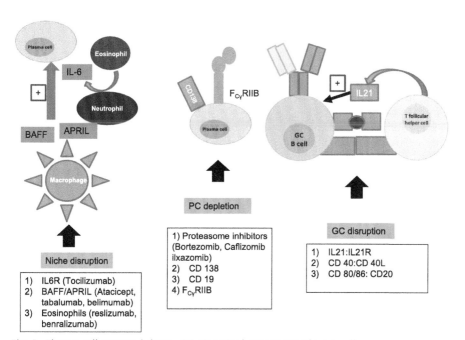

Fig. 3. Plasma cell-targeted drugs. GC, Germinal center; PC, Plasma cell.

cells induce B-cell immunoglobulin production, and this could be inhibited by an IL21R antagonist. The IL21-IL21R axis may, therefore, also be a useful target in transplantation.

Plasma cell depletion

Bispecific T-cell-engager antibodies, such as blinatumomab, that have dual specificity for CD19 and CD3, have been used for the treatment of B-cell leukemia.[45] These agents transiently induce a cytolytic synapse between a cytotoxic T cell and malignant B cell, causing granzyme and perforin release to effectively destroy the targeted cells. To date, there are no trials of these agents in solid organ transplantation.

Plasma cell-specific mAbs have been developed to treat multiple myeloma, including an anti-CD138 mAb.[46] These plasma cell-specific mAbs are currently used to carry radioactive isotopes to malignant plasma cells, but there may be a future in adapting them for use in transplantation.

Niche disruption

Several cytokines provide support for plasma cells within the bone marrow niche, including IL-6 and a proliferation-inducing ligand (APRIL). Tocilizumab, a humanized anti-IL6 receptor IgG1 mAb used in rheumatoid arthritis, has been used recently in a small phase 1/2 trial in transplantation.[47] Tocilizumab reduced DSA titers such that 5 of the 10 patients that were transplanted, and 6-month protocol biopsies, showed no evidence of ABMR. The trial did not identify any significant safety concerns with this approach. A larger randomized controlled trial is yet to be conducted.

Eosinophils are thought to be key producers of IL-6 within the bone marrow niche.[48] IL-5 blockade (aimed at inhibiting eosinophil survival) showed some utility in experimental models.[49] This area may be interesting to explore in transplantation, because IL-5-targeted therapies, such as mepolizumab or reslizumab, or the IL-5Ra inhibitor benralizumab, are already being trialed in asthma.[49,50]

Neutralizing BAFF and APRIL with atacicept, a fusion protein with the extracellular domain of a transmembrane activator (transmembrane activator and calcium modulating cyclophilin ligand interactor), a receptor for these cytokines, has shown promising effects on the development of DSAs in nonhuman primate models.[51] There have been 2 studies in which anti-BAFF antibodies were used in attempts to reduce DSAs in sensitized patients. One, a phase 2a single-arm study investigating the effect of giving tabalumab (a BAFF inhibitor) monthly for 6 months as monotherapy to 18 sensitized patients demonstrated a statistically significant, but clinically marginal, reduction in DSAs.[52] Similarly, a trial using the anti-BAFF antibody belimumab as monotherapy for desensitization was terminated because of a lack of efficacy (clinicaltrials.gov identifier: NCT01025193). These 2 negative studies are perhaps unsurprising, because BAFF is only one of several proplasma cell survival factors.

EMERGING DRUGS TO TARGET COMPLEMENT IN TRANSPLANTATION
Terminal Complement Blockade

Eculizumab, a humanized mAb against C5 that binds with high affinity and prevents the generation of the membrane attack complex (MAC), has been proposed as a therapeutic option for ABMR.[53] The rationale for its use is based on the theory that DSAs cause less harm to endothelial cells of the graft if the classical complement pathway is blocked. In fact, the beneficial effects of eculizumab may be 2-fold: preventing MAC-formation and reducing the proinflammatory effects of C5a.[54] However, evidence for the clinical validity of the concept of terminal complement blockade as a strategy to counteract ABMR is scarce and, as yet, limited to case reports and observational studies[55,56]

C1 Inference

Anti-C1s monoclonal antibody BIVV009

Another interesting therapeutic approach may be the selective blockade of the enzymatic C1 subcomponent C1s to prevent the formation of the Classic Pathway (CP) C3 convertase. In a single-arm pilot trial, 10 kidney transplant recipients diagnosed with late DSA-positive ABMR were included to receive a short course of anti-C1s antibody treatment (4 weekly doses of BIVV009 at 60 mg/kg).[57] The results showed that BIVV009 was able to effectively block alloantibody-triggered classical pathway activation, although the treatment had no effect on indices of activity in late ABMR. Nonetheless, this pilot trial provides a valuable basis for future studies designed to clarify the therapeutic value of CP blockade in transplantation.

C1-INH

Another promising approach may be the therapeutic use of purified C1-INH, a serine-protease inhibitor (serpin) blocking C1r and C1s activation and dissociating the C1 complex.[58] In a recent placebo-controlled trial, 18 kidney allograft recipients with acute ABMR were included to receive C1-INH (n = 9) or placebo (n = 9) as an add-on to standard treatment (intravenous immunoglobulin, plasmapheresis, and/or rituximab).[59] Endogenous C1 INH measured before and after PP demonstrated a decrease in functional C1 INH serum concentration by 43.3% ($P<.05$) for both cohorts (C1 INH and placebo) associated with PP. Intravenous administration of C1 INH was well tolerated overall and, importantly, exogenous C1 INH-treated patients achieved supraphysiological levels throughout. This new finding suggests that C1 INH replacement may be useful in the treatment of ABMR. However, further studies with larger groups and longer follow-up will be needed to confirm the safety and assess the potential reduction of transplant glomerulopathy, and 2 clinical trials using C1 INH inhibition to treat AMR are currently recruiting patients.[60,61]

SUMMARY

Emerging drugs/compounds to target T cells, alloantibody-producing B cells, plasma cells, and complement in transplantation continue to represent a powerful class of drugs to prevent and treat kidney allograft rejection. Their use should be deliberate and justified by a clear clinical indication and a favorable risk-benefit analysis.

REFERENCES

1. Agarwal A, Ally W, Brayman K. The future direction and unmet needs of transplant immunosuppression. Expert Rev Clin Pharmacol 2016;9(7):873–6.
2. Lamb KE, Lodhi S, Meier-Kriesche HU. Long-term renal allograft survival in the United States: a critical reappraisal. Am J Transplant 2011;11(3):450–62.
3. Stegall MD, Gaston RS, Cosio FG, et al. Through a glass darkly: seeking clarity in preventing late kidney transplant failure. J Am Soc Nephrol 2015;26(1):20–9.
4. Vella JP, Sayegh MH. Current and future immunosuppressive therapies: impact on chronic allograft dysfunction. J Nephrol 1997;10(5):229–31.
5. Aspeslet L, Freitag D, Trepanier D, et al. ISA(TX)247: a novel calcineurin inhibitor. Transpl Proc 2001;33(1–2):1048–51.

6. Busque S, Cantarovich M, Mulgaonkar S, et al. The PROMISE study: a phase 2b multicenter study of voclosporin (ISA247) versus tacrolimus in de novo kidney transplantation. Am J Transplant 2011;11(12):2675–84.

7. Wojciechowski D, Vincenti F. Tofacitinib in kidney transplantation. Expert Opin Investig Drugs 2013;22(9):1193–9.

8. Busque S, Leventhal J, Brennan DC, et al. Calcineurin-inhibitor-free immunosuppression based on the JAK inhibitor CP-690,550: a pilot study in de novo kidney allograft recipients. Am J Transplant 2009;9(8):1936–45.

9. Vincenti F, Tedesco Silva H, Busque S, et al. Randomized phase 2b trial of tofacitinib (CP-690,550) in de novo kidney transplant patients: efficacy, renal function and safety at 1 year. Am J Transplant 2012;12(9):2446–56.

10. Vincenti F, Silva HT, Busque S, et al. Evaluation of the effect of tofacitinib exposure on outcomes in kidney transplant patients. Am J Transplant 2015;15(6):1644–53.

11. O'Connell PJ, Vincenti BS. Tofacitinib in renal allograft recipients: long-term efficacy and safety in an active-comparator-controlled extension trial. Transplantation 2016;100(7S):S84–5.

12. Evenou JP, Wagner J, Zenke G, et al. The potent protein kinase C-selective inhibitor AEB071 (sotrastaurin) represents a new class of immunosuppressive agents affecting early T-cell activation. J Pharmacol Exp Ther 2009;330(3):792–801.

13. Weckbecker G, Pally C, Beerli C, et al. Effects of the novel protein kinase C inhibitor AEB071 (Sotrastaurin) on rat cardiac allograft survival using single agent treatment or combination therapy with cyclosporine, everolimus or FTY720. Transpl Int 2010;23(5):543–52.

14. Bigaud M, Wieczorek G, Beerli C, et al. Sotrastaurin (AEB071) alone and in combination with cyclosporine A prolongs survival times of non-human primate recipients of life-supporting kidney allografts. Transplantation 2012;93(2):156–64.

15. Tedesco-Silva H, Kho MM, Hartmann A, et al. Sotrastaurin in calcineurin inhibitor-free regimen using everolimus in de novo kidney transplant recipients. Am J Transplant 2013;13(7):1757–68.

16. Russ GR, Tedesco-Silva H, Kuypers DR, et al. Efficacy of sotrastaurin plus tacrolimus after de novo kidney transplantation: randomized, phase II trial results. Am J Transplant 2013;13(7):1746–56.

17. Andre P, Prasad KS, Denis CV, et al. CD40L stabilizes arterial thrombi by a beta3 integrin–dependent mechanism. Nat Med 2002;8(3):247–52.

18. Okimura K, Maeta K, Kobayashi N, et al. Characterization of ASKP1240, a fully human antibody targeting human CD40 with potent immunosuppressive effects. Am J Transplant 2014;14(6):1290–9.

19. Vincenti FYH, Klintmalm G, Steinberg S, et al. Clinical outcomes in a Phase 1b, randomized, double blinded, parallel group, placebocontrolled, single dose study of ASKP1240 in de novo kidney transplantation. Am J Transplant 2013; 13(suppl5):86.

20. Harland R, Klintmalm G, Yang H, et al. ASKP1240 in de novo kidney transplant recipients. Am J Transplant 2015;15(Suppl3).

21. Liu D, Krummey SM, Badell IR, et al. 2B4 (CD244) induced by selective CD28 blockade functionally regulates allograft-specific CD8+ T cell responses. J Exp Med 2014;211(2):297–311.

22. Adams AB, Ford ML, Larsen CP. Costimulation blockade in autoimmunity and transplantation: the CD28 pathway. J Immunol 2016;197(6):2045–50.

23. Poirier N, Dilek N, Mary C, et al. FR104, an antagonist anti-CD28 monovalent fab' antibody, prevents alloimmunization and allows calcineurin inhibitor minimization in nonhuman primate renal allograft. Am J Transplant 2015;15(1):88–100.

24. Kawai T, Cosimi AB, Spitzer TR, et al. HLA-mismatched renal transplantation without maintenance immunosuppression. N Engl J Med 2008;358(4):353–61.
25. Pruett TL, McGory RW, Wright FH, et al. Safety profile, pharmacokinetics, and pharmacodynamics of siplizumab, a humanized anti-CD2 monoclonal antibody, in renal allograft recipients. Transplant Proc 2009;41(9):3655–61.
26. Getts DR, Kramer WG, Wiseman AC, et al. The pharmacokinetics and pharmacodynamics of TOL101, a murine IgM anti-human alphabeta T cell receptor antibody, in renal transplant patients. Clin Pharmacokinet 2014;53(7):649–57.
27. Flechner SM, Mulgoankar S, Melton LB, et al. First-in-human study of the safety and efficacy of TOL101 induction to prevent kidney transplant rejection. Am J Transplant 2014;14(6):1346–55.
28. Vincenti F, Mendez R, Pescovitz M, et al. A phase I/II randomized open-label multicenter trial of efalizumab, a humanized anti-CD11a, anti-LFA-1 in renal transplantation. Am J Transplant 2007;7(7):1770–7.
29. Rostaing L, Charpentier B, Glyda M, et al. Alefacept combined with tacrolimus, mycophenolate mofetil and steroids in de novo kidney transplantation: a randomized controlled trial. Am J Transplant 2013;13(7):1724–33.
30. Sautenet B, Blancho G, Buchler M, et al. One-year results of the effects of rituximab on acute antibody-mediated rejection in renal transplantation: RITUX ERAH, a multicenter double-blind randomized placebo-controlled trial. Transplantation 2016;100(2):391–9.
31. Ai J, Advani A. Current status of antibody therapy in ALL. Br J Haematol 2015; 168(4):471–80.
32. Bachanova V, Frankel AE, Cao Q, et al. Phase I study of a bispecific ligand-directed toxin targeting CD22 and CD19 (DT2219) for refractory B-cell malignancies. Clin Cancer Res 2015;21(6):1267–72.
33. Mancianti N, Monaci G, Rollo F, et al. First case report of using Ofatumumab in kidney transplantation AB0 incompatible. G Ital Nefrol 2017;34(Nov-Dec) [pii: 2017-vol6].
34. Ye Q, Wang L, Wells AD, et al. BAFF binding to T cell-expressed BAFF-R costimulates T cell proliferation and alloresponses. Eur J Immunol 2004;34(10):2750–9.
35. Parsons RF, Yu M, Vivek K, et al. Murine islet allograft tolerance upon blockade of the B-lymphocyte stimulator, BLyS/BAFF. Transplantation 2012;93(7):676–85.
36. Thibault-Espitia A, Foucher Y, Danger R, et al. BAFF and BAFF-R levels are associated with risk of long-term kidney graft dysfunction and development of donor-specific antibodies. Am J Transplant 2012;12(10):2754–62.
37. Banham G, Prezzi D, Harford S, et al. Elevated pretransplantation soluble BAFF is associated with an increased risk of acute antibody-mediated rejection. Transplantation 2013;96(4):413–20.
38. Banham GD, Flint SM, Torpey N, et al. Belimumab in kidney transplantation: an experimental medicine, randomised, placebo-controlled phase 2 trial. Lancet 2018;391(10140):2619–30.
39. Dorner T, Kaufmann J, Wegener WA, et al. Initial clinical trial of epratuzumab (humanized anti-CD22 antibody) for immunotherapy of systemic lupus erythematosus. Arthritis Res Ther 2006;8(3):R74.
40. Winstedt L, Jarnum S, Nordahl EA, et al. Complete removal of extracellular IgG antibodies in a randomized dose-escalation phase I study with the bacterial enzyme IdeS–a novel therapeutic opportunity. PLoS One 2015;10(7):e0132011.
41. Jarnum S, Bockermann R, Runstrom A, et al. The bacterial enzyme IdeS cleaves the IgG-type of B cell receptor (BCR), abolishes BCR-mediated cell signaling, and inhibits memory B cell activation. J Immunol 2015;195(12):5592–601.

42. Lonze BE, Tatapudi VS, Weldon EP, et al. IdeS (Imlifidase): a novel agent that cleaves human IgG and permits successful kidney transplantation across high-strength donor-specific antibody. Ann Surg 2018;268(3):488–96.

43. Vincenti F, Rostaing L, Grinyo J, et al. Belatacept and long-term outcomes in kidney transplantation. N Engl J Med 2016;374(4):333–43.

44. de Graav GN, Dieterich M, Hesselink DA, et al. Follicular T helper cells and humoral reactivity in kidney transplant patients. Clin Exp Immunol 2015;180(2): 329–40.

45. Topp MS, Gokbuget N, Zugmaier G, et al. Long-term follow-up of hematologic relapse-free survival in a phase 2 study of blinatumomab in patients with MRD in B-lineage ALL. Blood 2012;120(26):5185–7.

46. Fichou N, Gouard S, Maurel C, et al. Single-dose anti-CD138 radioimmunotherapy: bismuth-213 is more efficient than Lutetium-177 for treatment of multiple myeloma in a preclinical model. Front Med (Lausanne) 2015;2:76.

47. Vo AA, Choi J, Kim I, et al. A phase I/II trial of the interleukin-6 receptor-specific humanized monoclonal (Tocilizumab) + intravenous immunoglobulin in difficult to desensitize patients. Transplantation 2015;99(11):2356–63.

48. Chu VT, Frohlich A, Steinhauser G, et al. Eosinophils are required for the maintenance of plasma cells in the bone marrow. Nat Immunol 2011;12(2):151–9.

49. Pavord ID, Korn S, Howarth P, et al. Mepolizumab for severe eosinophilic asthma (DREAM): a multicentre, double-blind, placebo-controlled trial. Lancet 2012; 380(9842):651–9.

50. Varricchi G, Bagnasco D, Borriello F, et al. Interleukin-5 pathway inhibition in the treatment of eosinophilic respiratory disorders: evidence and unmet needs. Curr Opin Allergy Clin Immunol 2016;16(2):186–200.

51. Kwun J, Page E, Hong JJ, et al. Neutralizing BAFF/APRIL with atacicept prevents early DSA formation and AMR development in T cell depletion induced nonhuman primate AMR model. Am J Transplant 2015;15(3):815–22.

52. Mujtaba MA, Komocsar WJ, Nantz E, et al. Effect of treatment with tabalumab, a B Cell-activating factor inhibitor, on highly sensitized patients with end-stage renal disease awaiting transplantation. Am J Transplant 2016;16(4):1266–75.

53. Stegall MD, Chedid MF, Cornell LD. The role of complement in antibody-mediated rejection in kidney transplantation. Nat Rev Nephrol 2012;8(11):670–8.

54. Ward PA. The harmful role of c5a on innate immunity in sepsis. J Innate Immun 2011;2(5):439–45.

55. Stegall MD, Diwan T, Raghavaiah S, et al. Terminal complement inhibition decreases antibody-mediated rejection in sensitized renal transplant recipients. Am J Transplant 2011;11(11):2405–13.

56. Bentall A, Tyan DB, Sequeira F, et al. Antibody-mediated rejection despite inhibition of terminal complement. Transpl Int 2014;27(12):1235–43.

57. Eskandary F, Jilma B, Muhlbacher J, et al. Anti-C1s monoclonal antibody BIVV009 in late antibody-mediated kidney allograft rejection-results from a first-in-patient phase 1 trial. Am J Transplant 2018;18(4):916–26.

58. Davis AE 3rd, Lu F, Mejia P. C1 inhibitor, a multi-functional serine protease inhibitor. Thromb Haemost 2010;104(5):886–93.

59. Montgomery RA, Orandi BJ, Racusen L, et al. Plasma-derived C1 esterase inhibitor for acute antibody-mediated rejection following kidney transplantation: results of a randomized double-blind placebo-controlled pilot study. Am J Transplant 2016;16(12):3468–78.

60. Behring C. Efficacy and safety of human plasma-derived C1-esterase inhibitor as add-on to standard of care for the treatment of refractory Antibody Mediated

Rejection (AMR) in adult renal transplant recipients (NCT03221842). 2017. Available at: https://clinicaltrials.gov/ct2/show/NCT03221842.

61. Shire. A multicenter study to evaluate the efficacy and safety of Cinryze® for the treatment of acute antibody-mediated rejection in participants with kidney transplant(ClinicalTrials.gov Identifier: NCT02547220). 2015. Available at: https://clinicaltrials.gov/ct2/show/NCT02547220.

Signaling Molecules in Posttransplantation Cancer

Murugabaskar Balan, PhD[1], Samik Chakraborty, PhD, Soumitro Pal, PhD*,[1]

KEYWORDS

- Posttransplantation cancer • CNI • Immunosuppression • Risk factor
- Signaling mechanisms

KEY POINTS

- Clinical data reveal that there is at least a 2-fold overall increased risk of cancer among transplant recipients compared with general population.
- Immunosuppression is essential to prevent graft rejection; however, it contributes to post-transplant cancer development.
- Molecular mechanisms of immunosuppressive agent-induced cell-intrinsic tumorigenic pathways are summarized.
- The role(s) of oncogenic virus infection in promoting transplant-related malignancies are discussed.
- Immunosuppression negatively impacts the host tumor immunosurveillance mechanisms, resulting in the unhindered growth of tumors.

INTRODUCTION

In solid organ transplantation (SOT), the short-term graft survival rate has significantly increased with the use of novel and better immunosuppressive agents. However, advent of malignancies after SOT drastically affects the long-term survival of the graft and the life expectancy of the recipients.[1] Epidemiologic studies from different regions of the world reveal that cancer development among transplant recipients is one of the major adverse outcomes after SOT and cancer-related mortality rates are much higher among organ transplant recipients.[2] For instance, a nested case-control study of kidney transplant recipients indicated that the major reason for deaths in patients with a functional renal graft was cancer.[3] Unfortunately, the second and fourth most common causes of death among liver and lung transplant recipients, respectively, is cancer.[4]

Disclosure Statement: This work is supported by National Institute of Health Grants R01 CA222355 and R01 CA193675 (to S.P.)

Division of Nephrology, Boston Children's Hospital, 300 Longwood Avenue, Boston, MA 02115, USA

[1] M. Balan and S. Pal are co-senior authors.

* Corresponding author.

E-mail address: soumitro.pal@childrens.harvard.edu

In the United States, a large-scale registry linkage study, comparing data from the Scientific Registry of Transplant Recipients (a federal registry) with several state and regional cancer registries, indicated a wide spectrum of cancer risk for 32 different malignancies among organ transplant recipients.[5] The study measured the relative risk of cancer in transplant recipients as the standardized incidence ratio (SIR) (ie, observed/expected cases), a statistical measure to compare the relative risk of cancer development among transplant recipients compared with the general population. The SIR risk measurements among kidney, liver, heart, and lung transplant recipients (among 175,732 transplants comprising 39.7% of US total from 1987 to 2008) revealed that cancer etiology and the type of cancer developed varies according to the organ transplanted. For example, liver cancer risk increased only among liver transplant recipients, whereas increased risk of kidney cancer was observed even among liver and heart transplant recipients.[5] Excluding squamous cell and basal cell skin cancer types, for which data are not collected by the cancer registries, the study observed a 2-fold overall increased risk of cancer among transplant recipients.[5]

The most common posttransplantation malignancy with increased risk was non-Hodgkin's lymphoma with a SIR of 7.54. The SIRs of the cancers of the lung and kidney were 1.97 and 4.65, respectively. Notably, renal cell carcinoma or kidney cancer risk during the first year after kidney transplantation was much higher with a SIR in the range of 7.28 to 10.28, indicating an accelerated risk of malignant transformation of the transplanted organ.[5] The SIRs for other cancers including liver, colorectal cancer, thyroid cancer, and myeloid neoplasms were also higher.[5]

Apart from known risk factors, such as recipient age, previous cancer, sun exposure (UV light) and donor-transmitted cancer, viral infections-related malignancies, such as non-Hodgkin's lymphoma (Epstein–Barr virus [EBV]), Kaposi sarcoma (human herpesvirus 8 [HHV8]) and liver cancer (hepatitis B virus [HBV] and hepatitis C virus [HCV]) have a higher rate of occurrence in organ transplant recipients.[2] Immunosuppression impairs the ability of the host immune system to control viral infection and decreases tumor immunosurveillance. Conceivably, the major risk factor for posttransplantation cancer arises from the indispensable need for long-term immunosuppression after SOT.

Interestingly, recent reports suggest that immunosuppressive agents can activate tumorigenic pathways independent of the involvement of the host immune system. It has also been reported that, with the use of immunosuppressive agents, preexisting cancer progress at much higher rate in transplant recipients.[2] Further, the life-long need for immunosuppressive agents to sustain the transplant limits the treatment options available for posttransplant cancer. This is because the tumorigenic pathways directly activated by immunosuppressive agents can potentially interfere with the efficacy of anticancer agents used to treat transplant recipients with cancer. The molecular mechanisms associated with the cancerous side effect of immunosuppressive agents are not completely understood. Therefore, a better understanding of the tumorigenic mechanisms that can solely be attributed to immunosuppressive agents will help us to define more effective cancer treatment strategies for organ transplant recipients.

In this review, we shed light on the cell-intrinsic tumorigenic pathways directly activated by immunosuppressive agents and the infection- and immune-mediated mechanisms of cancer development in organ transplant recipients.

HYPOXIA-RELATED SIGNALING MOLECULES IN POSTTRANSPLANT CANCER

In the process of procurement, preservation, and reperfusion, donor organs are subjected to hypoxia (lack of oxygen supply) and ischemic injury (lack of blood supply), commonly known as ischemia–reperfusion injury (IRI). Hypoxia and IRI are detrimental for preserving organ function and long-term graft survival.[6] The hypoxia-related signaling molecules involved in tumorigenic pathways are shown in **Fig. 1**.

In response to hypoxia, oxygen-sensitive transcription factors, termed as hypoxia-inducible factors (HIFs), regulate the transcription of hypoxia-responsive genes as a protective mechanism. A hypoxia-regulated α chain (1α, 2α, and 3α), bound to an oxygen-independent β chain, makes up the heterodimer complex of HIF. The cytoprotective function of HIF-1α and HIF-2α are well-studied. The activity of HIFs increases the expression of cytoprotective molecules including heat shock proteins, erythropoietin, and heme oxygenase-1 (HO-1). HO-1 catabolizes heme and the byproducts of this enzymatic reaction mediate cytoprotection.[7] Reports suggest that HO-1 promotes antiapoptotic pathways in response to IRI[8] and may play a significant role in the induction of tumorigenic pathways. Another molecule, vascular endothelial growth factor (VEGF), a downstream target of HIFs, also can contribute to tumor development when its levels increase, given that it plays a critical role in the formation of new blood vessels in tumor (tumor angiogenesis).[9]

Under normoxic conditions, the subunits of HIFs are targeted for polyubiquitination- and proteasome-mediated degradation by the tumor suppressor protein Von Hippel-Lindau (VHL).[6] VHL inactivation represents a pseudohypoxic condition and causes constitutive activation of HIFs, leading to an increased expression of cytoprotective molecules. Interestingly, germline mutations in VHL gene (known as VHL disease) are associated with the abnormal regulation of hypoxic response genes and predisposition to many malignancies including renal tumors, implying the role of hypoxia-related signaling pathways in posttransplant cancer.

Reactive oxygen species (ROS; such as superoxide, peroxide, and hydrogen peroxide) are reactive molecules derived from molecular oxygen and hydroxyl radical as a result of mitochondrial electron transport chain and the activity of nicotinamide adenine dinucleotide phosphate oxidases. Increase in ROS during IRI or pharmacologic agent-induced generation of ROS leads to oxidative stress and cell death.[8] However, cellular antioxidant enzymes, such as HO-1, manganese superoxide dismutase

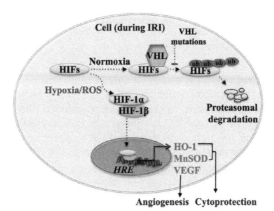

Fig. 1. Hypoxia-related signaling molecules in posttransplantation cancer. Under normoxic conditions, Von Hippel-Lindau (VHL) protein targets hypoxia-inducible factors (HIFs) for degradation. However, during ischemia–reperfusion injury (IRI), hypoxia and reactive oxygen species (ROS) generation activate HIFs. Activated HIFs translocate to nucleus and bind hypoxia response elements (HRE) in the promoter regions of hypoxia-inducible genes, such as HO-1 and manganese superoxide dismutase (MnSOD), and angiogenic factors (like vascular endothelial growth factor), leading to overexpression of these molecules.

and NAD(P)H dehydrogenase [quinone] 1, counteract ROS and mediate cytoprotection. Thus, a critical balance exists between the levels of ROS and the antioxidant system, and a shift toward an increased expression of cellular antioxidants can lead to oncogenic transformation of the cell.[7]

MOLECULAR TARGETS OF IMMUNOSUPPRESSIVE AGENTS

Immunosuppressive regimens are essential in SOT to suppress alloimmunity and prevent graft rejection. Understanding the molecular targets of immunosuppressive agents can shed light on protumorigenic mechanisms associated with immunosuppression. Effector T cells play a critical role in the immunologic rejection of transplanted graft. Immunosuppressive agents, used at various levels and combinations in SOT, inhibit the stimulation, activation, and expansion of effector T cells through different mechanisms.

Target genes of transcription factor nuclear factor of activated T cells (NFAT) are essential and contribute to the effector functions of T cell. T-cell receptor signaling increases intracellular calcium levels and activates calmodulin, which in turn binds and activates calcineurin. Phosphorylated NFAT is inactive and resides in the cytoplasm. Activated calcineurin, with its protein phosphatase activity, dephosphorylates NFAT and promotes the nuclear translocation of NFAT to activate transcription of NFAT target genes, including IL-2, IL-4, and IFN-γ, leading to T-cell activation.[10]

Calcineurin Inhibitors

CNIs such as tacrolimus (FK506) and cyclosporine, the most widely used immunosuppressive agent in transplant medicine, inhibit the activity of calcineurin, thereby suppressing NFAT-mediated transcription of cytokines necessary for the activation of T cells. Immunophilins such as cyclophilins and FK506-binding proteins (FKBPs) are cytosolic peptidyl-prolyl isomerases that catalyze cis-trans isomerization of proline residues and act as chaperones (proteins that regulate intermolecular and intramolecular interactions and govern proper protein folding and complex formation). Cyclosporine and tacrolimus form drug/immunophilin complexes by binding to cyclophilin and FKBP, respectively, and inactivate calcineurin.[10]

Mechanistic Target of Rapamycin Inhibitors

The mechanistic target of rapamycin (mTOR) signaling pathway regulates cell cycle progression, metabolism, and protein synthesis in response to a variety of stimuli including growth factors and nutrients. mTOR is a serine/threonine protein kinase and downstream effector molecule for growth factors-induced phosphoinositide 3-kinase (PI3K)-Akt signaling pathways. The tumor suppresser gene phosphatase and tensin homolog inhibits Akt activation through PI3K suppression and phosphatase and tensin homolog is lost or mutated in many cancer types, leading to hyperactivation of the mTOR pathway in cancer cells.

mTOR forms 2 distinct signaling complexes, namely the mTOR complex 1, containing RAPTOR, and mTOR complex 2, containing RICTOR. mTOR complexes regulate protein translation by modulating the activity of S6 kinase (known as p70S6K) and eukaryotic translation initiation factor 4E (through the regulation of el4E-bindng protein). mTOR inhibitors, such as rapamycin (sirolimus) and its derivatives (temsirolimus and everolimus), form drug/immunophilin complex by binding to FKBP12 and inhibit mTOR. IL-2/IL-2R and other growth factor-mediated signaling trigger mTOR pathway in T cells. mTOR inhibitors affect T-cell protein synthesis, leading to T-cell inactivation.[10]

Purine Analogues

Impeding DNA synthesis inhibits cell proliferation. Guanosine, a purine nucleoside, is an essential building block of DNA and RNA. Inosine-5'-monophosphate dehydrogenase is the enzyme involved in the de novo synthesis of guanosine. In contrast with many other cell types, which can also synthesize guanosine by recycled salvage pathways, T lymphocytes are dependent on inosine-5'-monophosphate dehydrogenase for the de novo synthesis of guanosine. Therefore, molecules (mycophenolate mofetil and mycophenolic acid) that inhibit IMDH activity and disrupt guanosine synthesis or purine analogues that interfere with the incorporation of endogenous purines (eg, azathioprine, 6-mercaptopurine) inhibit T-cell proliferation.[10]

Biologics

Biologic medicines, such as monoclonal antibodies, polyclonal antibodies, and recombinant fusion proteins, targeting key pathways involved in T-cell activation, are predominantly used either for induction therapy (the first phase of treatment) or in the treatment of acute rejection. Antibodies targeting IL2-R (basiliximab) have remarkable success in preventing graft rejection. Biologics targeting costimulatory pathways of T-cell activation are promising medicines in SOT. B7 family of ligands can bind to both CD28 and cytotoxic T-lymphocyte associated protein 4 (CTLA-4). In contrast with B7-CD28 interactions, which promote costimulatory signal, B7–CTLA-4 interactions inhibit T-cell activation. A recombinant CTLA-4 linked to an immunoglobulin frame, comparable with the soluble form of CTLA-4, can disrupt the B7-CD28 costimulatory interactions and inhibit T-cell activation.[11]

The mechanistic targets of different immunosuppressive agents used in SOT are depicted in **Fig. 2**. As discussed elsewhere in this article, biologics are mostly used in induction therapy, and among pharmacologic immunosuppressive agents, CNIs have been the standard of care in maintenance immunosuppression after SOT. However, malignancy is one of the important risks associated with the use of immunosuppressive agents, including CNIs.[12]

IMMUNOSUPPRESSIVE AGENT-INDUCED CELL-INTRINSIC TUMORIGENIC PATHWAYS

Recent reports suggest that immunosuppressive agents can directly promote tumorigenic pathways. The molecular events related to the immunosuppressive agent-induced growth and proliferation of cancer cells are represented in **Fig. 3**.

Role of Oncogene Ras

Activated Ras proteins transmit signals to other kinases including Raf family of kinases, resulting in the activation of mitogen-activated protein kinase and extracellular signal-regulated kinase. In addition to Raf, Ras also mediates its action through the activation of Rho and PI3K pathways. Therefore, sustained activation of Ras can transduce mitogenic signals and promote the growth of cancer cells. Raf kinase inhibitory protein, an inhibitor of Raf kinase, suppresses the Ras–Raf pathway. Carabin is an endogenous inhibitor of Ras. Interestingly, CNI treatment inhibits both Raf kinase inhibitory protein and carabin in cancer cells, leading to hyperactivation of the Ras–Raf pathway and promotion of tumor growth.[13]

Receptor Tyrosine Kinase–Mediated Signaling

RTKs are cell surface receptors that bind and respond to various factors, such as chemokines, cytokines and other growth factors (such as epidermal growth factor, insulin, and hepatocyte growth factor). RTKs play an important role in the regulation of cell

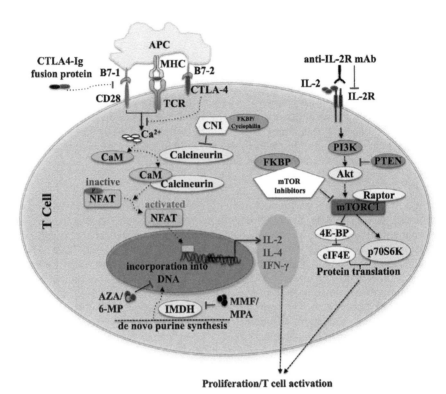

Fig. 2. Molecular targets of immunosuppressive agents. *Top left,* Antigen presentation via MHC on antigen-presenting cells (APCs) and costimulatory interactions (like B7-1/CD28) activate T-cell receptors (TCRs), and it leads to an increase in the intracellular calcium levels and activation of calmodulin (CaM), which in turn binds and activates calcineurin. Phosphorylated nuclear factor of activated T cells (NFAT) are inactive and reside in the cytoplasm. Activated calcineurin, with its protein phosphatase activity, dephosphorylates NFAT and promotes the nuclear translocation of NFAT to activate transcription of NFAT target genes, including IL-2, IL-4, and IFN-γ, leading to T-cell activation. Coinhibitory interactions like B7-2/cytotoxic T-lymphocyte associated protein 4 (CTLA)-4 suppress TCR-mediated signaling. Recombinant fusion CTLA4-Ig can disrupt B7-1/CD28 and other costimulatory signals necessary for T-cell activation. Calcineurin inhibitors (CNIs) form drug/FKBP (or cyclophilin) complex and inactivate calcineurin. *Right,* Mechanistic target of rapamycin (mTOR) is a serine/threonine protein kinase and is one of the downstream effector molecules for IL-2/IL-2R (and other growth factors)-induced phosphoinositide 3-kinase (PI3K)-Akt signaling pathways. Phosphatase and tensin homolog (PTEN) inhibits Akt activation through PI3K suppression. mTOR complex 1 (mTORC1), the functional protein complex containing RAPTOR, regulates protein translation by modulating the activity of p70S6K and eukaryotic translation initiation factor 4E (through eI4E-bindng protein [4E-BP]). mTOR inhibitors form drug/FKBP complex and inhibit mTOR. Anti–IL-2R antibody blocks the activation of IL-2R. *Bottom left,* Mycophenolate mofetil (MMF) and mycophenolic acid (MPA) inhibit IMDH-dependent de novo synthesis of guanosine nucleoside. Azathioprine (AZA) and 6-mercaptopurine (6-MP) antagonize endogenous purines and prevent the incorporation of guanosine into DNA. mAb, monoclonal antibody.

growth, differentiation and survival. Ligand binding to the extracellular domains of the RTKs induces cross-phosphorylation of specific tyrosine residues in the intracellular domains of the RTKs. Phosphotyrosine residues thus generated serve as docking sites of several Src homology 2 domain-containing signal transduction adapter

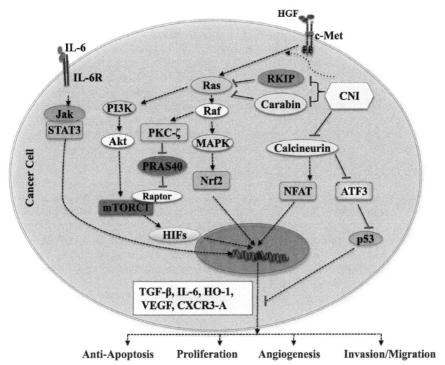

Fig. 3. Immunosuppressive agent-induced cell-intrinsic tumorigenic pathways. *Right*, RTK c-Met–mediated signaling promotes the activation of Ras-Raf–mitogen activated protein kinase (MAPK) pathways and the nuclear translocation of nuclear factor erythroid 2-related factor 2 (Nrf2), leading to overexpression of heme oxygenase-1 (HO-1). CNI enhances c-Met-induced Ras activation and HO-1 expression. Calcineurin inhibitors (CNI) inhibit Raf kinase inhibitory protein (RKIP) and carabin, the negative regulators of Ras, and contributes to sustained Ras activation in cancer cells. CNI promote the expression of activating transcription factor 3 (ATF3), and it can inhibit p53-mediated apoptotic pathways. *Center*, CNI increase the expression of vascular endothelial growth factor (VEGF) via the phosphoinositide 3-kinase (PI3K)-Akt–mechanistic target of rapamycin mTOR complex 1 (mTORC1) pathway channeled through hypoxia-inducible factors (HIFs). CNI-induced Ras-Raf-protein kinase C (PKC)-ζ activation inhibits proline-rich Akt substrate 40 (PRAS40), the negative regulator of mTORC1, and augments mTORC1 activity. CNI treatment increases the expression of transforming growth factor (TGF)-β, IL-6, and C-X-C motif chemokine receptor 3 [CXCR3]-A (the growth promoting CXCR3 isoform). *Left*, IL-6–mediated signaling activates Janus tyrosine kinase (JAK)–signal transducer and activator of transcription 3 (STAT3) pathway. Together, CNI-induced signaling activates cell-intrinsic protumorigenic pathways. HGF, hepatocyte growth factor.

molecules, which in turn relay the signaling to diverse downstream intracellular signaling pathways including Ras–Raf–mitogen-activated protein kinase and PI3K-Akt signaling pathways.[7]

RTK c-MET and its ligand hepatocyte growth factor play a significant role in the growth and progression of cancer cells. Transcription factors nuclear factor erythroid 2 [NF-E2]-related factor 2 (Nrf2) and BTB and CNC homology 1 (Bach1) regulate HO-1 expression in a positive and negative manner, respectively. In renal cancer cells, CNI treatment induces nuclear localization of Nrf2, leading to an overexpression of HO-1 and plays an important role in the growth and survival of cancer cells.[7]

Modulation of Chemokine Receptor Expression

Chemokines and their receptors play an important role in chemotaxis. Recent studies suggest a role in tumor growth as well. Chemokine receptor C-X-C motif chemokine receptor 3 (CXCR3), belonging to the family of G-protein–coupled receptors (GPCRs), exists as 2 isoforms namely CXCR3-A and CXCR3-B.[14] In contrast with CXCR3-A–mediated signaling, which promotes proliferative signals, CXCR3-B–mediated signaling inhibits the proliferation of cancer cells. In cancer cells, CNI treatment down-regulated the expression of the CXCR3-B isoform, whereas expression of CXCR3-A was not affected.[14] This report suggests that CNI-mediated modulation of alternative splicing of CXCR3 gene can play a significant role in the growth of tumors.[14]

Overexpression of Vascular Endothelial Growth Factor

Unphosphorylated proline-rich Akt substrate 40 negatively regulates mTOR complex 1 activity by sequestering RAPTOR from the complex. CNI-induced Ras activation pro-motes the phosphorylation of proline-rich Akt substrate 40 through protein kinase C and relieves the negative effect of proline-rich Akt substrate 40 on mTOR complex, leading to transcriptional activation of mTOR downstream target genes, including VEGF. Thus, CNI-induced cross-talk between Ras and mTOR increases the expres-sion of VEGF and promotes rapid progression of tumor.[15]

Role of Cytokines

It is well-established that cytokines, such as interleukins and interferons, modulate tumorigenic pathways. A notable cytokine involved in tumorigenesis is IL-6. The tumorigenic role of Janus tyrosine kinase/signal transducer and activator of transcrip-tion 3 activation in response to IL-6 has been well-described in many cancer types. CNI treatment increases IL-6 production in EBV-infected B cells and can play a potent role in cancer development.[1]

Transforming growth factor beta (TGF-β), a multifunctional polypeptide belonging to the TGF-β family of cytokines, while acting as a tumor suppressor during primary tu-mor development, promotes cancer cell migration and stimulates epithelial–mesenchymal transition, an invasive phenotype associated with metastasis. Reports suggest that CNI-induced TGF-β secretion can impart an invasive phenotype to non-transformed cells and promote tumor growth.[16]

Role of p53

p53, a tumor suppressor, induces cell cycle arrest and apoptosis in response to vari-ety of stimuli, including UV radiation (sunlight exposure), which cause DNA damage. CNIs downmodulate p53-dependent cell senescence in some cell types. Activating transcription factor 3 is negatively regulated by the calcineurin/NFAT pathway, and activating transcription factor 3 suppresses p53-dependent cell senescence. The CNI-mediated inhibition of calcineurin/NFAT increases the expression of activating transcription factor 3 and inhibits p53-dependent apoptotic pathways in cancer cells.[10]

Anticancer Effects of Mechanistic Target of Rapamycin Inhibitors

Although relatively less potent in terms of immunosuppression, reports suggest that the use of mTOR inhibitors have potent anticancer effects as evident from the decreased risk of cancer in transplant recipients treated with mTOR inhibitors (like rapamycin), either before or after a CNI regimen.[12] However, mTOR inhibition leads to the withdrawal of the negative regulatory loop between p70S6K and insulin receptor substrate 1, resulting in insulin receptor substrate 1–mediated Akt activation. Also, mTOR complex 2, which is mostly insensitive to rapamycin, can contribute to Akt activation. More research is needed to elucidate the tumor resistance mechanisms associated with mTOR inhibition.[12]

ONCOGENIC VIRAL INFECTIONS IN POSTTRANSPLANT MALIGNANCIES

Opportunistic and cotumorigenic viral infections, such as EBV, HHV8, and human papillomavirus, can promote certain types of cancer owing to immunosuppression in a transplant recipient. Cytomegalovirus infection, the most prevalent infection after transplantation, can lead to cytomegalovirus syndrome and end-organ disease. Although cytomegalovirus infection can be counteracted with prophylactic antivirals, it leads to other infections. In general, viral infections promote tumorigenesis through the disruption of apoptotic machinery of the infected cell, promoting escape of host immunosurveillance. Molecular mechanisms associated with viral infection-related malignancies in SOT are depicted in **Fig. 4**.

Epstein–Barr Virus

EBV infection poses a 20-fold increased risk for posttransplant lymphoproliferative disorder, including non-Hodgkin's lymphoma and Hodgkin's lymphoma.[2] Latent infection of EBV immortalizes B cells. Further, a lack of cytotoxic T cells, resulting from T-cell–depleting induction therapy for the treatment of acute graft rejection, fuels uncontrolled growth of EBV-infected B cells. Reports suggest that EBV infection results in the production of abnormally high levels of IL-6, leading to growth of B cells.[1] Thus, IL-6 plays a critical role in the pathogenesis of posttransplant lymphoproliferative disorder. In addition, EBV infection induced secretion of IL-10, a cytokine with immunosuppressive properties, aids in tumor development.[17]

Human Herpes Virus

HHV8 infection has been associated with increased risk of Kaposi's sarcoma after SOT with an SIR of 64.4.[5] HHV8-encoded viral Fas-associated death domain-like interleukin-1β-converting enzyme-inhibitory protein (vFLIP) suppresses CD95 (APO-1/Fas)-mediated apoptosis. Binding of CD95L to CD95 and association with Fas-associated death-domain containing protein leads to the formation of death-inducing signaling complex, which activates procaspase-8–mediated apoptosis. However, recruitment of cellular FLIP at death-inducing signaling complex inhibits procaspase-8 activation. vFLIP, comparable with cellular FLIP, disrupts death-inducing signaling complex activity and inhibits apoptosis. CD95-mediated apoptosis is essential for the immune-mediated elimination of virus-infected cells. Therefore, vFLIP expression helps HHV8-infected cells to evade host immunosurveillance.[18]

The B-cell lymphoma 2 family of proteins regulate both proapoptotic and antiapoptotic pathways. B-cell lymphoma 2 inhibits apoptosis and promotes cell survival. HHV-8–encoded viral GPCR (vGPCR) increases the expression of B-cell lymphoma 2 and inhibits apoptosis, leading to uncontrolled proliferation of the virus-infected cells.[19] Additionally, vGPCR is proangiogenic and increases the expression of many angiogenic factors, including VEGF and angiopoietin-2, as well as angiogenic receptors including VEGF and angiopoietin receptors.[20] Endothelial cells play a major role in angiogenesis and reports suggest that vGPCR activates VEGF receptors and promotes the proliferation of endothelial cells.[20] Remarkably, vFLIP also protects the endothelial cells from superoxide-induced apoptosis through the expression of antioxidant and antiapoptotic manganese superoxide dismutase.[18]

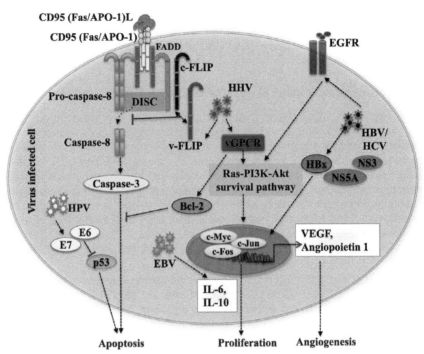

Fig. 4. Oncogenic viral infections in posttransplantation malignancies. *Top left*, Binding of CD95(Fas/APO-1)L to CD95(Fas/APO-1) initiates the formation of death-inducing signaling complex (DISC) involving pro-caspase-8 and Fas-associated death-domain containing protein (FADD) resulting in the activation of pro-caspase-8. Subsequent activation of other caspases promotes apoptosis. Human herpesvirus (HHV)-encoded viral Fas-associated death domain-like interleukin-1β–converting enzyme-inhibitory protein (vFLIP) interferes with the activation of pro-caspase-8 at DISC and inhibits apoptosis. HHV-encoded viral G protein-coupled receptor (vGPCR) promotes Ras-PI3K-Akt survival pathway and increases the expression of antiapoptotic Bcl-2. *Right*, Hepatitis B virus (HBV)-encoded HBx and hepatitis C virus (HCV)-encoded NS3 and NS5A proteins activate Ras-PI3K-Akt survival pathway. HBx and NS5A modulate RTK epidermal growth factor receptor (EGFR)-mediated signaling. HBx modulates the transcriptional activity of c-Myc, c-Fos and c-Jun and increases the expression of angiogenic factors, such as vascular endothelial growth factor (VEGF) and angiopoietin-1. *Bottom*, Human papillomavirus (HPV)-encoded E6 and E7 proteins inhibit p53-mediated apoptosis. Epstein–Barr virus (EBV) infection increases the secretion of IL-6 and IL-10. Together, oncogenic virus infection disrupts the apoptotic machinery of infected cells and also promotes angiogenesis, resulting in the malignant transformation of the infected cell.

Human Papillomavirus

Human papillomavirus-encoded E6 and E7 proteins inhibit p53-mediated apoptosis and promote malignant proliferation of host cells.[21]

Hepatitis B Virus and Hepatitis C Virus

Reports suggest that HBV and HCV infections are risk factors in posttransplant liver cancer. HBV-encoded HBx protein and HCV-encoded NS3 and NS5A proteins play a critical role in hepatic carcinogenic mechanisms. HBx promotes Ras activation, and both HBx and NS5A promote the PI3K–Akt survival pathway. Interestingly, HBx and NS5A modulate RTK epidermal growth factor receptor expression and ligand-binding activity, respectively, leading to the enhancement of the PI3K-Akt downstream signaling pathway. HBV infection leads to increased expression of VEGF and angiopoietin-1 and modulates liver angiogenesis. HBV and HCV viral proteins also modulate the transcriptional activity of protooncogenes c-Myc, c-Fos, and c-Jun and promote cell proliferation.[22]

IMMUNOSUPPRESSION-RELATED IMPAIRED TUMOR IMMUNOSURVEILLANCE

Tumor immunosurveillance is a complex interplay between tumor-intrinsic/-derived factors and the ability of host immune system to recognize and eliminate tumor cells. When tumor cells escape the attack of immune cells, tumor development is favored. Besides promoting cell-intrinsic protumorigenic pathways, immunosuppressive agents can also modulate host tumor immunosurveillance and contribute to posttransplant malignancies.

In addition to inhibiting T-cell functions, immunosuppression changes the phenotype of other immune cells. In transplant recipients with cancer, CD8$^+$ T cells have increased expression of CD57, a marker of T-cell immunosenescence. T-bet is a

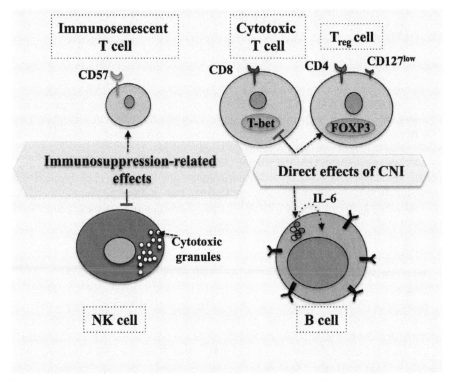

Fig. 5. Immunosuppression-related impaired tumor immunosurveillance. Important changes observed in the immune phenotype of transplant recipients, as a result of immunosuppression, are summarized. A calcineurin inhibitor (CNI) regimen has been associated with an increase in T regulatory (T$_{reg}$) cells and increased production of IL-6 from B cells. Increase in immunosenescent T cells and impaired natural killer (NK) cell cytotoxicity were observed in organ transplant recipients treated with CNI. Also, CNI treatment downregulated T-bet expression in CD8$^+$ T cells and drastically affected its cytotoxic effector functions in vivo. Taken together, immunosuppression alters the phenotype and functions of immune cells, leading to impaired tumor immunosurveillance.

key transcription factor regulating cytotoxic CD8[+] T-cell functions. Interestingly, CNI treatment, but not mTOR inhibition, downregulated T-bet expression in CD8[+] T cells and drastically affected cancer cytotoxicity in vivo.[23] Regulatory T cells, a subset of T cells (CD4[+]FOXP3[+]CD127[low]), suppress activation, proliferation, and cytokine production of effector T cells. Regulatory T cells are essential to check uncontrolled/ excessive immune reactions and to maintain immune homeostasis. However, abnormal increases in regulatory T cells suppresses effector T-cell functions and aids tumor cells escape of immune-mediated attack. CNI use has been associated with higher levels of regulatory T cells in the peripheral blood of kidney transplant recipients.[1] CNI treatment affects T-cell motility and migration of dendritic cells in response to chemokines in vitro.[24] Natural killer cells can recognize and eliminate tumor or virus infected cells through the release of cytotoxic granules. Decreased numbers of natural killer cells and reduced natural killer cell function are associated with cancers in organ transplant recipients.[1] In addition, CNI-induced secretion of immunomodulatory factors, such as TGF-β and IL-6 (which regulate B-cell activation and proliferation), and other host-derived immunosuppressive factors, such as IL-10 and adenosine, can negatively affect tumor immunosurveillance involving both the innate and the adaptive immunity system.[1] Potential mechanisms associated with immunosuppression-related impaired tumor immunosurveillance are schematically shown in **Fig. 5**.

SUMMARY

The incidence and mortality of cancers among transplant recipients are at least 2-fold higher when compared with the general population. This increased risk for cancer can be attributed to the burden of immunosuppressive regimens, infection, and altered immune phenotype. We have summarized the molecular mechanisms associated with the direct influence of immunosuppressive agents on cell-intrinsic tumorigenic pathways. Future research and clinical studies will reveal the efficacy of novel immunosuppressive agents (like Janus tyrosine kinase inhibitor) and the success of development of new concepts of immunomodulatory strategies, such as targeting T-cell glycolysis, T-cell cosignaling molecules, and the purinergic signaling axis. The goal is to achieve long-term graft survival while mitigating the risk of posttransplant cancer.

REFERENCES

1. Au E, Wong G, Chapman JR. Cancer in kidney transplant recipients. Nat Rev Nephrol 2018;14(8):508–20.
2. Sprangers B, Nair V, Launay-Vacher V, et al. Risk factors associated with post-kidney transplant malignancies: an article from the Cancer-Kidney International Network. Clin Kidney J 2018;11(3):315–29.
3. van de Wetering J, Roodnat JI, Hemke AC, et al. Patient survival after the diagnosis of cancer in renal transplant recipients: a nested case-control study. Transplantation 2010;90(12):1542–6.
4. Hall EC, Pfeiffer RM, Segev DL, et al. Cumulative incidence of cancer after solid organ transplantation. Cancer 2013;119(12):2300–8.
5. Engels EA, Pfeiffer RM, Fraumeni JF Jr, et al. Spectrum of cancer risk among US solid organ transplant recipients. JAMA 2011;306(17):1891–901.
6. Akhtar MZ, Sutherland AI, Huang H, et al. The role of hypoxia-inducible factors in organ donation and transplantation: the current perspective and future opportunities. Am J Transplant 2014;14(7):1481–7.

7. Balan M, Chakraborty S, Flynn E, et al. Honokiol inhibits c-Met-HO-1 tumor-promoting pathway and its cross-talk with calcineurin inhibitor-mediated renal cancer growth. Sci Rep 2017;7(1):5900.
8. Akhtar MZ, Henderson T, Sutherland A, et al. Novel approaches to preventing ischemia-reperfusion injury during liver transplantation. Transplant Proc 2013; 45(6):2083–92.
9. Basu A, Contreras AG, Datta D, et al. Overexpression of vascular endothelial growth factor and the development of post-transplantation cancer. Cancer Res 2008;68(14):5689–98.
10. Jung JW, Overgaard NH, Burke MT, et al. Does the nature of residual immune function explain the differential risk of non-melanoma skin cancer development in immunosuppressed organ transplant recipients? Int J Cancer 2016;138(2): 281–92.
11. Perez CP, Patel N, Mardis CR, et al. Belatacept in solid organ transplant: review of current literature across transplant types. Transplantation 2018;102(9):1440–52.
12. Gaumann A, Schlitt HJ, Geissler EK. Immunosuppression and tumor development in organ transplant recipients: the emerging dualistic role of rapamycin. Transpl Int 2008;21(3):207–17.
13. Datta D, Contreras AG, Basu A, et al. Calcineurin inhibitors activate the proto-oncogene Ras and promote protumorigenic signals in renal cancer cells. Cancer Res 2009;69(23):8902–9.
14. Datta D, Contreras AG, Grimm M, et al. Calcineurin inhibitors modulate CXCR3 splice variant expression and mediate renal cancer progression. J Am Soc Nephrol 2008;19(12):2437–46.
15. Basu A, Banerjee P, Contreras AG, et al. Calcineurin inhibitor-induced and Ras-mediated overexpression of VEGF in renal cancer cells involves mTOR through the regulation of PRAS40. PLoS One 2011;6(8):e23919.
16. Hojo M, Morimoto T, Maluccio M, et al. Cyclosporine induces cancer progression by a cell-autonomous mechanism. Nature 1999;397(6719):530–4.
17. Martinez OM, de Gruijl FR. Molecular and immunologic mechanisms of cancer pathogenesis in solid organ transplant recipients. Am J Transplant 2008;8(11): 2205–11.
18. Thurau M, Marquardt G, Gonin-Laurent N, et al. Viral inhibitor of apoptosis vFLIP/K13 protects endothelial cells against superoxide-induced cell death. J Virol 2009;83(2):598–611.
19. Abboud ER, Shelby BD, Angelova M, et al. Kaposi sarcoma-associated herpesvirus g protein-coupled receptor enhances endothelial cell survival in part by up-regulation of bcl-2. Ochsner J 2013;13(1):66–75.
20. Jham BC, Montaner S. The Kaposi's sarcoma-associated herpesvirus G protein-coupled receptor: lessons on dysregulated angiogenesis from a viral oncogene. J Cell Biochem 2010;110(1):1–9.
21. Tomaic V. Functional roles of E6 and E7 oncoproteins in HPV-induced malignancies at diverse anatomical sites. Cancers (Basel) 2016;8(10) [pii:E95].
22. Zemel R, Issachar A, Tur-Kaspa R. The role of oncogenic viruses in the pathogenesis of hepatocellular carcinoma. Clin Liver Dis 2011;15(2):261–79, vii–x.
23. Rovira J, Renner P, Sabet-Baktach M, et al. Cyclosporine A inhibits the T-bet-dependent antitumor response of CD8(+) T cells. Am J Transplant 2016;16(4): 1139–47.
24. Datta A, David R, Glennie S, et al. Differential effects of immunosuppressive drugs on T-cell motility. Am J Transplant 2006;6(12):2871–83.

Immunologic Effects of the Microbiota in Organ Transplantation

Kevin Rey, BSc[a,b], Jonathan C. Choy, PhD[a,b,*]

KEYWORDS

- Microbiota • Transplantation • Immune regulation

KEY POINTS

- The gut microbiota controls immune activation and regulation.
- Immunosuppressive drug activity may be affected by the gut microbiota.
- The presence of microbiota in graft recipients and donors can exacerbate transplant rejection.
- The gut microbiota has immune regulatory effects that prevent transplant rejection.

INTRODUCTION

Organ transplantation is the most effective treatment for end-stage organ failure but its success is limited by the eventual immune-mediated rejection of most grafts.[1] The current therapy for preventing graft rejection is life-long treatment with immunosuppressive drugs but this is associated with increased risk of malignancy and opportunistic infection. Future advances in the management of patients will require a better understanding of how the immune system is activated and regulated in response to transplanted organs.

The immune system senses environmental conditions in order to tailor the host response to specific exposures. As such, there is an intimate relationship between the immune system and microbes that colonize body surfaces. The microbiota is a community of bacteria, viruses, and fungi that inhabit the surfaces of the body. With

Funding: This work was funded by a grant from the Heart and Stroke Foundation of Canada (J. C. Choy). J.C. Choy is the recipient of a Michael Smith Foundation for Health Research Scholar award.
Disclosures: The authors have nothing to disclose.
a Department of Molecular Biology and Biochemistry, Simon Fraser University, 8888 University Drive, Burnaby, BC V5A 1S6, Canada; b Centre for Cell Biology, Development and Disease, Simon Fraser University, 8888 University Drive, Burnaby, BC V5A 1S6, Canada
* Corresponding author. Department of Molecular Biology and Biochemistry, Simon Fraser University, 8888 University Drive, Burnaby, BC V5A 1S6, Canada
E-mail address: jonathan.choy@sfu.ca

specific regard to the immune system, these microbes influence development and activation of this physiologic system.[2] As such, understanding the influence of the microbiota on immune responses that cause transplant rejection is an exciting and nascent field of study.

IMMUNOLOGIC REJECTION OF ORGAN TRANSPLANTS

The surgical introduction of a foreign organ into the body is an acutely powerful stimulus that causes activation of the host immune system. Early inflammatory and innate immune signals are essential for immune activation that causes graft rejection. The release of endogenous "danger" signals, such as High Mobility Group Box 1 and heat shock proteins, leads to their binding to innate immune receptors.[3] This results in the secretion of inflammatory cytokines that stimulate the recruitment of leukocytes into the transplanted organ.[4] Neutrophils, macrophages, and natural killer cells infiltrate transplanted organs early after surgery. They are directly cytotoxic, increase the production of cytokines and aid in recruitment of additional immune cells.[5–10]

Inflammatory signals also prime the activation of antigen presenting cells, such as dendritic cells and macrophages, which enable these cells to activate T cells that recognize antigens expressed by the donor.[11–15] These effector T cells then infiltrate the graft and cause rejection via killing or cytokine-mediated dysfunction of graft cells.[16–18] T cells also support the generation of antibodies generated toward grafts and this contributes to transplant rejection.[19,20]

In order to prevent rejection, recipients take life-long immunosuppressive agents. Drugs that inhibit calcineurin signaling, such as tacrolimus and cyclosporine, are most commonly used in combination with steroids.[21] These drugs work to inhibit pathways essential for T-cell activation. Cell cycle inhibitors, such as azathioprine and mycophenolate mofetil, can also be used to inhibit lymphocyte proliferation. Unfortunately, these drugs act broadly as immunosuppressive agents and have detrimental nonimmunologic side effects.

Immune activation is specifically opposed by the action of regulatory T cells (Tregs). These cells develop in the thymus or in peripheral tissues and inhibit immune responses by expressing inhibitory cell surface molecules, secreting immune inhibitory cytokines and metabolites, and depleting local levels of interleukin 2 (IL-2).[22] In transplantation, depletion of Tregs exacerbates rejection of grafts and increasing their numbers increases graft survival.[23–26] In addition to Tregs, other immune regulatory cell types, such as plasmacytoid dendritic cells and myeloid-derived suppressor cells, also inhibit T-cell responses and may prevent transplant rejection.[27–29] Development of cell therapy approaches using these regulatory cell types are in clinical trials for the management of organ transplant rejection (ONE Study, NCT02129881).

IMMUNOLOGIC EFFECTS OF THE MICROBIOTA

Microbes colonize all body surfaces and the gut microbiota is the most extensively studied microbial community affecting human health.[30,31] Importantly, the impact of the gut microbiota extends beyond that of the biology of the intestinal tract because it influences extraintestinal tissues.[32–34] Studies in which the gut microbiota is absent, depleted with antibiotics, or selectively reconstituted have shown that it controls protective and pathologic immune responses.[35,36] As a protective influence on human health, signals from this microbial community increase immune responses against several pathogens by supporting the tonic activation of neutrophils and monocytes.[37–40] Mechanistically, this may involve the induction of type I interferon (IFN) responses.[41] Signals from these microbes also increase the lifespan of neutrophils.[42]

The microbiota also increases IgG production in response to some vaccines and induces innate lymphoid cells to produce cytokines that keep pathogenic bacteria contained to the intestine.[43–45] The abovementioned immunologic effects of this microbial community contribute to healthy immune development.

In addition to protective immune responses, the composition of the gut microbiota also influences immunopathologic responses. Mice that receive fecal microbiota transplants (FMTs) from patients suffering from rheumatoid arthritis and multiple sclerosis (MS) experience increased disease severity compared with those that receive FMT from healthy controls, highlighting the causative effect of the gut microbiota in these disease processes.[46,47] This was associated with a relative decrease in several species of Clostridia in patients with MS.[48]

The effect of the gut microbiota on host immune responses is mediated by the ability of host cells to sense these microbes. Intestinal and immune cells express receptors, such as toll-like receptors (TLRs) and NOD-like receptors, which are activated by binding to microbial ligands. Sensing of these signals by cells in the intestine is essential for immune homeostasis by controlling the expansion and composition of gut microbes.[49] These signals also control the differentiation of immune regulatory cells.[50] Microbial antigens from the gut microbiota also affect immune development and activation.[51] Alterations in these immune regulatory properties of the gut microbiota influences immunopathologic processes.[52]

The gut microbiota has been shown to exacerbate disease in experimental autoimmune encephalomyelitis (EAE), a mouse model of MS, by inducing the development of Th17 cells that migrate to the central nervous system.[53,54] Also, accelerated development of spontaneous EAE in mice is associated with an increase in fecal IgM, which indicates gut dysbiosis, suggesting that proinflammatory signals from the gut accelerate some forms of autoimmunity.[55] Studies have also shown that type 1 diabetes (T1D) in mice is influenced by the composition of the gut microbiota and there may be some effect of the MHC haplotype, indicating that microbial antigens are important.[56,57]

In addition to exacerbating immunopathologic processes, the gut microbiota also induces essential immune regulatory effects that inhibit some immune-mediated diseases. This includes the induction of Tregs and production of immune regulatory metabolites. Several species in the genera *Clostridia* induce Tregs.[58–60] This seems to be a result of antigen-stimulation of Tregs because dendritic cells cocultured with heat-inactivated *Clostridia* are sufficient to elicit this effect.[61] These Tregs are capable of regulating immunopathologies in vivo as indicated by decreased eosinophil infiltration in mice fed with *Clostridium leptum* in a mouse model of airway allergy.[62]

The microbiota exerts a considerable portion of its influence on immune function via by-products of fiber fermentation. Fiber is broken down in the large intestine into the short-chain fatty acids (SCFAs), butyrate, acetate, and propionate, and these metabolites diffuse into the circulation.[63] SCFAs affect intestinal cells as well as immune cells by acting as ligands for receptors or via inhibition of histone deacetylases.[64] High-fiber diets or direct supplementation with SCFAs reduces the severity of food allergy, asthma, and colitis in mouse models.[65–67] This is associated with the generation of Tregs and the modification of inflammasome signaling.[65,67] Specifically, butyrate induces Tregs and increases IL-10 production while also decreasing proinflammatory cytokine production by colonic macrophages.[68,69] Butyrate has also been shown to have a developmental effect on immune regulation because rats born to mothers treated with butyrate while pregnant were resistant to developing virally induced T1D.[70] Acetate is also immunoregulatory through its ability to inhibit neutrophil responses via binding to GPR43.[71,72] However, an immunoregulatory effect of acetate may be context dependent because GPR43 sensing of this SCFA increases the severity of gout and is associated with an increase in reactive oxygen species production by macrophages.[73]

Polysaccharide A (PSA) produced by *Bacteroides fragilis* is another immunoregulatory bacterial metabolite that induces the development of Tregs via TLR2 signaling and increases dendritic cell antigen uptake in mesenteric lymph nodes.[74,75] PSA may also have activity as a ligand for MHCII on the surface of dendritic cells.[76] Tregs induced by PSA-treated dendritic cells have increased suppressive ability and IL-10 production.[77] *B fragilis* colonization protects against EAE induction in mice only if PSA synthesis is intact.[78]

Because the immune response is "educated" by its exposure to environmental stimuli, early life colonization by the gut microbiota has long-lasting effects on health. Temporary treatment with antibiotics that disrupts the composition of the gut microbiota early in life worsens psoriasis; this was partially reversed in antibiotic treated mice by cohousing with untreated mice.[79] Also, mice that develop in the absence of microbiota or that are exposed to certain antibiotics early in life have exacerbated systemic Th2 responses and local pathologic Th2 and Th17 immune responses in the lung.[80–82] Mice born to mothers treated with antibiotics have defective CD8 responses against vaccinia, including impaired IFNγ production.[83] In humans, dysbiosis of the gut microbiota early in life, caused by antibiotics or delivery by caesarean section, is associated with a significantly increased risk of developing childhood asthma.[84,85] These findings emphasize the importance of microbial colonization early in life as a component of immune education that effects responses later in life.

THE GUT MICROBIOTA IN ORGAN TRANSPLANTATION

The clear link between immune regulation and the microbiota suggests that it may be an important consideration when understanding immune responses that cause transplant rejection. Currently the most extensive evidence of the involvement of the microbiota in transplant rejection is in the intestinal inflammation that arises from graft versus host disease (GVHD). Studies in mice showed that GVHD modifies the composition of the gut microbiota and that germ-free or antibiotic-treated mice have more severe GVHD.[86,87] Both the donor and the recipient gut microbiota are influential, because decreased donor microbial diversity and increased recipient exposure to antibiotics increases the risk for aggravated GVHD and 1 year mortality, respectively.[88,89] This may be related to SCFA production because butyrate supports intestinal epithelial cell survival in mice and low butyrate levels after bone marrow transplantation predicts development of GVHD in humans.[90,91] The effects of the gut microbiota on GVHD are likely a result of combined influences on immune activation and the biology of the gut epithelium.

In addition to bone marrow transplantation, the microbiota may affect solid organ transplant rejection (**Fig. 1**). Clinical studies in kidney transplant recipients showed that a reduction in microbial diversity, *Clostridiales* and *Bacteroidiales*, in the gut microbiota is associated with increased posttransplant diarrhea and acute rejection.[92,93] However, there is extensive variability between individuals, which may make it challenging to translate observations into a diagnostic method for predicting acute rejection.[92] The composition of the gut microbiota may also influence immunosuppressive drug action. In kidney transplant recipients, increased relative abundance of *Faecalibacterium prausnitzii* is associated with an increase in tacrolimus dose at 1 month posttransplant.[94] Also, the microbiota of mice that are treated with tacrolimus is protective against skin transplant rejection, likely through the induction of Tregs.[95]

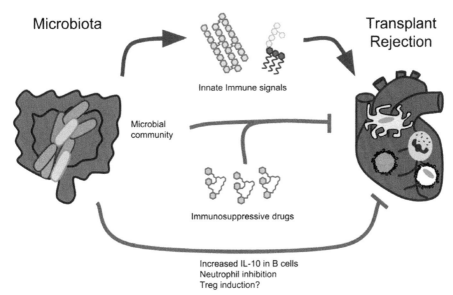

Fig. 1. Effects of the microbiota on organ transplant rejection. The microbiota is a source of microbial components that provides tonic immune-activating signals that exacerbates immune-mediated rejection of transplanted organs. In contrast, this microbial community also has immune regulatory effects and influences the activity of immunosuppressive drugs that can oppose organ transplant rejection.

These studies suggest that the microbiota influences immunosuppressive drug action and may have implications for immunosuppression of patients in the future.

A handful of experimental studies have also directly examined how the gut microbiota influences immune responses that lead to transplant rejection. Lei and colleagues[96] showed that presence of the gut microbiota in both the recipient and donor increases immune activation and transplant rejection using mouse models of skin and heart transplantation. Graft lifespans were increased if both the donor and recipient were germ free or treated with antibiotics. Elimination of microbes shortly before transplantation was sufficient for this effect, which was associated with a reduction in type I IFN and nuclear factor-κB pathway activation in dendritic cells.[96] This indicates that microbiota components provide tonic inflammatory signals that amplify immune rejection of transplanted organs.

In addition to immune-activating effects, the microbiota also has regulatory effects that prevent rejection. These microbes increase the development of transitional B cells that produce IL-10 that prevents tumor necrosis factor alpha production by T cells, increases T-cell derived IL-10 secretion and prolongs allogeneic skin graft survival.[97] Further, signals provided from the gut microbiota to graft recipients early in life have long-lasting effects that inhibit acute rejection later in life. In murine studies, the temporary ablation of the gut microbiota in recipients for only the first 3 weeks of life increased acute rejection of vascular grafts that were placed into these recipients later in life at 8 to 12 weeks of age. This indicates that disruption of the gut microbiota during early life development may have persistent effects on immune regulation that increases the development of immune responses that cause acute rejection.[98] The abovementioned studies taken together show that complex relationships exist between the gut microbiota and immune response that have varied effects on transplant rejection. Future studies are needed to identify ways to precisely target gut microbiota to prolong graft survival.

SUMMARY AND FUTURE DIRECTIONS

Studies over the past decade have established an important role for the gut microbiota in controlling immune development and activation. It is becoming evident that these microbes also affect many immunologic processes that affect organ transplantation. Further studies are needed to examine the mechanistic relationship between the gut microbiota and alloimmune responses as well as to identify therapeutic interventions that can delay or prevent transplant rejection. It will be important to determine the specific components of the microbiota that are protective and those that are pathologic. Also, the effectiveness of probiotics, diet, and other approaches to restore a healthy microbiota will need to be determined in organ transplantation. These approaches may provide safe and effective ways to treat detrimental immune responses in conjunction with immunosuppressive drugs. Lastly, studies that show the long-lasting effect of antibiotics early in life may inform antibiotic use in children.

REFERENCES

1. Lund LH, Khush KK, Cherikh WS, et al. The registry of the International Society for Heart and Lung Transplantation: thirty-fourth adult heart transplantation report-2017; focus theme: allograft ischemic time. J Hear Lung Transplant 2017;36(10):1037–46.
2. Macpherson AJ, de Agüero MG, Ganal-Vonarburg SC. How nutrition and the maternal microbiota shape the neonatal immune system. Nat Rev Immunol 2017;17(8):508–17.
3. Braza F, Brouard S, Chadban S, et al. Role of TLRs and DAMPs in allograft inflammation and transplant outcomes. Nat Rev Nephrol 2016;12(5):281–90.
4. Ishii D, Schenk AD, Baba S, et al. Role of TNFα in early chemokine production and leukocyte infiltration into heart allografts. Am J Transplant 2010;10(1):59–68.
5. Fukuzawa N, Schenk AD, Petro M, et al. High renal ischemia temperature increases neutrophil chemoattractant production and tissue injury during reperfusion without an identifiable role for CD4 T cells in the injury. Transpl Immunol 2009;22(1–2):62–71.
6. Iida S, Tsuda H, Tanaka T, et al. IL-1 receptor signaling on graft parenchymal cells regulates memory and de novo donor-reactive CD8 T cell responses to cardiac allografts. J Immunol 2016;196(6):2827–37.
7. Setoguchi K, Hattori Y, Iida S, et al. Endogenous memory CD8 T cells are activated within cardiac allografts without mediating rejection. Am J Transplant 2013;13(9):2293–307.
8. King CL, Devitt JJ, Lee TDG, et al. Neutrophil mediated smooth muscle cell loss precedes allograft vasculopathy. J Cardiothorac Surg 2010;5:52.
9. So M, Lee TDG, Hancock Friesen CL. Neutrophils are responsible for impaired medial smooth muscle cell recovery and exaggerated allograft vasculopathy in aortic allografts exposed to prolonged cold ischemia. J Hear Lung Transplant 2013;32(3):360–7.
10. Zhang Z-X, Huang X, Jiang J, et al. Natural killer cells play a critical role in cardiac allograft vasculopathy in an interleukin-6–dependent manner. Transplantation 2014;98(10):1029–39.

11. Steptoe RJ, Patel RK, Subbotin VM, et al. Comparative analysis of dendritic cell density and total number in commonly transplanted organs: morphometric estimation in normal mice. Transpl Immunol 2000;8(1):49–56.

12. Ueta H, Shi C, Miyanari N, et al. Systemic transmigration of allosensitizing donor dendritic cells to host secondary lymphoid organs after rat liver transplantation. Hepatology 2008;47(4):1352–62.

13. Celli S, Albert ML, Bousso P. Visualizing the innate and adaptive immune responses underlying allograft rejection by two-photon microscopy. Nat Med 2011;17(6):744–9.

14. Kabelitz D, Herzog WR, Zanker B, et al. Human cytotoxic T lymphocytes. I. Limiting-dilution analysis of alloreactive cytotoxic T-lymphocyte precursor frequencies. Scand J Immunol 1985;22(3):329–35.

15. Herrera OB, Golshayan D, Tibbott R, et al. A novel pathway of alloantigen presentation by dendritic cells. J Immunol 2004;173(8):4828–37.

16. Su CA, Iida S, Abe T, et al. Endogenous memory CD8 T cells directly mediate cardiac allograft rejection. Am J Transplant 2014;14(3):568–79.

17. Setoguchi K, Schenk AD, Ishii D, et al. LFA-1 antagonism inhibits early infiltration of endogenous memory CD8 T Cells into cardiac allografts and donor-reactive T cell priming. Am J Transplant 2011;11(5):923–35.

18. Walch JM, Zeng Q, Li Q, et al. Cognate antigen directs CD8+ T cell migration to vascularized transplants. J Clin Invest 2013;123(6):2663–71.

19. Gorbacheva V, Fan R, Wang X, et al. IFN-γ production by memory helper T cells is required for CD40-independent alloantibody responses. J Immunol 2015;194(3):1347–56.

20. Vaughn GR, Law YM, Jorgensen NW, et al. Antibody mediated rejection is associated with worse outcome than acute cellular rejection after pediatric heart transplant. J Hear Lung Transplant 2016;35(4):S413.

21. Wiseman AC. Immunosuppressive medications. Clin J Am Soc Nephrol 2016;11(2):332–43.

22. Wood KJ, Bushell A, Hester J. Regulatory immune cells in transplantation. Nat Rev Immunol 2012;12(6):417–30.

23. Benghiat FS, Graca L, Braun MY, et al. Critical influence of natural regulatory CD25+ T cells on the fate of allografts in the absence of immunosuppression. Transplantation 2005;79(6):648–54.

24. Wolf D, Schreiber TH, Tryphonopoulos P, et al. Tregs expanded in vivo by TNFRSF25 agonists promote cardiac allograft survival. Transplantation 2012;94(6):569–74.

25. Lal G, Yin N, Xu J, et al. Distinct inflammatory signals have physiologically divergent effects on epigenetic regulation of Foxp3 expression and Treg function. Am J Transplant 2011;11(2):203–14.

26. Jones ND, Brook MO, Carvalho-Gaspar M, et al. Regulatory T cells can prevent memory CD8 + T-cell-mediated rejection following polymorphonuclear cell depletion. Eur J Immunol 2010;40(11):3107–16.

27. Ochando JC, Homma C, Yang Y, et al. Alloantigen-presenting plasmacytoid dendritic cells mediate tolerance to vascularized grafts. Nat Immunol 2006;7(6):652–62.

28. Dugast A-S, Haudebourg T, Coulon F, et al. Myeloid-derived suppressor cells accumulate in kidney allograft tolerance and specifically suppress effector T cell expansion. J Immunol 2008;180(12):7898–906.

29. Lan YY, Wang Z, Raimondi G, et al. "Alternatively Activated" dendritic cells preferentially secrete IL-10, expand Foxp3+CD4+ T cells, and induce long-term

organ allograft survival in combination with CTLA4-Ig. J Immunol 2006;177(9): 5868–77.

30. Nicholson JK, Holmes E, Kinross J, et al. Host-gut microbiota metabolic interactions. Science 2012;336(6086):1262–7.

31. Rooks MG, Garrett WS. Gut microbiota, metabolites and host immunity. Nat Rev Immunol 2016;16(6):341–52.

32. Hunt KM, Foster JA, Forney LJ, et al. Characterization of the diversity and temporal stability of bacterial communities in human milk. PLoS One 2011;6(6):1–8.

33. Rehbinder EM, Lødrup Carlsen KC, Staff AC, et al. Is amniotic fluid of women with uncomplicated term pregnancies free of bacteria? Am J Obstet Gynecol 2018; 219(3):289.e1-e12.

34. Del Rio D, Zimetti F, Caffarra P, et al. The gut microbial metabolite trimethylamine-N-oxide is present in human cerebrospinal fluid. Nutrients 2017;9(10):2–5.

35. McKenney PT, Pamer EG. From hype to hope: the gut microbiota in enteric infectious disease. Cell 2015;163(6):1326–32.

36. Shamriz O, Mizrahi H, Werbner M, et al. Microbiota at the crossroads of autoimmunity. Autoimmun Rev 2016;15(9):859–69.

37. Schubert AM, Sinani H, Schloss PD. Antibiotic-induced alterations of the murine gut microbiota and subsequent effects on colonization resistance against clostridium difficile. MBio 2015;6(4):1–10.

38. Schuijt TJ, Lankelma JM, Scicluna BP, et al. The gut microbiota plays a protective role in the host defence against pneumococcal pneumonia. Gut 2016;65(4):575–83.

39. Clarke TB, Davis KM, Lysenko ES, et al. Recognition of peptidoglycan from the microbiota by Nod1 enhances systemic innate immunity. Nat Med 2010;16(2): 228–31.

40. Fagundes CT, Amaral FA, Vieira AT, et al. Transient TLR activation restores inflammatory response and ability to control pulmonary bacterial infection in germfree mice. J Immunol 2012;188(3):1411–20.

41. Kernbauer E, Ding Y, Cadwell K. An enteric virus can replace the beneficial function of commensal bacteria. Nature 2014;516(729):94–8.

42. Cappon A, Babolin C, Segat D, et al. Helicobacter pylori-derived neutrophil-activating protein increases the lifespan of monocytes and neutrophils. Cell Microbiol 2010;12(6):754–64.

43. Oh JZ, Ravindran R, Chassaing B, et al. TLR5-mediated sensing of gut microbiota is necessary for antibody responses to seasonal influenza vaccination. Immunity 2014;41(3):478–92.

44. Gury-BenAri M, Thaiss CA, Serafini N, et al. The spectrum and regulatory landscape of intestinal innate lymphoid cells are shaped by the microbiome. Cell 2016;166(5):1231–46.e13.

45. Sonnenberg GF, Monticelli LA, Alenghat T, et al. Innate lymphoid cells promote anatomical containment of lymphoid-resident commensal bacteria. Science 2012;336(6086):1321–5.

46. Maeda Y, Kurakawa T, Umemoto E, et al. Dysbiosis contributes to arthritis development via activation of autoreactive T cells in the intestine. Arthritis Rheumatol 2016;68(11):2646–61.

47. Berer K, Gerdes LA, Cekanaviciute E, et al. Gut microbiota from multiple sclerosis patients enables spontaneous autoimmune encephalomyelitis in mice. Proc Natl Acad Sci U S A 2017;11:201711233.

48. Miyake S, Kim S, Suda W, et al. Dysbiosis in the gut microbiota of patients with multiple sclerosis, with a striking depletion of species belonging to clostridia XIVa and IV clusters. PLoS One 2015;10(9):1–16.

49. Biswas A, Petnicki-Ocwieja T, Kobayashi KS. Nod2: a key regulator linking micro-biota to intestinal mucosal immunity. J Mol Med 2012;90(1):15–24.

50. Wang J, Shirota Y, Bayik D, et al. Effect of TLR agonists on the differentiation and function of human monocytic myeloid-derived suppressor cells. J Immunol 2015; 194(9):4215–21.

51. Soto R, Petersen C, Novis CL, et al. Microbiota promotes systemic T-cell survival through suppression of an apoptotic factor. Proc Natl Acad Sci U S A 2017; 114(21):5497–502.

52. Hugot J-P, Chamaillard M, Zouali H, et al. Association of NOD2 leucine-rich repeat variants with susceptibility to Crohn's disease. Nature 2001;411(6837): 599–603.

53. Ivanov II, Frutos RDL, Manel N, et al. Specific microbiota direct the differentiation of IL-17-producing T-helper cells in the mucosa of the small intestine. Cell Host Microbe 2008;4(4):337–49.

54. Lee YK, Menezes JS, Umesaki Y, et al. Proinflammatory T-cell responses to gut microbiota promote experimental autoimmune encephalomyelitis. Proc Natl Acad Sci U S A 2011;108(Suppl):4615–22.

55. Yadav SK, Boppana S, Ito N, et al. Gut dysbiosis breaks immunological tolerance toward the central nervous system during young adulthood. Proc Natl Acad Sci U S A 2017;114(44):E9318–27.

56. Yurkovetskiy L, Burrows M, Khan A, et al. Gender bias in autoimmunity is influenced by microbiota. Immunity 2013;39(2):400–12.

57. Silverman M, Kua L, Tanca A, et al. Protective major histocompatibility complex allele prevents type 1 diabetes by shaping the intestinal microbiota early in ontogeny. Proc Natl Acad Sci U S A 2017;114(36):9671–6.

58. Atarashi K, Tanoue T, Oshima K, et al. Treg induction by a rationally selected mixture of Clostridia strains from the human microbiota. Nature 2013; 500(7461):232–6.

59. Atarashi K, Tanoue T, Shima T, et al. Induction of colonic regulatory T cells by indigenous clostridium species. Science 2011;331(6015):337–41.

60. Narushima S, Sugiura Y, Oshima K, et al. Characterization of the 17 strains of regulatory T cell-inducing human-derived Clostridia. Gut Microbes 2014;5(3):333–9.

61. Li YN, Huang F, Cheng HJ, et al. Intestine-derived Clostridium leptum induces murine tolerogenic dendritic cells and regulatory T cells in vitro. Hum Immunol 2014;75(12):1232–8.

62. Li YN, Huang F, Liu L, et al. Effect of oral feeding with Clostridium leptum on regulatory T-cell responses and allergic airway inflammation in mice. Ann Allergy Asthma Immunol 2012;109(3):201–7.

63. Priyadarshini M, Thomas A, Reisetter AC, et al. Maternal short-chain fatty acids are associated with metabolic parameters in mothers and newborns. Transl Res 2014;164(2):153–7.

64. Park J, Kim M, Kang SG, et al. Short-chain fatty acids induce both effector and regulatory T cells by suppression of histone deacetylases and regulation of the mTOR–S6K pathway. Mucosal Immunol 2015;8(1):80–93.

65. Tan J, McKenzie C, Vuillermin PJ, et al. Dietary fiber and bacterial SCFA enhance oral tolerance and protect against food allergy through diverse cellular pathways. Cell Rep 2016;15(12):2809–24.

66. Thorburn AN, McKenzie CI, Shen S, et al. Evidence that asthma is a developmental origin disease influenced by maternal diet and bacterial metabolites. Nat Commun 2015;6:7320.

67. Macia L, Tan J, Vieira AT, et al. Metabolite-sensing receptors GPR43 and GPR109A facilitate dietary fibre-induced gut homeostasis through regulation of the inflammasome. Nat Commun 2015;6:1–15.

68. Smith PM, Howitt MR, Panikov N, et al. The microbial metabolites, short-chain fatty acids, regulate colonic treg cell homeostasis. Science 2013;341(6145): 569–73.

69. Chang PV, Hao L, Offermanns S, et al. The microbial metabolite butyrate regulates intestinal macrophage function via histone deacetylase inhibition. Proc Natl Acad Sci U S A 2014;111(6):2247–52.

70. Needell JC, Ir D, Robertson CE, et al. Maternal treatment with short-chain fatty acids modulates the intestinal microbiota and immunity and ameliorates type 1 diabetes in the offspring. PLoS One 2017;12(9):e0183786. Mounier C, ed.

71. Kamp ME, Shim R, Nicholls AJ, et al. G protein-coupled receptor 43 modulates neutrophil recruitment during acute inflammation. PLoS One 2016;11(9):1–15.

72. Maslowski KM, Vieira AT, Ng A, et al. Regulation of inflammatory responses by gut microbiota and chemoattractant receptor GPR43. Nature 2009;461(7268): 1282–6.

73. Vieira AT, Macia L, Galvão I, et al. A role for gut microbiota and the metabolite-sensing receptor GPR43 in a murine model of gout. Arthritis Rheumatol 2015; 67(6):1646–56.

74. Round JL, Mazmanian SK. Inducible Foxp3+ regulatory T-cell development by a commensal bacterium of the intestinal microbiota. Proc Natl Acad Sci U S A 2010; 107(27):12204–9.

75. Mazmanian SK, Cui HL, Tzianabos AO, et al. An immunomodulatory molecule of symbiotic bacteria directs maturation of the host immune system. Cell 2005; 122(1):107–18.

76. Cobb BA, Wang Q, Tzianabos AO, et al. Polysaccharide processing and presentation by the MHCII pathway. Cell 2004;117(5):677–87.

77. Telesford KM, Yan W, Ochoa-Reparaz J, et al. A commensal symbiotic factor derived from Bacteroides fragilis promotes human CD39 + Foxp3 + T cells and T reg function. Gut Microbes 2015;6(4):234–42.

78. Ochoa-Reparaz J, Mielcarz DW, Ditrio LE, et al. Central nervous system demyelinating disease protection by the human commensal bacteroides fragilis depends on polysaccharide a expression. J Immunol 2010;185(7):4101–8.

79. Zanvit P, Konkel JE, Jiao X, et al. Antibiotics in neonatal life increase murine susceptibility to experimental psoriasis. Nat Commun 2015;6:8424.

80. Hill DA, Siracusa MC, Abt MC, et al. Commensal bacteria-derived signals regulate basophil hematopoiesis and allergic inflammation. Nat Med 2012;18(4): 538–46.

81. Russell SL, Gold MJ, Willing BP, et al. Perinatal antibiotic treatment affects murine microbiota, immune responses and allergic asthma. Gut Microbes 2013;4(2): 158–64.

82. Russell SL, Gold MJ, Reynolds LA, et al. Perinatal antibiotic-induced shifts in gut microbiota have differential effects on inflammatory lung diseases. J Allergy Clin Immunol 2015;135(1):100–9.e5.

83. Gonzalez-Perez G, Hicks AL, Tekieli TM, et al. Maternal antibiotic treatment impacts development of the neonatal intestinal microbiome and antiviral immunity. J Immunol 2016;196(9):3768–79.

84. Bokulich NA, Chung J, Battaglia T, et al. Antibiotics, birth mode, and diet shape microbiome maturation during early life. Sci Transl Med 2016;8(343):1–14.

85. Arrieta M-C, Stiemsma LT, Dimitriu PA, et al. Early infancy microbial and metabolic alterations affect risk of childhood asthma. Sci Transl Med 2015;7(307):307ra152.

86. Jenq RR, Ubeda C, Taur Y, et al. Regulation of intestinal inflammation by microbiota following allogeneic bone marrow transplantation. J Exp Med 2012; 209(5):903–11.

87. Tawara I, Liu C, Tamaki H, et al. Influence of donor microbiota on the severity of experimental graft-versus-host-disease. Biol Blood Marrow Transplant 2013; 19(1):164–8.

88. Liu C, Frank DN, Horch M, et al. Associations between acute gastrointestinal GvHD and the baseline gut microbiota of allogeneic hematopoietic stem cell transplant recipients and donors. Bone Marrow Transplant 2017;52(12):1643–50.

89. Farowski F, Bücker V, Vehreschild JJ, et al. Impact of choice, timing, sequence and combination of broad-spectrum antibiotics on the outcome of allogeneic haematopoietic stem cell transplantation. Bone Marrow Transplant 2017;53(1):52–7.

90. Mathewson ND, Jenq R, Mathew AV, et al. Gut microbiome–derived metabolites modulate intestinal epithelial cell damage and mitigate graft-versus-host disease. Nat Immunol 2016;17(5):505–13.

91. Romick-Rosendale LE, Haslam DB, Lane A, et al. Antibiotic exposure and reduced short chain fatty acid production after hematopoietic stem cell transplant. Biol Blood Marrow Transplant 2018. https://doi.org/10.1016/j.bbmt.2018.07.030.

92. Fricke WF, Maddox C, Song Y, et al. Human microbiota characterization in the course of renal transplantation. Am J Transplant 2014;14(2):416–27.

93. Lee JR, Muthukumar T, Dadhania D, et al. Gut microbial community structure and complications after kidney transplantation: a pilot study. Transplantation 2014; 98(7):697–705.

94. Lee JR, Muthukumar T, Dadhania D, et al. Gut microbiota and tacrolimus dosing in kidney transplantation. Stepkowski S, ed. PLoS One. 2015;10(3):e0122399.

95. Zhang Z, Liu L, Tang H, et al. Immunosuppressive effect of the gut microbiome altered by high-dose tacrolimus in mice. Am J Transplant 2018;18(7):1646–56.

96. Lei YM, Chen L, Wang Y, et al. The composition of the microbiota modulates allograft rejection. J Clin Invest 2016;126(7):2736–44.

97. Alhabbab R, Blair P, Elgueta R, et al. Diversity of gut microflora is required for the generation of B cell with regulatory properties in a skin graft model. Sci Rep 2015; 5:1–12.

98. Rey K, Manku S, Enns W, et al. Disruption of the gut microbiota with antibiotics exacerbates acute vascular rejection. Transplantation 2018;102(7):1085–95.

Moving?

Make sure your subscription moves with you!

To notify us of your new address, find your **Clinics Account Number** (located on your mailing label above your name), and contact customer service at:

Email: journalscustomerservice-usa@elsevier.com

800-654-2452 (subscribers in the U.S. & Canada)
314-447-8871 (subscribers outside of the U.S. & Canada)

Fax number: 314-447-8029

Elsevier Health Sciences Division
Subscription Customer Service
3251 Riverport Lane
Maryland Heights, MO 63043

*To ensure uninterrupted delivery of your subscription, please notify us at least 4 weeks in advance of move.

Printed and bound by CPI Group (UK) Ltd, Croydon, CR0 4YY

03/10/2024

01040403-0019